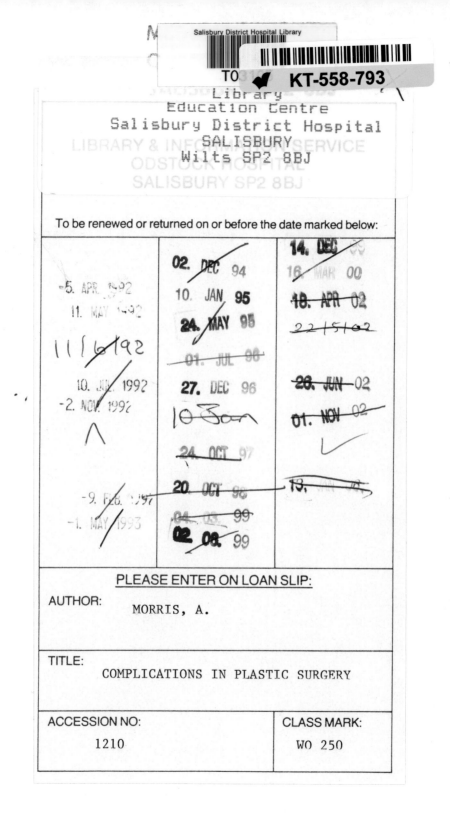

To be renewed or returned on or before the date marked below:

-5. APR. 1992	02. DEC 94	14. DEC 99
11. MAY 1992	10. JAN 95	16. MAR 00
11/6/92	24. MAY 95	18. APR 02
	01. JUL 96	22/5/02
10. JUL 1992	27. DEC 96	28. JUN 02
-2. NOV. 1992	10 Jan	01. NOV 02
	24. OCT 97	
-9. FEB. 1997	20. OCT 98	13. JAN
-1. MAY 1993	04. 03. 99	
	02. 08. 99	

PLEASE ENTER ON LOAN SLIP:

AUTHOR: MORRIS, A.

TITLE: COMPLICATIONS IN PLASTIC SURGERY

ACCESSION NO:	CLASS MARK:
1210	WO 250

Complications of
Plastic Surgery

Complications in Surgery Series
Edited by John A. R. Smith

Other volumes in this series

Complications of Plastic Surgery

A. McG. Morris
MA, FRCS(Ed), FRCS(Eng)

Consultant Plastic Surgeon to Tayside Health Board and
Honorary Senior Lecturer in Surgery, Dundee University

J. H. Stevenson
FRCS(Ed)

Consultant Plastic Surgeon to Tayside Health Board and
Honorary Senior Lecturer in Surgery, Dundee University

A. C. H. Watson
FRCS(Ed)

Consultant Plastic Surgeon to Lothian Health Board and
Part-time Senior Lecturer, Department of Clinical Surgery,
Edinburgh University

Baillière Tindall
London Philadelphia Toronto Sydney Tokyo

Baillière Tindall   24–28 Oval Road
W. B. Saunders   London NW1 7DX

The Curtis Center
Independence Square West
Philadelphia, PA 19106-3399

1 Goldthorne Avenue
Toronto, Ontario M8Z 5T9, Canada

Harcourt Brace Jovanovich
Group (Australia) Pty Limited
32–52 Smidmore St
Marrickville, NSW 2204, Australia

Harcourt Brace Jovanovich Japan Inc.
Ichibancho Central Building, 22-1 Ichibano
Chiyoda-ku, Tokyo 102, Japan

First published 1989

British Library Cataloguing in Publication Data
Morris, A. McG.
  Complications of plastic surgery.—
  (Complications in surgery).
  1. Medicine. Plastic surgery
  I. Title   II. Stevenson, J. H.   III. Watson,
  A.   IV. Series
  617′.95

  ISBN 0–7020–1360–9

Typeset by Latimer Trend & Company Ltd, and printed in Great
Britain by Mackays of Chatham PLC, Letchworth

Contents

Series Foreword

All doctors who are involved in the care of surgical patients are all too aware of the hazards of the operation and the morbidity and mortality that can result from an ill considered or ill managed procedure, and of the complications, whether related directly to the operation, the disease process, the patient or even to the hospital environment. It is also true to say that many hospitals are now mindful of these difficulties and have introduced a pattern of regular medical audit through which the extent and the significance of the problem can be identified and which, when necessary, can point to the remedy.

The majority of complications are of course preventable by careful preoperative preparation, by skilled operative technique and by proper postoperative care, but when they do occur, it is the early recognition, the immediate and correct investigation, and the awareness of the operative treatment that will decide the eventual outcome and the likelihood of early recovery.

Obviously every surgeon would like to believe that in his own practice complications will be, at the least, occasional events and hopefully this is the case in most hospitals. The corollary of this is, however, that the personal experience of many surgeons in these serious potential or actual problems is not great and the opportunities for the trainee surgeon to learn about them, and about their clinical significance and management, are less than adequate.

This deficiency of experience in the average surgeon, whether general surgeon or specialist, has now been appreciated and John Smith in this series of texts has set out to provide what has been termed a 'reference point' from which the surgeon will be able to increase his awareness of the problems and increase his knowledge in areas where he is unlikely to gain experience from clinical practice. The prime aim of the series has been to ensure that knowledge of the existence of complications increases, that prevention can become more widely accepted and that the recognition and management of established complications can be undertaken with skill and competence.

Each of the volumes in the series considers a specific area of surgical practice and, in each, authorities in the field have presented their experience and their views in such a way that it will not only instruct but will also stimulate the reader to study the subject further.

It is undoubtedly an area of surgical practice that is of major importance and which has been somewhat neglected in the past. This is the first time that there has been an attempt to present a comprehensive account covering all aspects of practice and it will undoubtedly be a significant contribution to patient care in its broadest interpretation.

Sir James Fraser Bt, PRCS(Ed)
Nicolson Street
Edinburgh

Editor's Foreword

Most textbooks of surgery acknowledge that postoperative complications exist and some describe methods of prevention or options for their further management. However, it is clear to me from conversations with junior staff, candidates for higher degrees and trainees in all branches of surgery that there is no reference to which they can turn where the complex problem of complications is adequately considered, i.e. covering details of aetiology, predisposition and methods of prevention, together with advice on which complications are likely to be encountered and how they may be recognized, investigated and managed.

This series is directed at all surgical trainees and also at the consultant working outside specialist referral centres. The latter may not often encounter the complications which are under consideration, but when they are encountered the surgeon needs advice on what to do, what not to do and, finally, when specialist referral is indicated.

The authors in this series are all consultants with a specialist practice in teaching hospitals. Each has been asked to provide the necessary information and to be dogmatic where that is possible, but to advise on the options where the situation is less clear. Points of persisting controversy have been identified.

Each volume is self-sufficient, except that *Complications of Surgery in General* deals with all general surgical complications to avoid detailed repetition in the other, more specialist, volumes. Inevitably there is some overlap between volumes but I feel this to be preferable to omitting topics that may be important. Detailed references have not been included. as a deliberate policy of the series, but suggestions for further reading are provided.

Finally, not all the complications described have been created by the authors; the selection of topic reflects, rather, their ability to deal with such problems as are referred to them!

The concept of a single volume on *Complications in Surgery* arose in discussions involving, on separate occasions, Mrs Ann Saadi (lately of Baillière Tindall), Mr R. M. Kirk (Royal Free Hospital, London) and myself. The volume has grown into a series but acknowledgements are due to Mrs Saadi and Mr Kirk for the idea and to Mrs Saadi for the enthusiasm which ensured the launch. The artistic talent of Mr Pat Elliott is clear for all to see and is greatly appreciated. Finally, I am happy to acknowledge the support and encouragement of my wife and family.

John A. R. Smith
Northern General Hospital
Sheffield

Preface

Plastic surgery is a very wide-ranging specialty. The typical
workload crosses boundaries into other specialties and impinges
onto them. The basic aims of plastic surgery are to build up
tissues or restore lost parts, but the specialty also encompasses
cosmetic surgery in which the aim is to improve or restore the
quality of the body shape or image. These two objectives are not,
of course, mutually exclusive and the aims of cosmetic treatment
should be applied widely to all surgical specialties. There is no
merit in leaving an unsightly scar, for example, if, with a little
thought and careful planning, a better standard of result could
be obtained.

The prevention and management of complications in plastic
surgery are different in some respects from those in other
specialties. There are more variables to be taken into account.
Counselling is in some instances extremely difficult and
persuading the patient that an operation is neither indicated nor
required can be a very trying process.

The aim of this book is to help the surgeon training in plastic
surgery as well as other branches of 'surgery in general'. It
should also help the specialist in other disciplines. The problems
encountered during basic techniques in the major branches of
plastic surgery are discussed and a range of solutions to various
problems is presented. There is a strong emphasis on
consultation with, and the need for referral back to, a plastic
surgeon. A common source of referral to plastic surgeons is
complications that arise during procedures done by other
specialties. If referral of problems is timely, as soon as they
become evident, it may be possible to find a simpler solution
than if there is delay and complications become compounded by
exposure and desiccation of soft tissues, stiffness or swelling.
The essence of plastic surgery repair is an artistic and sensitive
use of combinations of methods that is difficult to learn from a
book. There is no substitute for experience and a period
observing or working with an expert is recommended.

The first five chapters cover the complications of the basic
techniques of patient assessment, management of wound
healing and trauma, skin grafts, skin flaps and scars. The
remainder of the book is then devoted to detailed consideration
of problems in specific areas.

In this litigious era, there is a tendency to fudge the issue
when complications are discussed, in case negligence is implied.
Such terms as 'unfavourable results' are used to distinguish the
less than ideal result from the 'inevitable result' such as a scar,
that must occur when skin is cut. In this volume, 'complications'

are discussed in the true meaning of a disease or diseases concurrent with another disease. Inevitable or avoidable problems are discussed as complications.

We should like to acknowledge the secretarial help of Helen Stein, Anne Henderson, Sheena Bremner, Sandra Findlay, Elsie Jeffrey, Linda Brown and Tom Morris. Thanks are also due to the photographers at the Royal Hospital for Sick Children Edinburgh, Bangour General Hospital, Dundee Royal Infirmary and Bridge of Earn Hospital, and to Mr Patrick Elliott for line drawings and the production staff at Baillière Tindall. We also wish to thank our wives and families for forbearance at a prolonged labour but sturdy outcome.

A. M. Morris,
J. H. Stevenson,
A. C. H. Watson

1 General Complications of Plastic Surgery

The scope of plastic surgery is so wide that inevitably a large number and variety of complications can arise. The specialty falls into two natural divisions: reconstructive surgery, and aesthetic or cosmetic surgery. Reconstructive surgery is the repair of defects arising, for example, from congenital abnormalities, trauma and tumour excision. Cosmetic surgery is treatment to restore or enhance the patient's appearance. In reality these categories are merely ends of a spectrum and there is no true dividing line between them (Fig. 1.1).

The complications can be divided into three groups:

1 General complications common to all surgery, which are discussed in 'Complications of Surgery in General'.
2 The specific complications for each technique, which are discussed in the relevant chapters of this book.
3 Complications unique to plastic surgery, which arise in large part from the name, reputation and mystique of the specialty. To the lay person, 'plastic surgery' frequently implies some form of 'invisible mending'. The patient may have an extremely high expectation of possible improvements, reinforced by strong media publicity. The net effect is that there may be a disproportionate degree of dissatisfaction with the result. For example, a minor complication might be regarded as a disaster. It is essential that the patient about to undergo plastic surgery should be fully aware of the limitations of available techniques. There is no more difficult complication to deal with than a patient who asks, after a long course of treatment, 'when am I going to get the plastic surgery?'

Figure 1.1
The spectrum of plastic surgery. It is not a simple linear scale, but is blurred, depending on the patient's reaction to the deformity.

Reconstructive surgery

Cosmetic surgery

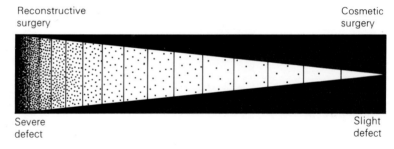

Severe defect

Slight defect

Predisposing factors

As plastic-surgical techniques improve, the number of complications should decrease, but there are a number of factors that will prevent this happening.

The increasing complexity of available procedures

With the advances in surgical techniques and therapeutic skills in associated specialties (for example, anaesthesia), the increased range and scope of plastic surgery will lead to a paradoxical increase in complications, as patients with more severe diseases and older patients are operated on. The more major procedures involving teams of surgeons from different specialities, and prolonged operating times, will tend to magnify the number of complications. It will also become increasingly difficult to attribute the complications to a particular specialty.

Patient expectation

Plastic surgery is performed using standard surgical technique and does not imply an extraordinary or miraculous quality of result. No effort must be spared to give the patient a full and frank explanation of the available procedures and likely result. However, the patient may already expect too much because he has been referred for 'plastic surgery' by a general practitioner or another specialist. It is extremely important that the surgeon, particularly the inexperienced surgeon, does not promise the patient that he will do 'a little plastic surgery' without full explanation about its limitations. Unrealistic expectation by the patient is a potent cause of postoperative dissatisfaction.

The extent of a patient's reaction to a deformity is surprisingly variable. Highly suspicious or complaining individuals will demand treatment of the most minor deformities (Fig. 1.2). Such pernickety individuals will tend to be more dissatisfied with results, however good the final outcome. On the other

Figure 1.2
Over-reaction to a defect. This patient complained bitterly about the disfigurement caused by this lump at the corner of the mouth, which was only visible when the mouth was open.

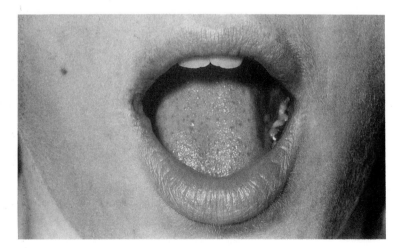

hand, some people show a seemingly total disregard for their own appearance, possibly as a defence mechanism about being thought foolish if they complain. They excuse themselves for 'bothering the surgeon' and yet have problems that are interfering with their appearance (Fig. 1.3).

Failure to refer for specialist advice

Late referral for consultation by a surgeon after the defect has been made denies the patient two lines of treatment. First, prior consultation with full evaluation in elective cases affords the chance to perform a combined procedure in which reconstruction can proceed at the time of primary treatment. This will avoid two anaesthetics and avoid complications that may supervene between the two treatment episodes and shorten the hospitalization time. Secondly, in emergency cases, it is essential to call in the plastic-surgical team at the outset, before general anaesthesia is given, so that the full extent of the trauma can be gauged. This allows full examination of the extent of devitalization and undermining, which is essential information in planning wound repair. It also permits a joint approach to the surgical exposure that might be required for orthopaedic or neurosurgical procedures, when preservation of as much tissue as possible may be vital to reconstruction.

The complication referred

A large part of the case load in plastic surgery is the treatment of complications referred from other specialties. Sometimes the complication is referred later by the general practitioner. The presence of an untreated wound or scar indicates previous trauma when there may have been loss of tissue or previous infection, causing induration. This compromises the corrective surgery, and correct timing of the repair attempt is crucial. If vital structures are threatened, rapid repair is necessary, but, if

Figure 1.3
Under-reaction to a massive lipoma of the neck. The patient apologized effusively for wasting the surgeon's time at the initial consultation.

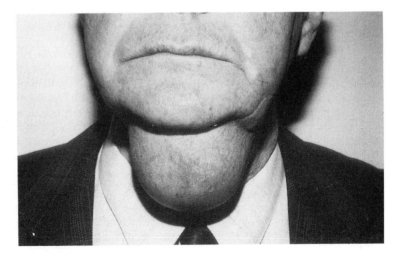

at all possible, delay should allow oedema and induration to settle, helping to avoid subsequent complications.

Prevention of complications

Patient selection and assessment

Before undertaking to treat a patient, the plastic surgeon must satisfy himself, after taking a full history and performing relevant examinations, that there are adequate answers to three vital questions:

1 Does the patient have a problem?
2 Is the problem correctly identified?
3 Is the problem amenable to treatment?

1 In the majority of cases, the problem will be clear and easily defined, for example, a severe congenital defect or deformity after trauma. However, particularly at the right-hand end of the spectrum of treatment (Fig. 1.1), where the defect may be slight, it is essential that the surgeon and patient can both define and agree the extent and degree of the deformity. If the patient has a complaint about his appearance that the surgeon cannot see, it may be an indication that the patient has a distorted body image, perhaps from psychotic disease. Surgical intervention is contra-indicated and psychiatric assessment and treatment would be more appropriate.

2 The patient may have a clearly defined complaint but his lack of technical expertise may make it difficult for him to appreciate the exact nature of the problem. Full pre-operative assessment and counselling enables the surgeon to define the true nature of the problem and establish a plan of correction. For example, a patient may complain of a large nose and request a rhinoplasty. If there is a relative underdevelopment of the jaw and chin, a more appropriate form of treatment might be advancement osteotomy of the mandible or chin augmentation (Fig. 1.4). To operate on the nose in such circumstances might be inappropriate and result in a dissatisfied patient.

3 In all surgical treatment, a balance has to be struck between the overall benefit to the patient and the risk of complications that inevitably accompany all surgical procedures. The surgeon therefore has to establish not only that the problem is correctable but that there will be an overall tangible benefit not offset by the various complications and side effects of treatment. For example, a patient with a scar that is causing cosmetic but no functional deformity may decide, after full consultation, that the expected improvement of a scar revision is so slight that it does not justify the risk.

Operative treatment not indicated

Treatment by a surgeon does not necessarily involve a surgical operation. It is very important to keep in mind that it is a person who is being treated, not a disease. However it can be extremely

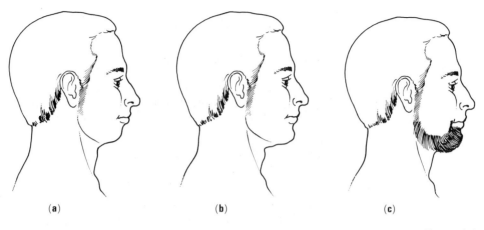

(a)　　　　　　　　　　(b)　　　　　　　　　　(c)

Figure 1.4

Relationships to other facial features can alter the apparent size of an anatomical structure. In this figure, the noses are all the same size. The relatively large nose in (a) can be 'corrected' by augmenting the chin (b), or by growing a beard (c).

difficult to handle the patient when an operation is neither indicated nor desirable. If a problem is not amenable to surgery it does not mean that 'nothing can be done'. A whole range of conservative measures may be available including dressing, splintage, physiotherapy, occupational therapy, cosmetic camouflage and specific measures such as in the management of a scar (see Chapter 5). The provision of careful advice and repeat follow up consultation is a vital part of treatment and will help to prevent patient dissatisfaction. For example, in the treatment of a child with a strawberry haemangioma or hypertrophic scar which will improve spontaneously, the parents can be very distressed if a policy of wait and see is advocated. The benefits of conservative management must be stressed and non-operative management should be presented in a positive reassuring manner.

When the defect is particularly complex and involves structures such as the eye, eyelids, ear and nose that are extremely difficult to reconstruct, consideration must be given to providing a prosthesis. This can give a very realistic appearance and, by avoiding surgery, complications can be prevented (Fig. 1.5a, b, c).

Patients' age

The age of the patient is another important factor. While it is true that the incidence of operative complications is increased in the aged, old age *per se* is not a contra-indication to surgery. The physiological rather than chronological age is a better guide, but each case must be judged on its own merits. Children,

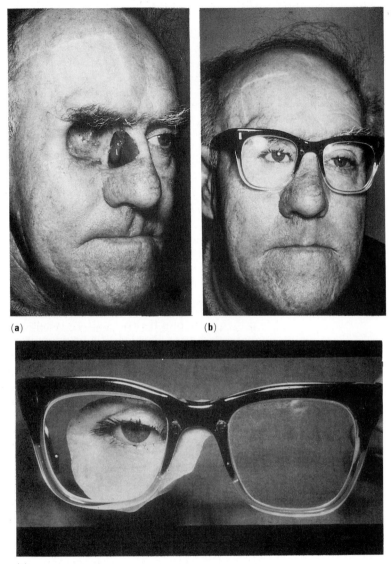

(a)   (b)

(c)

similarly, should not be barred from surgery that is needed. The
correction of a defect in the young patient should be timed
carefully to try to avoid any adverse psychological effects.
Major defects should, where possible, be corrected before the
child has to mix with peer groups at nursery or infant school. It
may be prudent to delay treatment of a minor complaint in an
infant until it can be done under local anaesthetic in later
childhood if it is not causing embarrassment. Surgery on the
face should be avoided at the toddler stage, if possible, because
frequent falls and knocks can cause wound breakdown.

Plan the procedure with the patient Once a patient has been selected for treatment, it is essential to discuss the possible methods to be used and the various alternative operative techniques. All relevant steps of surgery should be described, paying particular attention to possible complications as well as the likely associated problems, for example the problem of secondary donor site scarring if a graft or flap procedure is to be employed. A useful technique is to ask patients what they hope will be the outcome of the treatment. This may reveal a totally unrealistic expectation that can be discussed and corrected at this stage. Many patients believe that skin grafts are a method of covering up scars so that they disappear. If this mistaken impression is left uncorrected, there is likely to be an unfavourable result and a dissatisfied patient, even if the procedure is carried out faultlessly. At this stage patients should have the opportunity to think again, reconsider the pros and cons, and decide whether they still require treatment. If there is any serious doubt in the patient's or surgeon's mind it is better to wait and consider the problem at a later consultation, rather than to press for a rapid decision.

Discuss recovery time All operations, however minor, have postoperative problems and the patient should be warned about them so that they can make appropriate arrangements. Swelling, redness, and bruising is likely to occur and will last for at least two weeks. The patient may feel tired and will probably have to arrange a spell off work. A housewife will require help in the home if she is to be discharged early. An outline of the time spent with dressings on will help planning of social and other engagements. Some patients are quite unrealistic about their ability to return to full activities and a little time spent discussing this problem pre-operatively can prevent a lot of anguish postoperatively'.

Patient consent If the process outlined in the previous sections has been carried out fully, it will form the basis for the patient to give 'informed' consent. The patient or his parent or guardian, should sign a declaration to this effect. It is not necessary in Britain to have a comprehensive list of every conceivable possible complication, but a reasonable explanation should be given of the common or serious complications. In North America, however, it is customary to have a comprehensive document listing all described complications drawn up for the consent form.

If the patient is a minor, but old enough and fully able to understand the treatment (usually from seven years old) it is best to ask for his or her co-operation and consent also. This is especially wise if a long-term complicated series of procedures is to be undertaken that relies heavily on patient compliance.

Pre-operative preparation A patient in the fittest possible pre-operative condition is likely to withstand surgery better. All steps should therefore be taken to eliminate any concomitant disease or other adverse factors.

In elective surgery in particular, there is usually adequate time to prepare fully and ensure that all factors are favourable. Associated illness should be controlled as far as possible. All medication that might affect the operation or anaesthetic should be known. Consideration should be given to stopping the contraceptive pill for eight weeks to minimize the chance of deep-vein thrombosis in high-risk operations. Hypertension should be controlled and it is not advisable to operate within six months following a coronary thrombosis. The obese patient should lose weight prior to surgery, and marked anaemia (haemoglobin less than 10 Gm.%) should be corrected by a course of iron therapy.

Clean operations should not be carried out in the presence of general or local sepsis, particularly if a prosthetic implant is to be used. In emergency cases a balance must be struck between the need for adequate preparation and the likely deterioration that may occur if surgery is delayed. In general, provided shock is treated, plastic surgical treatment to give skin cover can usually be delayed until major neurosurgical, thoracic, and abdominal emergencies have been corrected (Fig. 1.6).

Figure 1.6
While potentially life threatening injuries to the head and neck following a road traffic accident must take priority, the treatment of this severe injury to the lower lip must not be neglected. Early primary repair is indicated.

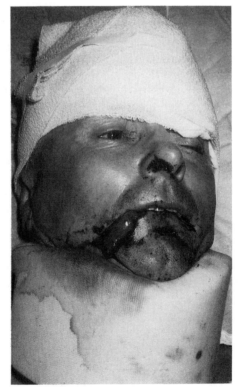

A history of allergy to drugs or anaesthetic agents should be obtained and enquiry should also be made about problems with dressings or bandages. Allergy to a particular type of surgical tape, for example, can lead to problems of pain and irritation, particularly if prolonged splintage is required. Early premature removal of such a dressing, to change it, can give rise to increased complications.

Anaesthesia   Good anaesthesia is essential if surgery is to be performed safely.

Local anaesthesia
In a large proportion of plastic-surgical cases it is appropriate to use local anaesthesia with or without sedation. The amount of local anaesthesia used should be very carefully monitored so as not to exceed the safe dose. A vasoconstrictor can be used in the local anaesthetic, but it must not be used in a ring block procedure for fear of causing permanant damage to the circulation. Similarly, local anaesthesia with a vasoconstrictor should be used sparingly, if at all, when flap surgery is to be performed, as it may interfere with flap viability. Hyaluronidase to spread the local anaesthetic should not be used in the presence of malignant disease or infection, for fear of causing dissemination.

General anaesthesia
Steady anaesthesia, with hypotension if necessary, is extremely helpful in performing safe surgery. The anaesthesia must continue until after the dressing is in place. Coughing should be avoided, if possible, on waking as this predisposes to haematoma formation.

Plan the operation   Planning begins at the time of the initial consultation and proceeds in stages. It is essential that the final operative plan is not worked out for the first time 'on the table'; it should be considered carefully beforehand and worked out by measurement and marking on the patient before premedication is administered. This is particularly true when there is a postural factor, such as in breast or abdominal surgery.

It is not always possible to predict and plan for all eventualities, so a defensive approach to planning should be adopted and suitable alternative strategies should be discussed with the patient beforehand (see Chapter 2 on wound healing).

During operation planning should follow a logical pattern:

1 plan;
2 mark;
3 check.

Marking must be performed using an absorbable dye, for example Bonney's Blue, which will not leave a permanent tattoo. Mark before local anaesthetic is injected, as distention distorts the tissues. Before surgery is commenced, the marking must be checked for accuracy. Reverse planning using a pattern of non-extensible material such as paper, bandage, or jaconet will help to check the plans.

Once the defect to be repaired is established, another check is made to ensure that the proposed repair is feasible. A modification or a change to an alternative second-line plan at this stage will save needless error and complication.

Surgical technique

1 The surgeon, assistants, and nursing assitant should be as comfortably positioned as possible and preferably seated (Fig. 1.7).
2 The patient should be prepared and towelled in an aseptic manner to decrease the risk of infection. The draping of the patient should be carefully performed to expose the whole operative field and the important local anatomical landmarks (Fig. 1.8). In particular, the use of keyhole drapes should be avoided as it is very easy to lose orientation and end up with the incision out of alignment.
3 Minimize tissue trauma by gentle tissue-handling with fine instruments. Use as few and as fine sutures as possible to

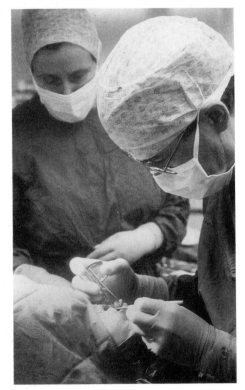

Figure 1.7
A comfortable sitting position is essential if accurate surgery is to be performed. In this case, with the patients head almost in the surgeon's lap, a good central view of the patient's face allows accurate planning. The forearms resting on the operating table stabilize the hands.

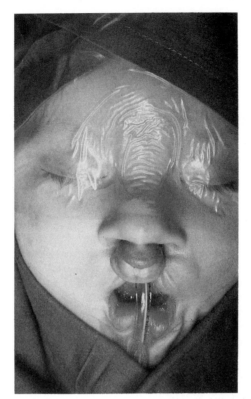

achieve the required result. The tissues should be treated with respect and kept moist to prevent desiccation. This is particularly a problem when working under tourniquet, as the circulation is stopped and the continued effect of the heat from the operating lights and evaporation caused by air currents from the air-conditioning can kill tissue.

4 Ensure a good view with adequate lighting aided by adequate homeostasis. An assistant using suction to follow the scalpel prevents flooding of the operative field. If it is not possible to use a tourniquet, local injections of a vasoconstrictor in local anaesthetic or hypotensive anaesthesia will help keep the field relatively avascular. Haemostasis is best achieved by fine bipolar diathermy (Fig. 1.9), with ligatures for the larger bleeding points.

5 Team work is used whenever possible in the more extensive operations: one team carries out the resection, the other the reconstruction. This may allow overlap of the two components of the operation, saving the patient anaesthetic time and reducing fatigue of the operator. Similarly, breaks in the operation should be taken where appropriate to allow rest for the surgical team. A convenient time, for instance, is after

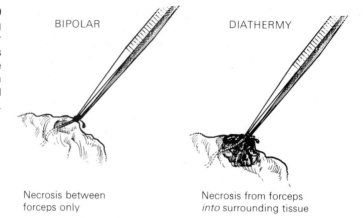

Figure 1.9
Haemostasis using fine tipped bipolar coagulation causes much less tissue necrosis than conventional diathermy.

BIPOLAR

DIATHERMY

Necrosis between forceps only

Necrosis from forceps *into* surrounding tissue

release of the tourniquet or while the hypotensive anaesthesia is being reversed. A pause will allow bleeding points to be identified without the risk of initial reactive haemorrhage into the wound, and haematoma formation. During breaks, all wounds must be covered with suitable moist dressings of physiological fluid, for example isotonic saline. After careful haemostasis, the wound is sutured.

6 If there is any appreciable dead space, closed suction drainage is advisable to prevent haematoma formation. This reduces the risk of tissue necrosis and infection. The risk of infection can be further reduced using prophylactic antibodies where necessary if the wound is potentially contaminated.

7 The application of a dressing, when indicated, is an integral part of the operation and is best performed by a member of the surgical team. Although some situations demand support and pressure, excessive pressure that would restrict the circulation should be avoided.

Postoperative care

The after-care is as important as the planning and the operation itself. Clear instructions should be given to the specialist nursing team. If the patient is nursed in a general ward, there is a heavier responsibility on the medical staff to supervise care. Monitoring for adequate circulation in an extremity or flap is particularly important. Haematoma should be diagnosed and released as soon as detected.

Dressings should generally be left undisturbed and clear instructions should be given about them to the patient and nursing staff. Change of dressings should be performed by members of the surgical team or trained nursing staff.

Keep accurate records

Make sure you have an accurate note of the patient's present complaint as well as the findings on examination. A good accurate sketch is frequently more valuable than a prose description and accurate operation notes should be made. Pre-operative photographs are invaluable as a record. They can be used to remind the patient of the pre-operative condition and can sometimes satisfy a complaining patient who may have forgotten the extent of the original deformity.

Day-case surgery   Plastic surgery procedures of increasing complexity are per-formed as day cases. Patient selection of fit individuals is extremely important and those with special risks should be eliminated by adequate pre-operative assessment at the initial consultation. It is most unwise to operate on both hands at the same time when the patient is allowed home early. All but minor lower-limb surgery is contra-indicated because of problems associated with early dependancy causing bruising, oedema, and slow wound healing. After-care will be particularly difficult and the patient should be given clear written instructions about postoperative care and notified whom to contact in case of unforeseen difficulties.

If general anaesthetic has been used, the patient must be accompanied home by a responsible person and not allowed to drive a motor vehicle for twenty-four hours.

Cosmetic Surgery—the Unfavourable Result

In most respects, cosmetic surgery is an integral part of plastic surgery, with similar complications. However, it is at the right-hand end of the plastic-surgery spectrum, and the patient's presenting complaints are usually less in magnitude though no less important to the patient. There is a finer balance to be maintained and considered and the differences are more in degree than substance. In some instances there has not been any tangible complication, yet the patient is dissatisfied with the result. The term 'unfavourable result' is a useful concept when considering these complications of cosmetic surgery, and it is important to be able to predict and avoid operating on those patients in whom an unfavourable result is likely (Table 1.1).

Table 1.1
Criteria for predicting
unfavourable results in
cosmetic surgery.

1 Minimal physical defect
2 Patient is unable to localize defect accurately
3 Patient is over-demanding with multiple complaints, bearing long lists and diagrams
4 Previous unsuccessful cosmetic surgery
5 Surgeon has difficulty establishing rapport
6 Male patient—particularly for facial surgery
7 During times of emotional stress, e.g. separation, bereavement
8 Obesity, with patient making no effort to comply with pre-operative instructions to lose weight

Careful patient selection and assessment are even more important. The patient's problem must be very clearly established. If
there is a history of psychiatric disturbance, the help of a
psychiatrist should be enlisted with the particular aim of screening out patients with psychosis. The lesser defect may mean that
only a smaller improvement can be gained and therefore the
risks of harm are relatively exaggerated. This is particularly
true when the defect is minimal, and it is necessary to steer the
patient away from surgery if the defect is so small that the
chance of improvement is negligible.

It is very important in the assessment not to promise a
particular result or shape and it is not wise to show photographs
of other results to patients, as their expectation may be heigh-
tened. The aim is to operate on a patient who has a realistic
expectation of the likely result and improvement.

Management of the unfavourable result
1 Follow-up consultation will allow the chance for the patient
   to inform the surgeon if he or she is not happy with the result.
   The surgeon should acknowledge that there is a problem and
   must not ignore or dismiss the complaint without proper
   evaluation. If possible identify the nature of the complaint.
   Reference to the pre-operative record, especially photographs,
   at this stage will sometimes allow the problem to be resolved.
2 When the complaint is of swelling, a later follow-up consultation is recommended. Bruising and oedema can be quite
   alarming to patients and their relatives if they have not been
   forewarned.
3 If there is a genuine problem that is agreed by the patient and
   surgeon, re-operation can be performed. The detailed treatment of complications is contained in subsequent chapters of
   this book.
4 Difficulty arises when the patient is not happy with a result
   that is technically satisfactory. Full discussion should be
   developed to see whether there is any underlying cause of
   dissatisfaction. The patient may be depressed and not amenable to counselling. A further consultation after a few months
   may allow the patient to settle and accept the new appearance. If all else fails, suggest that the patient should seek a
   second opinion.
5 A paradoxical situation exists in which the patient is happy
   with the result and the surgeon is not. The wise surgeon
   should resist the temptation to 'gild the lily' and should not
   try to persuade the patient to undergo further treatment.

Conclusion

Most patients are pleased with the results of reconstructive
surgery for congenital or traumatic defects. Similarly, the

majority of cosmetic surgery patients have satisfying results. Careful pre-operative selection, assessment and counselling of the patient should allow an operation to proceed in favourable circumstances by eliminating possible adverse factors. A patient who enters treatment in a relaxed frame of mind with realistic expectations is likely to derive most benefit from surgery. Open communication between doctor and patient, if complications develop, helps to resolve most disputes.

Persisting controversies
- The role of the psychiatrist in patient assessment.
- Experience and training requirements for cosmetic surgeons.
- Informed consent, the extent of a surgeon's duty to explain particular complications and risks inherent in an operation.

Further reading
Goldwyn, R.M. (Ed) (1984) *The Unfavourable Result in Plastic Surgery: Avoidance and Treatment*. Boston: Little Brown.

Regnault, P. & Daniel, R.K. (1984) *Aesthetic Plastic Surgery: Principles and Techniques*. Boston: Little Brown.

2 Complications of Wound Healing

A major part of reconstructive plastic surgery is devoted to soft-tissue repair. Treatment after trauma is particularly difficult, with potential complications arising from the wound itself, the systemic complications of trauma, or the general complications of surgery.

Impaired wound healing
The chief complication of all surgery is impaired wound healing which may present as:

1 complete failure to heal with progression to a chronic ulcer or discharging sinus,
2 delayed healing, which inevitably leads to greater oedema, stiffness, fibrosis and scarring, can occur in one or more of many layers in a complex wound,
3 poor quality of healing. While some form of scar is inevitable, from an incised wound of the skin, a severely distorted or contracted scar is an unfortunate complication (see Chapter 5).

Adverse Factors in Wound Healing

General factors

Nutrition A wide variety of nutritional and metabolic factors influence wound healing and infection. Also complex metabolic and nutritional disturbances follow serious injury or infection. These processes are interrelated and difficult to quantify, but deficiencies should be corrected.

Vitamin A. Vitamin A influences wound healing, and experimentally induced deficiency retards epithelialization of wounds.

Vitamin C. Ascorbic acid is essential for collagen synthesis, and deficiency causes scurvy with impaired wound healing, increased capillary fragility and decreased resistance to infection (Fig. 2.1). Vitamin C is not stored in the body so that in severe injury, for example extensive burns, vitamin C supplements of 1 g of ascorbic acid should be given daily prophylacti-

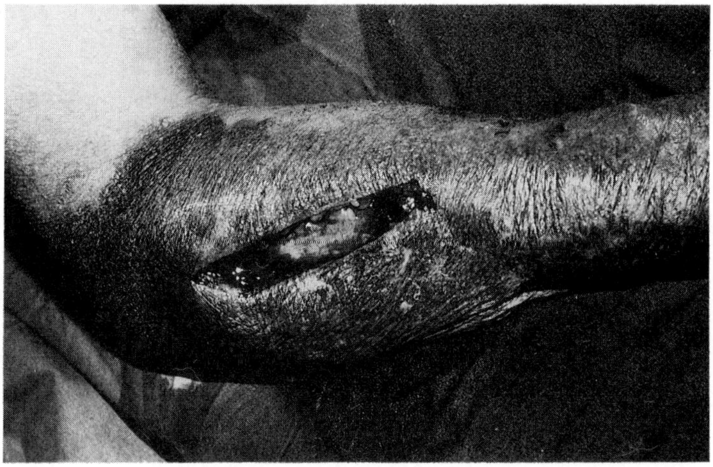

Figure 2.1
Scurvy impairs wound
healing. There is no
sign of improvement in
this injury, which is
several days old. Note
the multiple scars from
numerous minor
injuries. There was a
rapid response to
vitamin C therapy.

cally. There is, however, no evidence that large doses accelerate healing in the patient with normal ascorbic acid levels.

Protein. In severe injury, negative nitrogen balance (catabolism) may develop with breakdown of body protein, particularly if there is additional loss in the form of exudates as in extensive burns. Deficiency of protein impairs growth and healing. Special care should be taken to supply adequate nutrition with high calorific value to minimize catabolism.

Trace elements. Zinc deficiency is associated with impaired healing. If long-term parenteral nutrition is required, supplements of zinc must be given.

Anaemia   There is a widely held belief that if the haemoglobin level is less than 10 g%, healing will not occur or that grafts will not take. This is not entirely true, but healing may be delayed. A very low haemoglobin level should be corrected if chronic blood loss is occurring—particularly in burns, when the taking of skin grafts causes further blood loss.

Steroid therapy   Glucocorticoids in any dosage, given long term, interfere with wound healing in several ways:

1 The skin becomes thinner and softer and is more vulnerable to injury.
2 Increased capillary fragility causes haematoma formation.
3 Systemic or local steroids decrease resistance to wound infection. It is vital, however, not to stop steroids at the time of injury and booster doses will be needed.
4 Scars are weaker and tend to become atrophic.

Diabetes mellitus Diabetes predisposes the patient to infection that will delay wound healing. Major arterial disease or microangiopathy can cause spontaneous necrosis at the periphery and slow wound healing. Peripheral neuropathy adds a trophic element to the delay in wound healing.

Hypoxia Adequate tissue perfusion of oxygenated blood at physiological levels is vital for wound healing. It is doubtful whether breathing air with increased oxygen levels will promote wound healing, but there is evidence that hyperbaric oxygen is useful in treating anaerobic wound infections or preventing incipient necrosis of skin flaps.

Smoking By its strong vasoconstrictor action, smoking decreases tissue perfusion and may tip the balance, causing tissue necrosis where the blood supply is compromised.

Age Skin heals more rapidly in children, with a stronger scar, but clinically this can be a disadvantage and frequently gives rise to thick hypertrophic scarring that takes a long time to fade and is cosmetically less acceptable than the pale atrophic scar of the older patient.

Local factors

Wound environment There is considerable interest, at present, in the microenvironment of the healing wound. When a wound is completely closed by sutures or tapes, the type of dressing has little effect on the rate of healing. In open wounds, prevention of desiccation is vital, as dehydration causes tissue necrosis. Complete ranges of new dressings have been developed including semipermeable films, semiocclusive hydrogels and occlusive hydrocolloids. Studies comparing these new dressings with traditional gauze dressings suggest that wound healing, particularly epithelialization, is quicker. However there is the potential complication that the moist environment encourages infection. One advantage is greater patient comfort. This new epithelium is particularly vulnerable to trauma and a protective dressing should be kept on to avoid mechanical interference with the healing wound. Frequent dressing changes should be avoided at first for the same reason, unless infection occurs.

Exposure treatment or the application of a traditional dressing to a superficial burn, graze or split skin donor site gives some loss of superficial tissue in the surface scab. However, it does work in practice, allowing healing, and the new epithelium is more robust. It is very important that the dressing or scab is not forcibly removed and should be left in place for at least one week.

Wound infection   A wide variety of pathogens can infect wounds and delay
healing:

1 Haemolytic streptococcus infection is particularly serious, as
it causes wound healing to fail and may convert a superficial
burn into full thickness loss. It can disrupt skin grafts, which
are attacked by its enzymes.
2 *Pseudomonas pyocyaneas* is a danger in burn wounds and
thrives in a moist environment. It has systemic effects and
may cause Gram-negative septicaemic shock as well as local
wound infection.
3 Tetanus or gas gangrene can develop from contaminated
wounds.

Haematoma   A haematoma causes delay in wound healing in several ways:

1 It may act as a foreign body and focus for infection.
2 The physical presence of a haematoma separates tissue planes
or lifts a graft or flap from its bed, preventing vascularization.
3 Increased tension in a wound as a result of a haematoma may
contribute to vascular insufficiency.
4 An established haematoma produces localized oedema and
bruising that will slow wound healing, delay mobilization and
give rise to stiffness, fibrosis and scarring.

Ischaemia   Impaired arterial or venous blood supply can cause ischaemia,
delaying wound healing or causing tissue necrosis. Tight wound
closure as a result of poor suture technique, pressure from a
haematoma or dressing, and poor design of an incision or flap
can all cause ischaemia.

Wound type   1 Tidy wounds, i.e. clean incised, wounds, heal rapidly.
2 Untidy wounds with irregular, contused, dirty or contaminated edges heal less well. Wounds seen and treated late are
more likely to be contaminated or infected. Primary closure is
contra-indicated in any wound that is grossly contaminated
or seen more than eight hours after injury.

Site of wound   The rate of wound healing depends on the region of the body
affected. The thin skin of the eyelids heals very rapidly, whereas
the thicker back skin heals relatively slowly. The blood supply is
better in the head and neck and wounds there heal more rapidly.
Wounds in the leg heal slowly owing to a combination of poor
blood supply with venous stasis on dependancy and tension.

Foreign-body   Any foreign body such as fibre from clothing, glass, wood,
reaction   sutures, ligatures, glove powder, haematoma or slough can
cause chronic inflammation and delay healing (Fig. 2.2a, b).

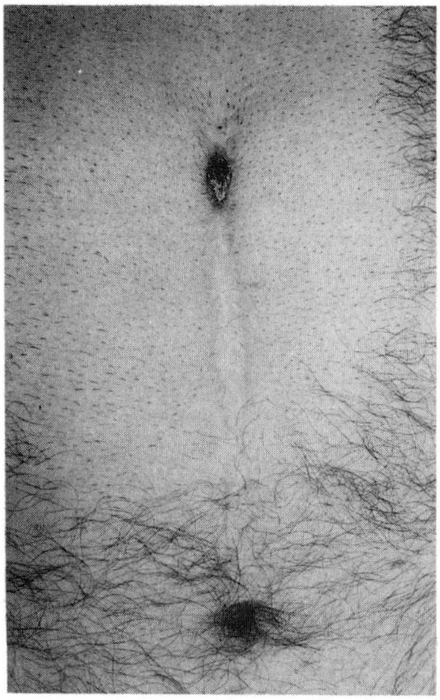

Figure 2.2
Chronic wound sinus
(a) caused by a large
buried knot of non-
absorbable suture (b).

(a)

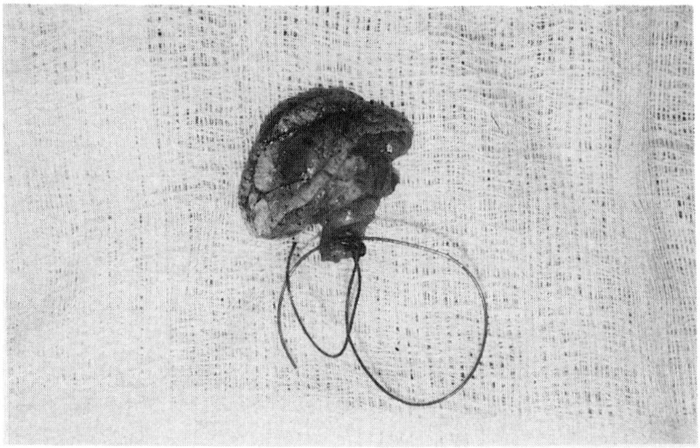

(b)

Figure 2.2
Chronic wound sinus
(a) caused by a large
buried knot of non-
absorbable suture (b).

Allergy to sutures and drugs

Some patients are allergic to catgut sutures, which are discharged from the wound in repeated chronic sterile abscesses. Allergy to topical preparations, tapes and bandages can cause severe blistering and superficial skin loss.

Movement, pressure and repeated trauma

Good postoperative care is very important to minimize early, repeated trauma to a healing wound. Splintage of adjacent joints will help to limit movement. Care must be taken to ensure that any dressing or splint is not so tight that it causes tissue necrosis or compartment compression syndromes.

When a wound is inexplicably slow to heal in spite of all reasonable precautions, and especially if chronic ulceration occurs in the absence of infection, patient interference causing dermatitis artefacta should be suspected.

Local irradiation   X-ray therapy produces progressive arterial damage and fibrosis that interferes with wound healing. Sutures should be left in longer than usual. Even minor trauma to an irradiated area can give rise to radionecrosis.

Prevention of impaired wound healing
Every care should be taken to maximize healing by recognizing and avoiding, or treating where possible, any adverse factors. Tactics of wound management should be based on sound general principles.

Emergency or trauma surgery   The wound must be treated in the context of the total injury. The overall health and survival of the patient must be ensured, but an order of priority should be established without forgetting the wound. Once survival is ensured the patient often judges the end result by the external defect, such as quality of scarring. Nothing should be done in treatment that neglects the wound and prejudices wound healing.

Assess the situation   In major emergencies, with large numbers of casualties, compromises inevitably have to be made according to the circumstances. *Triage* (see Table 2.1) should be performed by an experienced surgeon, but ideally all specialties likely to be involved in the treatment of the patient should be notified

Table 2.1   Primary assessment of trauma

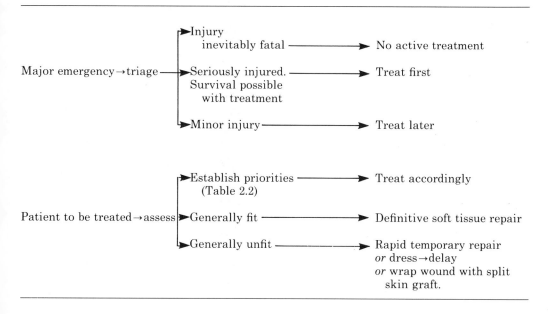

urgently. There is no reason, when small numbers of casualties are involved, why any specialty should be omitted. In particular, where burns or major soft-tissue injuries are concerned, the plastic-surgery team must be involved from the outset to partake in accurate assessment of the wound, so that definitive repair can be planned. It may be possible to combine treatment, thereby shortening total operating and anaesthetic time, speeding recovery and diminishing the chances of complications.

Order of priority   Resuscitation must be instituted immediately according to the list of priorities after an initial rapid appraisal has been made (Table 2.2).

There will be discussion about the exact order in a list of priorities, but restoration of skin cover is usually placed last. However, at all stages it is vital to consider emergency dressing of the wound to help with resuscitation by arresting haemorrhage, controlling pain and preventing further tissue damage by contamination or dehydration.

Exposed soft tissues, brain, gut, etc. must be covered with a waterproof dressing such as polythene film or saline gauze soaks to prevent desiccation and further damage. An outer layer of soft absorbent material such as a wound pad, bandage and a splint stabilizes wounds and fractures. An exposed eye devoid of eyelids should be covered with antiseptic eye ointment (Fig. 2.3) and polythene sheeting or watch glass to prevent corneal dehydration (Fig. 2.4). Toxic agents such as alcohol-based antiseptics should be kept off open wounds because they cause tissue necrosis.

Reassess the   It is important to continue the assessment *pari passu* with
patient   resuscitation, as the correction of one abnormality can bring another problem to light. For example, the administration of fluid to a shocked patient, by restoring the circulation, may restart haemorrhage, with calamitous results if it is not diagnosed and stopped.

Table 2.2 Management of trauma, order of priority.		
Immediate	Secure airway
	Restart heart
	Restore respiratory cycle
	Arrest haemorrhage*
Resuscitate	Restore fluid loss I.V.
	Decompress intracranial tension
	Correct abdominal/chest injuries
	Control pain*
Definitive	Reduce/fix fractures*
	Reconstitute injured vessels
	Repair nerve, muscle, tendon
	Restore skin cover*
***Remember**	Emergency wound care at each stage
	Cover with clean moist dressing

Figure 2.3
Apparent loss of
eyelid, causing severe
pain as the
conjunctiva becomes
dehydrated. The eye
should be completely
covered with eye
ointment (a) giving
immediate pain relief,
until the injury can be
explored. Removal of
the windscreen glass
pinning the eyelid to
the supra-orbital
ridge (b) allowed
primary closure of
the wound (c).

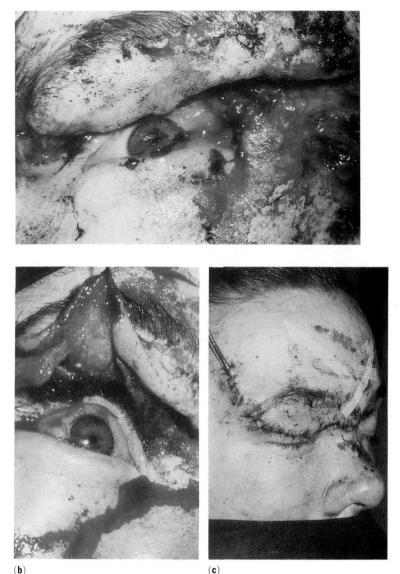

(b)   (c)

Assess the wound   The degree of damage and extent of loss or devitalization must be estimated before a plan for treatment can be made. Assessment of nerve injury must be made before any anaesthetic is administered.

The history of the cause of the accident gives vital information in helping to estimate the extent of injury.

1 Gunshot wounds give variable damage depending on the type of gun. High-velocity gunshot wounds should be treated with

Figure 2.4
Chemosis and corneal
ulceration resulting
from a severe burn (a).
A tarsorhaphy should
have been performed
to prevent this
complication.
Polythene sheet
mounted on a foam
ring prevents
dehydration (b) while
arrangements are
made for treatment.

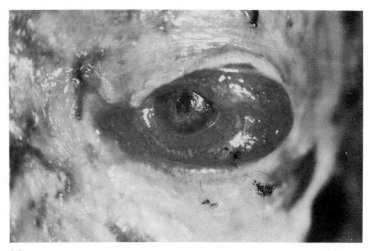

(**a**)

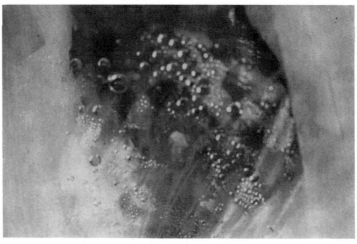

(**b**)

great care, as they can be very misleading. There may be extensive deep damage with little external evidence.

2 Run-over injuries, where the initial appearance may be reassuringly good, usually have extensive subcutaneous disruption with degloving leading to extensive tissue necrosis later (Fig. 2.5).

3 High-pressure injection injuries, especially if toxic chemicals have been injected, are notoriously difficult to interpret in the early phase of treatment.

If the patient is in generally poor condition, with shock or low blood pressure, it is impossible to make a complete assessment. Circulation must be fully restored before an accurate diagnosis of tissue viability can be made (see Table 2.3). A second examina-

Figure 2.5
Appearance of the wound three weeks after suture of a severe degloving laceration of the right leg. Widely undermined skin flaps from such a runover injury have lost their blood supply and direct primary repair is bound to lead to skin necrosis.

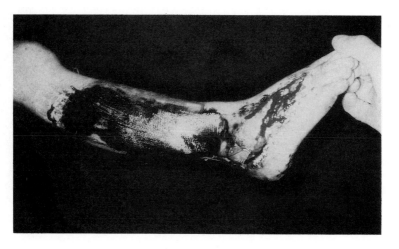

Table 2.3
Factors making wound assessment difficult.

- Patient shocked—Low blood pressure causing poor tissue perfusion
- Constricting clothing or dressings proximally
- Major vascular damage
- Unstable fracture
- Compartment compression
- Hypothermia—Systemic or local
- Poor lighting conditions

tion performed after an interval may clarify the position. When there is an extensive or complicated wound, final assessment can sometimes only be made under anaesthetic (Fig. 2.6).

Preparation for the operation   The wound and the surrounding skin should be cleaned thoroughly to remove dirt and contamination. The antiseptic should contain a detergent to aid cleansing and must not be spirit-based. It must also be light in colour so that skin staining does not interfere with the assessment of tissue viability. Hair-bearing areas can be shaved, but important landmarks such as eyebrows should be left so that they can be used to align the repair accurately. Drapes should be placed to give full exposure not just a 'keyhole' around the wound.

Tourniquet   In limb surgery a tourniquet is an extremely useful aid; the cuff should be placed on the limb pre-operatively but should not be inflated until required, as it might further impair tissue viability.

Debridement   Cleansing must extend into the depths of the wound. Ingrained dirt must be removed by copious irrigation or by scrubbing the tissues with a gauze or sterile brush (Fig. 2.7). Dermabrasion of heavily tattooed areas may be necessary and gives the best results when done at the time of primary surgery (Fig. 2.8).

Figure 2.6
Full assessment of this injury (a) from a potato harvester can only be made at operation under general anaesthetic. The wound is cleaned and debrided (b). Exploration revealed a defect of the skull which needed to have the dura secured (c) before the wound was repaired. (d) Appearance at four weeks showing wound repair supplemented by a small skin graft over exposed periosteum.

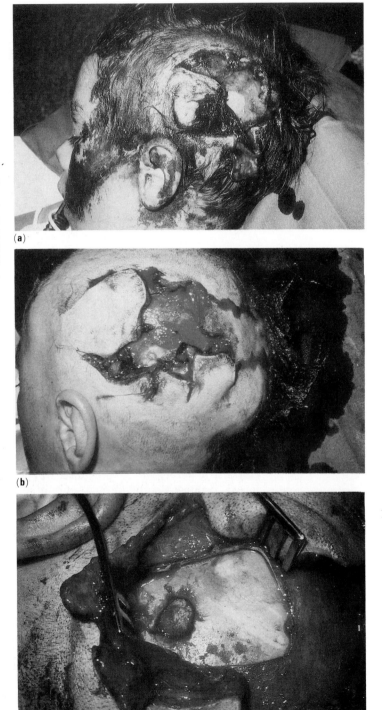

(a)

(b)

(c)

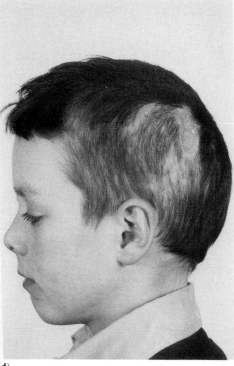

(d)

Figure 2.7
A heavily dirt-ingrained wound (a) must be thoroughly cleaned (b), before it is ready for suture to prevent a tattooed scar.

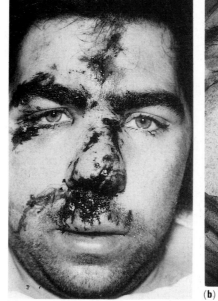

(a)

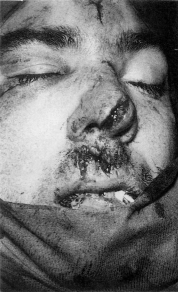

(b)

Figure 2.8
An explosive injury caused deeply ingrained dirt in this patient from a rubber tyre weld which exploded during testing (a). Dermabrasion (b) is excellent for removing the deeply ingrained dirt from flat skin surfaces. (c) The result after one hour's treatment. Note, dermabrasion must not be used on the eye lids or mucosal surfaces as there is a danger of tearing the tissues and therefore the remaining dirt must be individually picked out by sharp dissection.

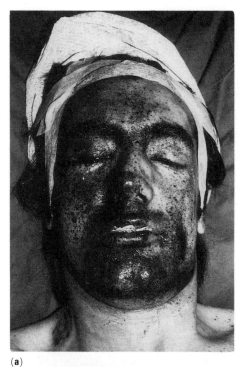

(**a**)

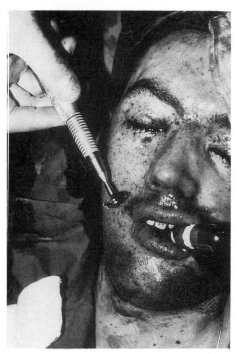

(**b**)

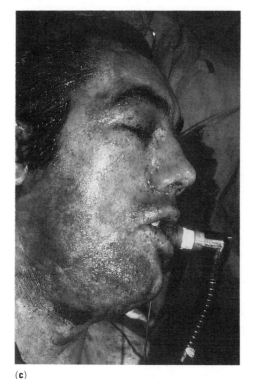

(c)

All haematoma and dead or devitalized tissue must be removed. Dead muscle that gives no contraction on pinching should be excised. Skin debridement of viable wound edges should be kept to an absolute minimum and is not necessary in areas with good blood supply such as the face or scalp. There is no place for routine excision of wide margins of viable skin even in contaminated wounds.

Haemostasis should be obtained using fine ligatures or bipolar coagulation in preference to diathermy, which causes greater tissue necrosis (Fig. 1.9).

The following tests of skin viability are useful at this stage (see Table 2.4).

1 Inspection of skin colour or capillary return.
2 Bleeding from the wound edge.
3 Fluorescein injected systemically gives staining of viable skin.

Time the repair
(see Table 2.5)

1 Before the surgeon proceeds to a definitive repair, the wound must be reassessed during the operation. If any tissues are of doubtful viability, especially in crush injuries or high-velocity wounds, primary suture is contra-indicated. The wound is dressed and inspected again a few days later.

Table 2.4 Assessment of skin viability.	● History	Nature of injury
	● Inspection	Capillary bleeding from wound edge
		Capillary return after release of pressure
		Colour
		Congestion
		Oedema
		Blistering
		Sensation

● Tourniquet release, reflex vasodilatation after release
● Doppler flowmeter
● Thermocouple, thermography
● Dye tests, e.g. fluorescein
● Clearance tests, radioisotope
● Direct percutaneous oxygen measurement

$$TCPO_2 > 20 \text{ mmHg viable, will heal}$$
$$< 20 \text{ mmHg variable, may not heal}$$

2 Delayed primary repair can be carried out within a few days after further debridement of any non-viable tissue. If the condition of the wound is again in doubt, it is best to delay. This not only gives a chance for tissue necrosis to declare itself but allows oedema to subside.

3 Secondary repair can be performed at a later operation when the condition of the wound is satisfactory.

4 Heavily contaminated, untidy wounds, those treated more than eight hours after injury, and infected wounds should not be closed primarily.

5 If in doubt, delay. It is sometimes difficult to assess tissue viability in the acute situation. As long as the wound is protected by an occlusive dressing, less harm will be caused by delay than by injudicious early wound closure.

6 If the condition of the patient is grave, rapid repair by wrapping the wound with a split skin graft may give a good temporary repair.

Treat or prevent infection

There is no substitute for adequate surgical debridement in preventing infection. Routine prophylactic antibiotic need not be given for clean, tidy wounds that are treated within six hours of injury. All other patients with contaminated, untidy wounds with devitalized tissue, or those treated late, should be given suitable antibiotic prophylaxis against gas gangrene and tetanus. The patient's immune status against tetanus should be determined and appropriate measures such as booster toxoid or antitetanus serum should be administered.

Build on a firm foundation

The inexperienced surgeon may be tempted to suture the skin only, as this is usually a deceptively easy part of the repair. However, access through an open wound judiciously extended is good and the opportunity must be taken to explore, clean and

Table 2.5   Summary flow chart of management of the trauma wound

Defect

Early
Clean
Tidy — <8 hr old — L.A. or G.A. — **Wound toilet** Debride → Clean → Adequate local tissue → Direct primary repair

Late
Dirty
Untidy
G.S.W. — >8hr — G.A. — Wound toilet Debride Dress → E.U.A. 48hr → Dirty / Clean

Old wound infected — G.A. — Toilet Debride Treat infection → E.U.A. or dress under sedation Debride → Repeat until clean → Adequate local tissue → Direct secondary repair

Tissue avulsed available → Replant by microvascular repair or graft

Tissue missing → Repair, see Table 2.6

repair all damage as necessary. The repair should be built up from below starting with reduction and fixation of fractures, followed by repair of vessels, nerves, tendons, muscle and other soft tissue. Finally, the skin can be closed.

Place normal tissue in a normal position

In complex skin wounds it is sometimes difficult to know where to begin. If possible, identify anatomical structures such as nostril or lip margin, eyebrow or eyelid and suture these first (Figs. 2.9, 2.10, 2.11). Once key landmarks are aligned, the rest of the wound falls more easily into place.

Never discard anything

All viable tissue must be preserved at first so that, after assessment, it can be put into its correct place (Fig. 2.12). Only rarely can or should 'excess' viable tissue be excised and certainly not until tension-free wound closure is obtained.

Replace like with like

If there is extensive tissue loss it is usually not possible to replace what is missing with identical tissue, except in the case of amputation if the part can be restored with revascularization by microvascular anastomosis. Care must be taken to ensure that appropriate repair is performed. For example, hair-bearing skin should not be applied by graft or flap to a non-hair-bearing area.

Prevent further damage

Throughout the treatment of a wound the first principle is to do no harm. Gentle handling of tissues with fine instruments will minimize further trauma. Dehydration should be prevented by keeping all open wounds moist either by repeated irrigation or by covering them with saline gauze soaks.

Figure 2.9
Identifiable landmarks are marked with ink dots to help wound alignment.

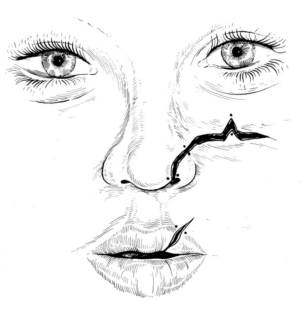

Figure 2.10
Notched scar caused by failure to align the nostril margin correctly.

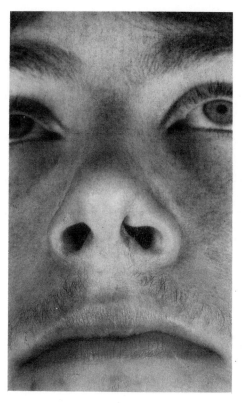

Figure 2.11
Before this wound was sutured, the eyebrow was shaved unnecessarily, making alignment more difficult.

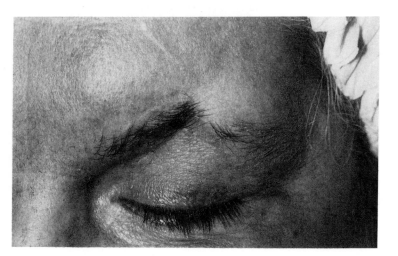

Figure 2.12
During wound debridement, especially on the face, there is no place for routine excision of wound margins and ragged tissue. If it had been done in this case (a), the loose tissue on the cheek might have been discarded. It was in fact the viable eyelids seen before they were sutured over the wired orbital fractures (b).

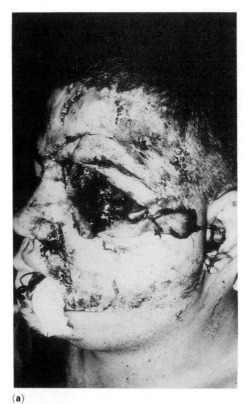

(a)

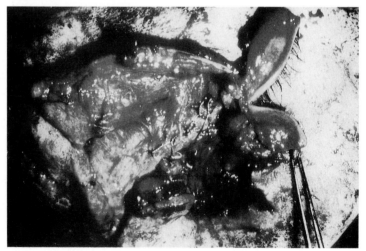

(b)

Techniques of Wound Repair

Prevention of Complications

Placing the incision
The trauma wound is predetermined by the nature and extent of the injury, which is beyond the control of the surgeon. However, in making extensions of wounds or elective incisions, the onus is on the surgeon to place them in such a way as to favour wound healing. There are three basic principles to be observed when placing a scar.

1 *Adequate exposure.* The incision must be placed in such a way and be sufficiently long that adequate exposure is obtained to do the operation intended. It should be capable of extension if necessary to enable unexpected problems to be tackled. An incision placed in an inconspicuous place, for example in the hair line, can be used to conceal the scar but it is essential that the design is such that the flap can be retracted far enough to approach the operation site.
2 *Maintain adequate blood supply.* Incision lines and flap design must take into account the local blood supply. Particular care is needed when planning extensions to traumatic wounds.
3 *Select the correct direction.* The decisive factor in production of a fine linear scar is not the method of closure but the direction of the incision in relation to skin cleavage lines. Scars placed in or parallel to natural skin crease lines generally heal better than those orientated in other directions.

Skin crease lines
There are many named skin crease lines but there are many discrepancies between them.

Relaxed skin tension lines (RSTL of Borges) are the most reliable in practice on the limbs and trunk. They follow the furrows that are formed when the skin is relaxed and are readily identified by flexing or pinching the skin lightly and observing the creases formed. In any particular part of the body there is one direction of pinch giving the biggest furrows. These are parallel to the relaxed skin tension lines (Fig. 2.13).

Wrinkle lines (Kraissl). The natural crease or wrinkle lines are the direction of choice for an incision on the face (Fig. 5.2). Not only is there a natural crease into which the scar will fall but the facial muscles are arranged at right angles to these lines and will tend to draw the wound together on facial movement, allowing better wound healing. If not obvious in younger patients, they can be seen by asking the patient to grimace.

Lines of Langer, though well known are not so reliable. Published diagrams show that in certain parts of the body, for example the antecubital fossa and outer canthus of the eye, they

Figure 2.13
Detection of the
relaxed skin tension
lines.

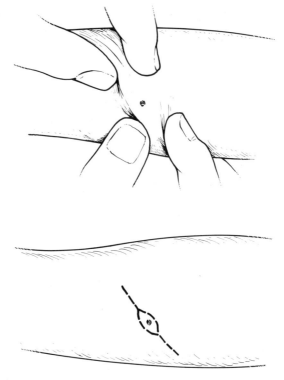

bear little relation to the lines of choice for making an incision to obtain the best scar. The method used to obtain them— observing the direction of round awl puncture marks in a cadaver, which become linear slits—means that they are inappropriate for clinical surgery! Langer found that the lines were not entirely consistent between subjects of different build.

Individual variation The most important point to remember in placing an incision is that every patient has a slightly different individual pattern of skin crease lines. They also vary with age, body build, sex and body position. Diagrams of stylized skin crease patterns can be very misleading and must not be used like maps. The individual pattern in the patient concerned must be marked out carefully before the incision is made.

Avoid haematoma Good haemostasis is vital before closure. Wound drainage should be used whenever there is likely to be bleeding or seepage of serum or lymph from under large flaps. Closed suction drainage is the method of choice, as it allows complete closure of the wound and the exudate is removed, preventing maceration of the wound.

Suture technique There are three prerequisites for good suture repair of a wound:

delicate instruments used atraumatically, fine suture materials, and accurate apposition of the tissues.

Instruments should be as fine as possible and appropriate for the task intended. Magnification is useful using loupes and for microvascular repairs, the use of an operating microscope necessitates suitable microinstruments. Fine-toothed forceps or skin hooks should be used to hold the skin. The use of crushing tissue forceps on the skin must be avoided as they can leave permanent marks.

Suture materials should be as fine as possible while strong enough for the intended purpose. Synthetic monofilament materials produce the least tissue reaction. Atraumatic needles with sharp cutting points leave less obvious marks in the skin.

Sutures that are to be left buried can be absorbable or non-absorbable, but coloured sutures must not be placed near the surface, as they will show. The knots and suture ends must be kept as neat as possible to limit the foreign body in the wound. The volume of a suture knot increases as the power of three of the suture diameter, to that subcutaneous suture numbers are kept to the minimum required to achieve accurate wound closure.

A rule of thumb for skin repair is that the distance between sutures should be the same as the size of the tissue bite on either side of the wound. If smaller bites are used more sutures will be required. A larger number of small sutures removed in stages causes less stitch marks.

Accurate tissue apposition should hold the wound edges in a normal anatomical relationship.
1 Repair proceeds from below outwards in layers to eliminate dead space (Fig. 2.14). If there is a large complex wound, one or more suction drains can be inserted in different layers. The skin should be slightly everted. Inverted wound edges tend to heal with a permanently depressed scar. Ideal suture tension is sufficient to approximate the wound without blanching the skin. Tight sutures cut through, increasing stitch marks.
2 Adhesive skin tapes can be used in addition to sutures or may replace skin sutures entirely in less complex wounds (Fig. 2.15). Tapes should be microporous to prevent maceration of the wound edge. They are less traumatic to the tissues, leave no skin marks and are easier to remove in children, but they have a tendency to invert the wound edge.
3 Oblique wounds are difficult to close. Where skin loss is not a problem the wound can be excised to give vertical edges. If the removal of further skin is not possible a smaller suture bite should be taken on the acute angled side or a mattress suture can be used. In hair-bearing areas an oblique wound parallel to hair follicles is desirable and edges should not be trimmed vertically as a large bald strip will result.

Figure 2.14
(a) Wound repair
should proceed in
layers from below,
suturing anatomical
layers. (b) Fat sutures,
if used, tend to cut out
or crush the tissue
and should be loosely
tied taking small bites.

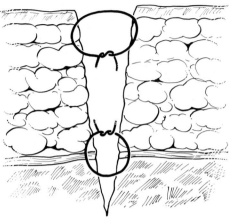

(**a**)

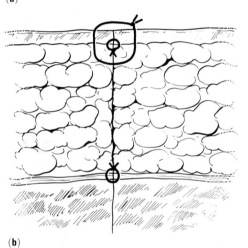

(**b**)

4 When skin of two different thicknesses is sutured the surface level of the wound may not align well. It can sometimes be adjusted by moving the suture knot over to the lower side.

Tissue excess and the dog ear

If an excised wound defect is closed by direct approximation, there will be tension at the middle of the wound with relative excess at each end. This bulge or dog ear can be unsightly and is a well-recognized complication of excisional surgery or when skin flaps are rotated. They tend to settle postoperatively and flatten.

Management. If the dog ear is prominent it can be removed by marking out a further triangle of skin and excising it to make the angle more acute. Alternatively, the dog ear can be lifted in a skin hook and trimmed along one side. This flap is then held across to judge the excess and is trimmed accordingly (Fig. 2.16). These manoeuvres will increase the length of the scar.

Figure 2.15
A method of wound repair using adhesive tapes in addition to sutures. Accurate repair of a curved wound (a) would require a large number of fine sutures. Steristrips used to supplement the repair (b) can be left in place when the sutures are removed at three days. This prevents stitch marks in the wound seen in a red hypertrophic phase at one year's follow up (c), and on full maturation of the scar four years later (d).

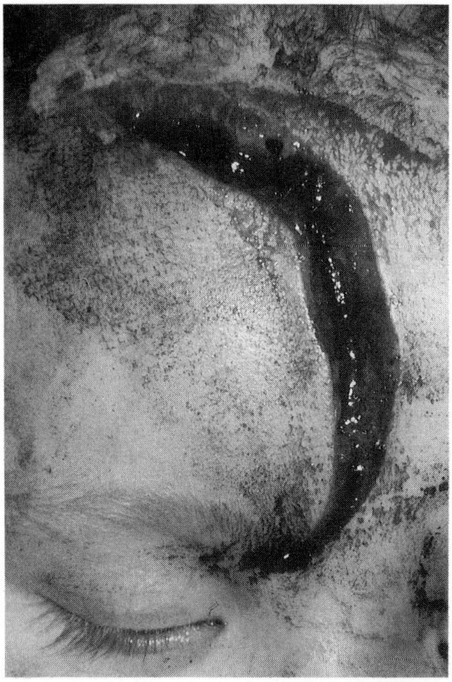

(a)

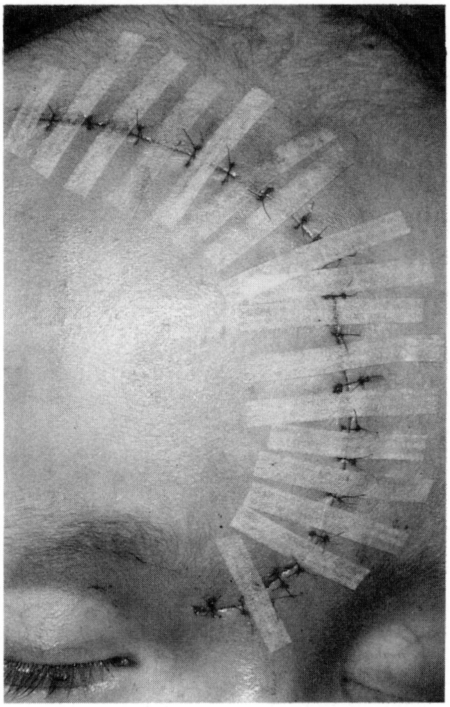

(b)

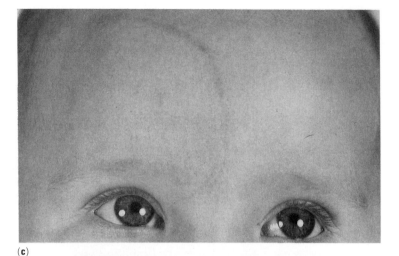

(c)

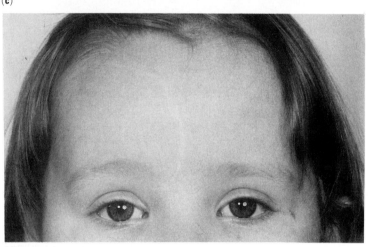

(d)

Postoperative care   Careful postoperative management is essential to back up any operative measures. The basic principle is to rest the injured part in the acute oedematous phase and then to mobilize once fractures have stabilized and the oedema has begun to settle.

Dressings may not be required or even desirable. The inner layer should be non-adherent with a gauze transmitting layer in the middle topped off with an absorbent layer and conforming bandage. Care must be taken when pressure dressings are applied to ensure that they are not too tight or restricting the circulation. If possible a digit or part of a flap should be left exposed so that the circulation can be monitored. Elevation of an injured limb will minimize oedema formation. Oedema is very difficult to disperse once it has set in and the aim should be prevention. Pressure sores can easily develop in a shocked or

Figure 2.16
Method used to
remove a 'dog ear'.

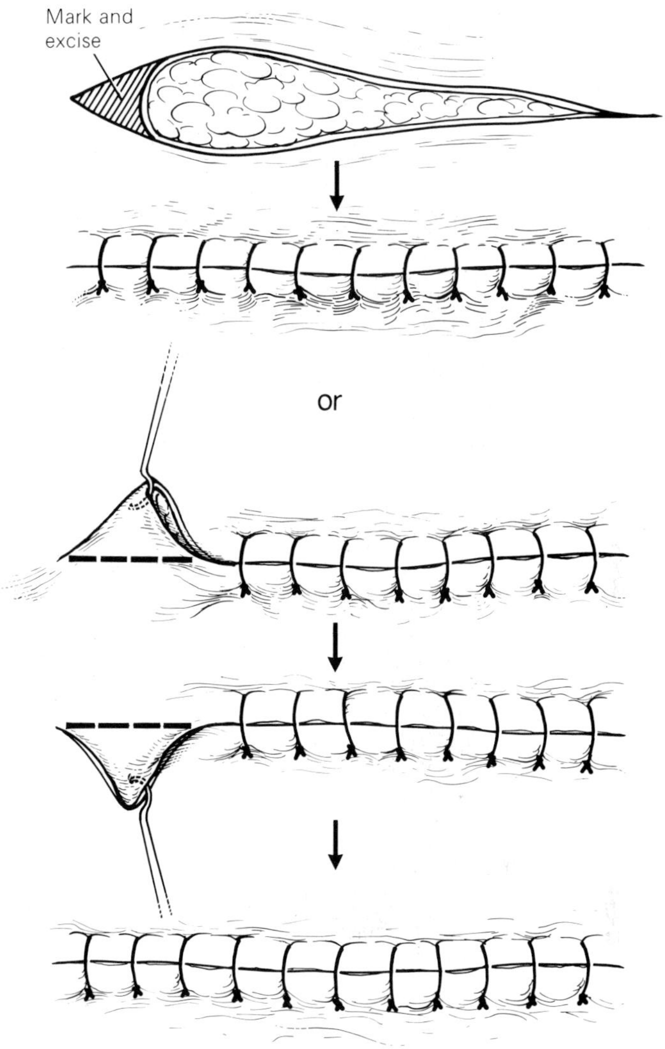

Mark and
excise

or

injured patient if preventive measures such as regular turning are neglected. The damage may not be revealed until several days later. The most vulnerable time is immediately after the accident, even before the patient is taken to hospital, when severe pain causes shock and restricts mobility.

Early suture removal   Skin sutures left in place for more than 48 hours may cause permanent scarring (Fig. 2.17). Sutures should therefore be removed as soon as possible consistent with wound healing. The timing of suture removal varies depending on the site, tension and direction of the wound, age, obesity or any other factor likely to delay healing. On the face, alternate sutures can be removed after 48 hours and replaced with skin tapes. The

Figure 2.17
Suture marks resulting from deep tension sutures used to repair an infected wound of the shin in a child. They are permanent and grow in pace with the patient.

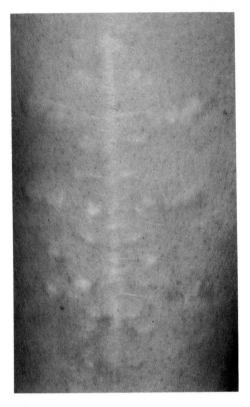

remainder can come out at 5 to 7 days. Trunk and limb wounds heal much more slowly and sutures should be left in longer.

Suture removal can be distressing for young children and before putting them in thought should be given to the problem of removal. Alternative techniques are to use subcutaneous sutures with skin tapes, a subcuticular monofilament suture that slides out easily (Fig. 2.18), or fine absorbable sutures that do not need to be removed. If a complex wound has been repaired it may be better to sedate the child or give a general anaesthetic when removing the sutures.

Wound Management When Tissue is Missing

Unless the defect is small, reconstruction by tissue transfer will have to be considered. It is vital, if there is going to be excessive tension, not to suture the wound directly. Signs of excessive tension are inability to approximate the wound edges or blanching when they are closed. Care should be taken in repairing a wound of a limb under conditions of exsanguination and tourniquet. The volume of the subcutaneous tissues is reduced and may give deceptively easy wound closure. Once the tourniquet is

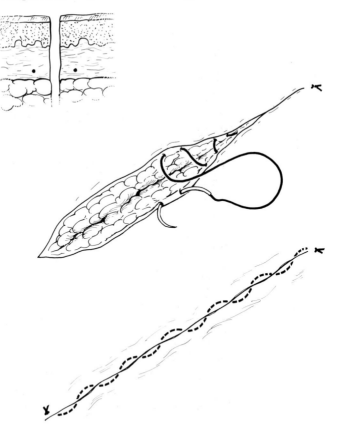

released the inflow of blood with return of tissue turgor and
oedema may cause excessive tension with wound breakdown or
skin necrosis. This problem is exacerbated if a Plaster of Paris
splint or compression dressing is applied.

Principles of management (see Table 2.5)

Avulsion injury:
tissue available

If the blood supply remains intact in partially avulsed wounds or
if it can be restored by microvascular anastomosis, replantation
and primary repair is possible (Fig. 2.19).

Degloving injuries
Degloving injuries need particularly careful treatment. The
commonest cause is in a runover injury when a pneumatic tyre
strips off large flaps of skin. The usual plane of injury is between
the fat and the deep fascia and all the arterial nutrient perforators are disrupted. The marginal blood supply coming into the
base of such a flap can only sustain about one inch breadth of
flap. The remainder of the flap will necrose (Figs. 2.5, 2.20).

Figure 2.19
Avulsion injury of the face (a, b). The blood supply was adequate and primary repair was possible (c). A crush injury of the chest necessitated positive pressure ventilation (d) and a small tarsorrhaphy was required to protect the eye as a result of the facial palsy. (e) Result at two months.

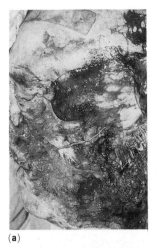

(a)

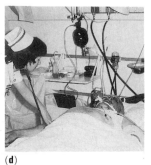

(d)

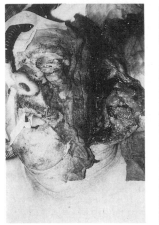

(b)

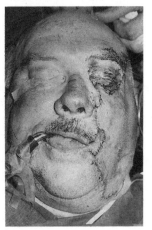

(e)

(c)

Figure 2.20
Flap laceration of the
leg with necrosis. Note
that even though the
flap is proximally
based the blood
supply is insufficient to
sustain more than the
proximal one inch of
skin. The remainder of
the flap is undergoing
various stages of
ischaemic necrosis.

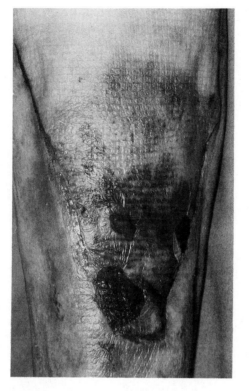

Diagnosis

The history of injury in machinery or a runover and tyre marks on the skin are a good pointer to a degloving injury (Fig. 2.21a). Open degloving injury is usually easily diagnosed by lifting the skin flap up to gauge the extent of undermining. A closed degloving injury can be very deceptive and difficult to detect, particularly in a shocked patient when bleeding under the flap may not occur. The skin will feel loose on the underlying fascia or muscle. Once resuscitation is obtained, haematoma will build up under a closed degloving injury.

Prevention of complications

The open degloving injury of a limb must not be repaired by direct suture. Extensive skin flap necrosis is inevitable. The extent of subcutaneous fat necrosis may be more than the loss of the overlying skin, giving rise to infection and further skin damage.

The closed degloving injury must be suspected and the diagnosis confirmed by incising into the centre of the degloved area through a small stab incision. A probe can then be easily passed into the degloved space. If it is small and the overlying skin is viable, the wound can be sutured but a suction drain must be inserted. Pressure dressing must be avoided as the external

Figure 2.21
Degloving injury
caused by a runover
injury of the leg. Note
that the initial
appearance is
deceptively normal (a),
but the bus tyre marks
should alert the
surgeon to the severity
of the injury and the
subcutaneous
disruption seen in the
thigh (b). All
devitalized skin is
removed and defatted.
It can then be
reapplied to the
debrided wound (c) as
a free skin graft.
Wounds of both legs
were treated in a
similar way and were
completely healed in
two weeks (d).
Contrast this result
with Figs. 2.5 and 2.20.

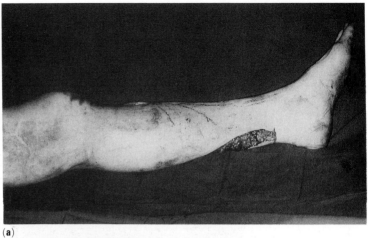

(a)

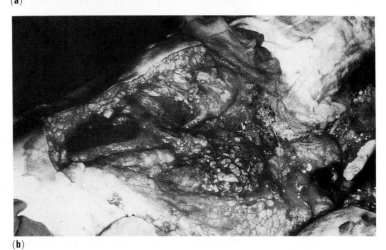

(b)

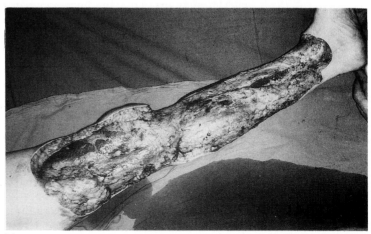

(c)

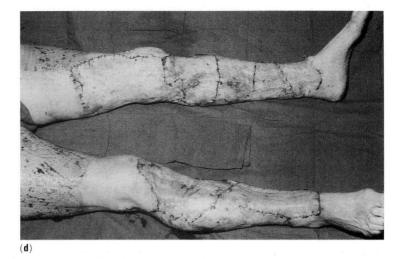

(d)

pressure added to the devitalization will further compromise the blood supply to the skin.

The large open or closed degloving injury must be treated radically, and early, if the skin is to be saved (Fig. 2.21). All undermined skin should be removed except for the attached marginal one-inch strip. After thorough debridement, the skin flap is defatted completely and can then be re-applied to the wound as a free skin graft if vital structures are not exposed and there is a good blood supply in the wound bed. This can be done as a primary procedure, but if there is any doubt about viability of the bed, a delayed procedure is recommended, and the wound is dressed with moist soaks. The skin graft is stored in a domestic refrigerator at 4°C in a sterile container. Delayed grafting is then performed when the wound is reinspected 48 hours later after further debridement as necessary.

If vital structures are exposed or there is a poor blood supply in the base of the wound, flap repair is required (see Chapter 4). Local flap skin is unlikely to be available in this type of injury. An alternative is to use local vascularized tissue such as muscle or fascia and cover it with a split skin graft.

Avulsion injury: tissue not available (See Table 2.6) Repair by the most appropriate method should be used, but in severe, complex injuries the decision requires great experience and surgical skill and referral to a specialist is essential. In limb trauma, amputation as a primary or secondary procedure should be considered in very severe injury as a convenient method to gain early healing, when the alternative is a long series of surgical procedures and the usefulness of the limb will be limited.

When a visible feature of the face, such as nose or ear, is irreparably lost, the wound should be closed primarily by direct suture of the wound edges, if possible, or graft repair; the

Table 2.6 Summary flow chart of wound repair of skin defect

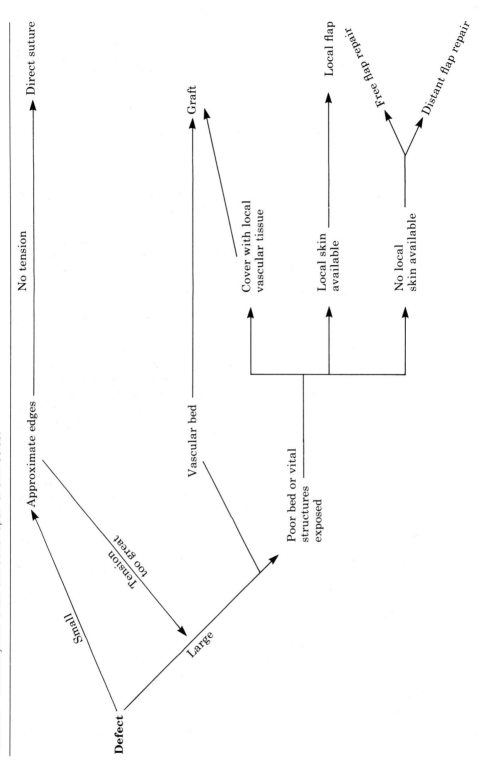

problem of secondary reconstruction can then be discussed at leisure. A temporary prosthesis can be supplied and in many instances a prosthetic replacement will be preferable to the surgical reconstruction (Fig. 1.5).

The Chronic Non-healing Wound

Predisposing factors

Initial trauma. A crushing injury with widespread tissue devitalization is more likely to result in a non-healing wound.

Foreign body. Any of a large range of foreign bodies in a wound can give rise to delayed healing and lead to chronic ulcer or sinus formation:

1 wound contaminants, such as shrapnel, clothing, glass, dirt and debris;
2 sutures; absorbable or non-absorbable material particularly thick sutures with large knots (Fig. 2.2);
3 implants such as a metal plate or infected joint prosthesis;
4 slough, for example dead skin or subcutaneous tissues;
5 granulation tissue. In general granulation tissue formation means there is a vascular response in the wound and repair is possible. However, excessive, exuberant granulation tissue can, in itself, act as a block to healing and prevent epithelialization or destroy epithelium by growing over it.

Infection. Chronic infection may contribute to delay in wound healing but usually in combination with retained foreign body. In specific instances, for example tuberculosis, infection alone causes non-healing.

Neoplasia. The history of trauma may be misleading in a chronic wound. Any ulcer that does not heal in spite of satisfactory treatment for a few months should be biopsied to exclude malignant disease (see Fig. 2.22).

Marjolin's ulcer is a squamous cell carcinoma that develops in a chronic wound after many years.

Vascular insufficiency. Major arterial or venous disease is a cause of non-healing, particularly in the lower limb. In practice it is sometimes very difficult to distinguish between the two problems.

Pressure. Excessive pressure whether caused by decubitus or from an external appliance, for example Plaster of Paris cast, can cause ulceration or contribute to non-healing in a wound (Fig. 2.23). Tissue damage is proportional to the pressure applied

Figure 2.22
A history of trauma can be misleading. This infected granulating wound resulting from 'a scratch' proved to be a basal carcinoma on biopsy.

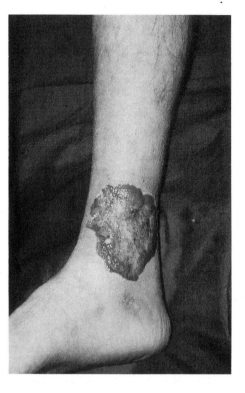

Figure 2.23
Pressure on the skin from a Plaster of Paris cast and the underlying displaced bone fragment (a) has caused a pressure sore at the fracture site, rendering it a compound injury (b).

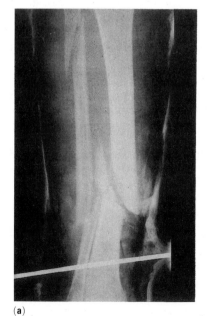

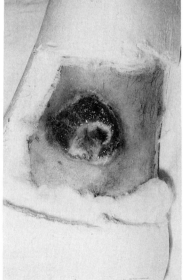

(a)   (b)

but also to the length of time of exposure. Patients lying in bed should be turned at least two-hourly if they are unable or unwilling to turn themselves. It is a wise precaution not to operate on more than one surface at a time if possible as the patient may have to lie on a wound, thereby delaying its healing.

Sensory loss. Skin devoid of protective sensation is very vulnerable to repeated trauma or pressure. Diabetic neuropathy is a particularly severe problem because absent sensation is allied to poor microvascular circulation and trophic ulcers are particularly common in diabetics.

Haematological disorders. Blood dyscrasias such as spherocytosis and sickle cell anaemia predispose to ulceration or poor healing in the lower limb.

Dermatitis artefacta. Bizarre wounds with delayed healing should give rise to the suspicion of patient interference. Wounds that heal in hospital or under occlusive dressings but break down repeatedly are particularly suspicious.

Prevention
Care should be taken to avoid, eliminate or treat predisposing factors of delayed healing.

1 Adequate debridement before wound closure is essential. If there is any doubt, delay. Avoid haematoma by suction drainage.
2 Implanted foreign materials should be used with care and should be avoided in the contaminated or infected wound.
3 Adequate pressure-relieving measures are essential in susceptible patients to prevent further pressure damage.

Investigation
1 Bacterial culture.
2 Haematological investigation for haemoglobin and blood dyscrasias.
3 Plain X-ray examination may reveal a foreign body, or a sinogram may show the extent of the wound.
4 Any chronically unhealed wound should be biopsied to exclude malignant disease if it fails to heal after adequate conservative management (Fig. 2.22).

Management

Debridement
At any stage, wound healing cannot progress in the presence of slough. Adequate debridement implies removing all the dead tissue. This is frequently done without anaesthetic by sharp dissection (Fig. 2.24).

Treat infection
Wounds infected with pathogenic organisms should be treated until clear of infection. Conservative management using

Figure 2.24
Debridement of
slough. This can be
done slowly with
repeated dressings or
by sharp dissection
(a, b). The split skin
graft placed over this
vascular achilles
tendon as a temporary
dressing took well and
gave long-term
repair (c).

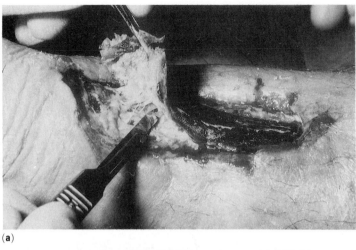

(a)

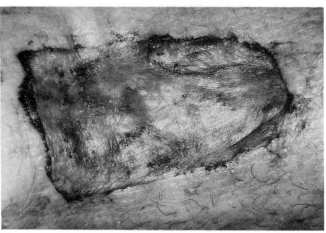

(b)

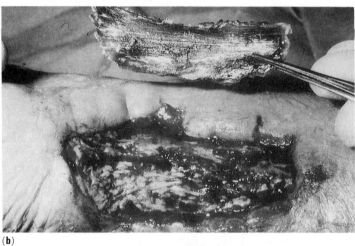

(c)

Figure 2.25
Conservative management of a chronic granulating wound. This pressure sore was the result of a fractured neck of femur (a). Once the patient was mobile following pinning of the fracture it was not advisable to close the sore surgically, even though a flap repair was possible, as it would have delayed rehabilitation and prolonged the stay in hospital. The ulcer was therefore treated as an out-patient. The silastic bung (b) is a useful method for treating cavities to allow healing from below.

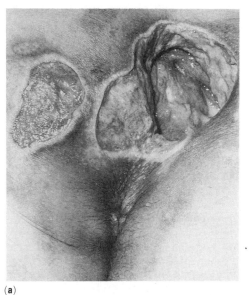

(**a**)

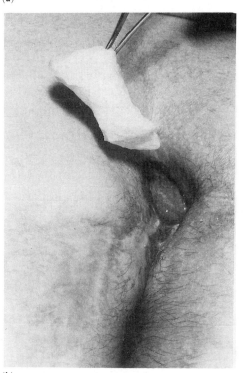

(**b**)

repeated dressings moistened with antiseptic solutions such as dilute Milton will clean most wounds satisfactorily. Systemic antibiotics may be required. Topical antibiotics should not usually be used as there is a risk of hypersensitivity developing.

Conservative treatment

After correction of predisposing factors, repeated dressing, splinting with elevation and rest encourages healing. If the wound is small and no vital structures are exposed, conservative management can be considered as an out-patient. Cavity wounds should be kept open so that healing can progress from below. A silastic foam bung dressing is particularly useful in out-patient management (Fig. 2.25).

Tissue transfer

Once the wound is clean and infection is treated, reconstruction can be performed (see Table 2.6).

Persisting controversies

- Do modern occlusive dressings speed up healing?
- The extent of debridement required in traumatic wounds.
- The place of skin tapes in wound closure and postoperative splinting.
- Which system of skin crease lines gives the best results?

Further reading

Bucknall, T.E. & Ellis, H. (1984) *Wound Healing for Surgeons*. London, Philadelphia: Baillière Tindall.

Montandon, D. (1977) Wound Healing. *Clinics in Plastic Surgery*, Vol. 4. Philadelphia, London: W.B. Saunders.

Gillies, H. & Millard, D.R. (1957) *The Principles and Art of Plastic Surgery*. Boston: Little Brown.

3 Complications of Free Grafts

A free graft is completely detached before transplantation to a new site. During the transfer it is severed from its blood supply and a successful result—'take'—depends on it picking up sufficient blood supply, by revascularization from the recipient bed, before tissue necrosis has occurred (Fig. 3.1). In practice, for this to be achieved free grafts must have a large surface area in proportion to their volume. Free skin grafts can therefore include only epidermis and dermis devoid of all subcutaneous tissue. In contrast, flap transfer involves the transportation of a piece of tissue attached at all times by one edge through which the blood supply must be maintained (Fig. 3.2). Free flap transfer is made possible by microvascular anatomosis of the nutrient blood supply (see Chapter 6).

Figure 3.1
The stages in the take of a split-thickness skin graft. The graft is vulnerable at all stages (a, b, c) to disruption of its attachment to the underlying bed until fibrous tissue connections have formed (d).

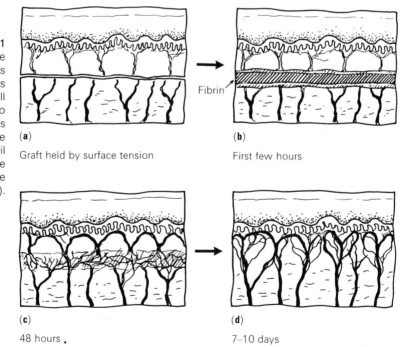

(a) Graft held by surface tension

(b) First few hours

Fibrin

(c) 48 hours .

(d) 7–10 days

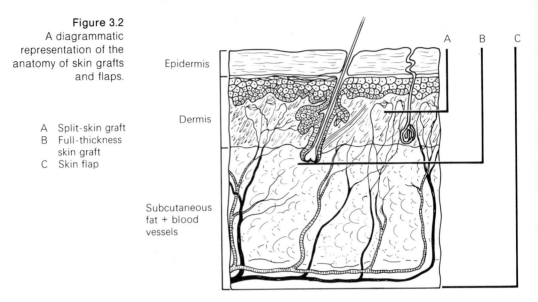

Figure 3.2
A diagrammatic
representation of the
anatomy of skin grafts
and flaps.

A   Split-skin graft
B   Full-thickness
    skin graft
C   Skin flap

Epidermis

Dermis

Subcutaneous
fat + blood
vessels

Complications of Free Skin Grafts

Free skin grafting is easier to perform, but the quality of result is usually less good than a flap procedure, which has a greater number of potential complications. As in all tissue transfers, there are additional problems that arise from the donor site. Immediate complications are usually the result of a technical error. The most important complication is failure to take, which is usually revealed within a few days, causing delayed healing or failure of the graft.

General complications
Problems arise in two main ways.

1 True complications of a skin graft procedure, which can develop at any stage of the process. These will be discussed in detail later in the chapter.
2 Results of normal uneventful graft healing can give rise to dissatisfaction. This is often a case of faulty selection of the most appropriate method or poor patient understanding of the possible results.

Predisposing factors

Recipient site
- Any area that is itself devoid or deficient of a nutrient blood supply is not able to support and sustain a viable graft and a flap procedure will be required.
- Interposition of any mechanical blockage between the blood supply in the bed and the graft, such as slough, haematoma,

pus, foreign body or surgical materials for example, sutures or drains—will prevent revascularization of the graft.
- Infection by β haemolytic streptococci of groups A, B, C and G or *Pseudomonas pyocyaneas* predisposes to graft failure.
- The shape of the recipient site determines the placing of the marginal scar and can affect the tendency for graft contraction to occur. Straight scars across the volar aspect of a joint may lead to flexion contracture.

The graft   If the viability of the graft has been compromised in any way it will fail to take or heal slowly.

- A graft that has been allowed to dry out will die.
- Storage of grafts is possible, but the viability gradually declines during storage. The conditions for successful storage will be discussed later.
- Contamination of the graft by pathogenic organisms interferes with healing.
- Mechanical damage for example crushing by careless handling can compromise the graft.

Surgical expertise   A skin graft is a very fragile, vulnerable structure until it is safely established, and inexperience in the surgical team of medical or nursing staff can cause complications during the operative phase or postoperatively.

Patient expectation   There is a tendency for lay people to consider that a graft is a form of invisible mending, so that there may be great disappointment even if the graft has taken perfectly. Referring clinicians may have given an over-optimistic impression of the likely result.

First impressions of the appearance of a newly healed graft can be misleading as it may look discoloured, bruised and irregular. This will improve to some extent with time, but if the patient is not warned of this initial ugly appearance disappointment can set in and is very difficult to dislodge. Chance remarks to relatives or friends, or even insensitive or ignorant medical and nursing staff can do irreparable damage at this vulnerable period of recovery.

Graft selection   The type of graft selected may be crucial in determining the final result. A graft taken from an inappropriate donor area may not be acceptable even if the take is perfect. There may be a poor colour match if the graft is taken from a distant part of the body. For example, grafts from the lower limb tend to be more deeply pigmented and should not be used on the face if it is possible to use a donor site nearby. In general the nearer the donor site is to the recipient site the better will be the result of the graft.

The choice between split-thickness or full-thickness skin grafts needs very careful consideration. Graft expansion methods such as meshing can also enhance the take but adversely affect the cosmetic results of the graft. Even if a graft is technically possible across the volar aspect of a joint, flap repair would have less tendency to contract.

Prevention of complications

Recipient site A graft will not take over avascular tissues such as bare cortical bone, exposed tendon or cartilage. It will take over areas with a good blood supply, for example subcutaneous fat, muscle, cancellous bone or bone covered by periosteum and over paratenon and perichondrium. In practice it is possible for a graft to 'bridge' over a small non-vascular area of up to 1 cm diameter. The blood supply is picked up from the surrounding tissue bed and travels horizontally in the graft. If larger avascular areas are exposed, flap repair is essential (Table 3.1).

Graft choice The better quality of full-thickness skin grafts (see Fig. 3.2), which contain all the elements of normal skin, makes them preferable to partial-thickness skin grafts in areas where good appearance or function is required (Table 3.2).

Small defects The decision to graft a small defect must be evaluated carefully, particularly towards the end of treatment of a larger wound. If a

Table 3.1
Comparison of the properties of free skin grafts and flaps.

	Free skin graft	*Flap*
Blood supply	Needs vascular bed	Carries own blood supply, will cover avascular bed
Availability	Large areas available	Limited availability
Donor defect	Variable Not usually marked	Full thickness defect usually leaves noticeable scar
Cosmesis	Variable	Good
Function	Variable	Good

Table 3.2
Comparision of the properties of split skin and full thickness skin grafts.

	SSG	*FTSG*
Availability	Readily available	Limited
Donor scar	Usually inconspicuous	Marked donor scar
Take	Good, early	Less reliable, longer to establish
Cosmesis	Variable	Good usually
Function	Variable Contracture a problem	Good Less contracture

graft is used, the necessary immobility required to allow a take may set back overall recovery and delay rehabilitation. The part slowest to heal is frequently in an area subjected to trauma or near a joint. Continued conservative management may well allow mobility to continue, avoiding stiffness.

Preoperative planning

It is essential to plan the operation with the full co-operation and consent of the patient. The pros and cons of alternative methods should be discussed, in particular the likely quality of the graft and its appearance. Discussion should also include the extent, site and likely appearance of the donor scar, care being taken to place the donor site in a functionally and aesthetically acceptable place.

Operative technique

There is no doubt that careful, gentle technique in preparing the recipient site, taking the graft and applying it, is essential to prevent many of the complications of free grafts. There is no substitute for experience. It is important that the surgeon should see grafting operations before doing them on his own. Careful adherence to basic techniques will help to ensure a good result. Good anaesthesia is vital and the patient must be comfortable and still. If general anaesthesia is used, gradual awakening, avoiding coughing, will help to prevent haematoma.

Haemorrhage

1 In general, skin grafts contract when they are cut, so that the donor site must be bigger in surface area than the defect to be covered. The bleeding from a split-skin donor site can be very rapid, as a vast number of capillaries are cut.

2 All staff, including the anaesthetist, should be fully aware that there may be a risk of haemorrhage and shock when large areas of skin graft are being taken. The patient should be blood-grouped and cross-matched and an intravenous drip should be set up and running before large grafts are cut.

3 Efficient, rapid surgery will decrease the operating time and therefore the time for bleeding. The operating theatre must be fully prepared with sufficient trained staff available and adequate dressings assembled to avoid delays, particularly when treating burns (see Chapter 10).

4 The surgeon must be sufficiently experienced to deal with any complications. This includes knowing when to cut short the operation before shock develops, applying compression dressings to limit blood loss, and planning a second stage. Grafts already cut can be stored and applied at secondary procedures.

5 When operating on a limb, a tourniquet helps to limit blood loss.

Anaesthesia

1 The patient may be old and unfit and vulnerable to

complications of anaesthesia and should be made as fit as possible before grafting is performed.

2 The anaesthetist must be sufficiently experienced to anticipate and prevent extra problems caused by blood loss.

3 For prolonged procedures when large surface areas are exposed, heat loss is a problem. The patient should be on a thermostatically controlled warming blanket and the operating theatre temperature should be increased. Children are particularly at risk.

4 Local anaesthesia can be useful when cutting skin grafts, but the safe dose must not be exceeded. Anaesthetic block technique in a limb with a tourniquet gives a good operative field. For local infiltration, dilute anaesthetic with adrenalin is preferred. Hyaluronidase used as a spreading factor, in the dose of one ampoule added to the local anaesthetic, aids diffusion (Fig. 3.3).

5 Topical local anaesthetic cream is an excellent method of preparing a donor site but it must be applied at least one hour in advance and covered with an occlusive dressing to be effective.

Postoperative care Good postoperative care is essential for successful grafting. The patient is best looked after by a trained team of specialist medical, nursing and ancillary staff. There should be continuity of care. For example, damage to a graft can easily occur during transfer from operating theatre to ward, if inexperienced staff are involved.

Figure 3.3
A technique to aid the infiltration of local anaesthetic into a split-skin graft donor site using hyaluronidase. The local anaesthetic is injected at one edge and can be rolled subcutaneously using a gauze swab into an extensive area.

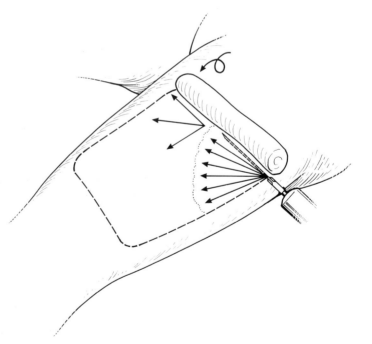

Prevention of technical complications

Full-thickness skin grafts

1 The size of graft required must be accurately marked out with a template of inelastic material using Bonney's Blue. The advantage of a full thickness graft will be prejudiced if it is cut so small that a patched graft is required (Fig. 3.4).
2 The graft should be marked under normal skin tension so that, when it is sutured into the defect, it is under normal tension.

Figure 3.4
The transfer of a full-thickness, post-auricular skin graft. Note the use of a pattern to gauge the size accurately, the complete removal of the subcutaneous fat, and the accurate placement of marginal sutures to approximate the graft edge to the recipient site skin edge.

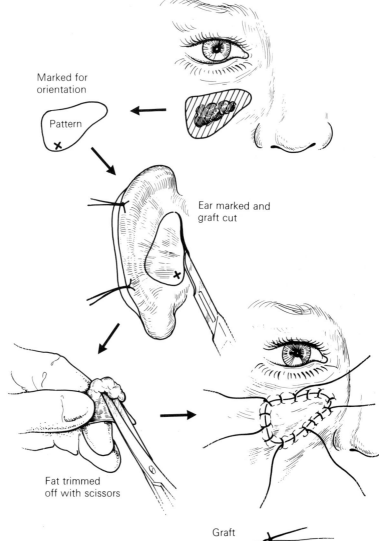

Marked for orientation

Pattern

Ear marked and graft cut

Fat trimmed off with scissors

Graft

Particular care is required when marking and taking a post-auricular graft. The ear has to be pulled forward. If it is stretched excessively before marking, the resulting graft will be too small when cut.

3 The graft can be taken by cutting it from the subcutaneous fat—alternatively, the graft can be defatted after it is taken. All fat must be removed. Care must be taken not to buttonhole or crush the skin.

4 Once taken, the graft must be kept moist in a saline gauze swab, until it is required, to prevent it drying out.

Split-thickness skin grafts

1 Theoretically, any area of intact skin will suffice as a donor site, but careful selection is required. The skin thickness varies in different parts of the body and it is important to consider what thickness of skin graft is required before deciding on the donor site.

2 Care must be exercised in older patients, as the skin gets thinner with age, particularly in post-menopausal females, and in babies whose skin is thin.

3 If donor sites are limited, grafts will have to be cut to a thickness determined by the donor-site availability.

4 The main problem in cutting split skin grafts is judging the depth and cutting accurately at that depth. As a sheet of graft of uniform thickness is usually required, a good working knowledge of the four main methods of cutting split skin grafts is essential.

Free knife method
Using a scalpel, razor blade or long unguarded knife (Blair knife), the split thickness graft is cut freehand. This method relies on high degrees of skill and practice and is not often used except for cutting small grafts. Control over the thickness of graft is very difficult, and patchy or irregular grafts can result. This method should not be used by the novice.

Guarded hand-held dermatome
The Humby modification of the original Blair knife has made it possible to control the depth of cut more easily by adjusting a round bar above and slightly in front of the blade. It is the most commonly used method of cutting a skin graft but still requires skill and experience in setting the blade and using the knife.

Mechanical dermatome
Modern dermatomes, driven by electric motor or compressed air, work on the principle of a fixed-depth gauge with reciprocating blade to cut the graft. They are generally easier to use than the hand-held dermatome and have the added advantage that grafts can be cut from concave donor sites, such as the abdomen and flanks. The width of graft is limited by the size of the instrument, usually to less than 3 inches.

Drum dermatome

This instrument removes a lot of the uncertainty from taking grafts. The donor site skin is stuck to the drum with contact adhesive or a double-sided adhesive tape on the drum. As the drum is rotated the skin is lifted and the knife blade moved from side to side cuts the skin graft. A predetermined size of graft can be cut by applying adhesive only to the desired area.

Complications arise in several ways.

1 If the adhesive is patchy an irregular graft will be cut.
2 The depth setting may not be accurate owing to damage to the instrument. The depth setting must always be checked before use.
3 Once learned, the technique is easy but experience is needed. Too much lift and the skin may come off the drum, causing holes or patches. Too little lift and the blade may cut into the full thickness of the surrounding skin. The drum dermatome method is slow and cumbersome but it is very effective in cutting grafts off concave areas such as the abdomen.
4 It is necessary to ensure that the guard is correctly fitted to prevent the blade injuring the surgeon's index finger.

Precautions when taking split skin grafts

Check the dermatome

1 The responsibility lies with the surgeon to check the dermatome, but it is essential that the theatre assistant or scrub nurse reminds him, when handing over the assembled knife, that the setting has not been checked.
2 The instrument must be assembled correctly. In a large institution using T.S.S.U. facilities there may be a large number of dermatomes in circulation and they may be dismantled for cleaning. The dermatome must be checked on each occasion it is used for correct assembly, normal functioning and absence of damage.
3 The blade must be sharp, preferably new if a disposable blade is used, and correctly seated in the dermatome.
4 Excessive wear or play in an instrument must be avoided. Check that all screws and lock-nuts are securely tightened.

Check the depth setting

1 Do not rely solely on the depth indicator. If the instrument is free of damage, the gauge of a drum dermatome will be more reliable. On a Humby knife there is considerable variation in the gauge accuracy, and because of the length of the blade the effect of any play will be exaggerated.
2 By holding the dermatome up to the light, the actual clearance between blade and guard can be seen and the setting can be adjusted accordingly. If the guard is bent, the knife should not be used.

With experience, the desired thickness can be judged accurately by eye. For the beginner, a useful indicator of setting is to use a disposable scalpel blade—thickness 0.7 mm—as a template for a medium-thickness split skin graft taken from an adult donor site.

3 With the Humby knife the thickness of graft cut depends on the individual operator. Such factors as pressure applied and the angle of the knife alter the depth of graft. The setting of a Humby knife is therefore individual to the surgeon, who will have to learn to judge the setting that suits him.

Prepare the donor site

1 The exact placing of the donor site should be agreed with the patient pre-operatively. In a hair-bearing area, a shave shortly before surgery is best. Shaving a day or two before can cause small septic scratches and spots that may contaminate the graft and donor site.

2 Place the assistants in the optimum position to help. A Humby knife is best used on the forehand. Left- and right-handed knives are obtainable. The best donor site is the flat surface of a limb. The whole area should be exposed and clear of drapes. The surgeon can work up or down the limb, whichever is more convenient, but the assistants should be on the opposite side of the limb leaving a clear space down the surgeon's forehand side.

3 Tension the donor site. It is impossible to cut a skin graft from a soft and floppy donor site. One assistant supports the limb from below to release any muscle tension and by flattening the palm spreads out the skin. The tips of the fingers and the thumb or thenar eminence are used to grip the skin to put it under slight circumferential tension to stop sideways wobble (Fig. 3.5). A second assistant puts tension on the skin in the longitudinal plane by counter-pressure just behind the blade with a hand or board (Fig. 3.6).

4 The assistants must maintain a steady position and correct tension throughout the cutting phase. Blood from previous donor sites may make the hold slippery. Gauzes over such areas will help to maintain a good grip.

5 Lubrication of the donor site is essential to stop the skin moving with the blade. Detergent-based antiseptics such as Betadine, liquid paraffin or vaseline are suitable lubricants.

Relax

If the donor site has been prepared correctly and if the assistants are well placed, cutting the graft is relatively easy. There is considerable knack and coordination required, but best results are obtained if the surgeon is confident and relaxed. The blade should move to and fro across the skin smoothly and steadily. A tense surgeon is likely to apply erratic pressure and a series of small cuts or chips of graft will result.

Check the thickness of the graft

This must be done as the first few millimetres of graft are cut.

1 Observe the graft. A thin graft is transparent and crinkly, a thick graft is opaque and stiff.

Figure 3.5
The donor site for a
split-skin graft must be
held flat and under
some tension if sheets
of graft of uniform
thickness are to be
cut.

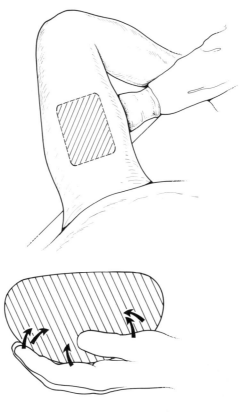

Figure 3.5
The donor site for a split-skin graft must be held flat and under some tension if sheets of graft of uniform thickness are to be cut.

2 Observe the donor site. The bleeding pattern varies according to the thickness of the graft. The donor site for a thin graft has a large number of fine bleeding points. When the graft is thick, the donor site has a smaller number of larger bleeding points. In extreme cases, subcutaneous fat will be observed.

Readjust any depth error

1 *Graft too thin.* Either stop, readjust the knife and start again, or, if the error is small, adjust the angle of the knife or press more firmly to increase the depth of cut.
2 *Graft too thick or donor site too deep.* Either stop, treat the wound as a laceration, suture it and start again; or, if the error is minor, adjust the angle of the knife or press down less firmly on it to decrease the depth.
3 It may be possible to keep the blade in place and readjust the setting. This requires experience, since it is then difficult to judge the thickness. When cutting restarts, a gap or thin area is easily produced.
4 Maintain momentum. If possible do not stop but adjust the thickness by minor alteration of pressure and angle of the

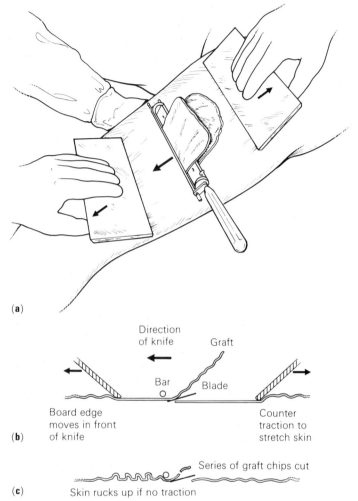

Figure 3.6
Cutting a split-skin
graft. Note (a and b)
that an assistant puts
tension behind the
knife to stretch the
skin. If this is not done,
the skin rucks up and
an irregular graft
results (c).

(**a**)

Direction
of knife   Graft

Bar   Blade

Board edge   Counter
moves in front   traction to
(**b**)   of knife   stretch skin

Series of graft chips cut

(**c**)   Skin rucks up if no traction

knife. If the knife stops it is likely to form a button-hole effect, a thin patch or a thick ridge in the graft.

Care of the graft   A skin graft is extremely vulnerable.

1 Keep the graft moist. Desiccation leads to rapid death and the graft should be placed in a gauze swab moistened with isotonic saline.
2 Identify the graft. At operation, grafts should be placed in a readily identifiable swab. For this purpose, coloured swabs are used to prevent the embarrassing complication of the graft being discarded with contaminated swabs.
3 *Storing the graft*. Any graft not used can be stored if kept moist and cool. It is folded with the cut surface inwards, covered in a saline gauze and placed in a sealed sterile jar,

labelled with the patient's name and the date of harvesting. It will keep for at least two weeks stored in a domestic refrigerator at +4°C. Thin grafts keep well, but thick partial-thickness and full-thickness grafts do not survive so readily.

Prepare the graft

For ease of handling, the skin can be spread onto a tulle gras backing, allowing its size to be gauged more easily. The graft must be spread *cut surface up* so that when it is applied to the defect the cut surface will be in contact with the bed. The cut surface can usually be identified as it is shiny and smooth and reflects the light better.

Donor-site complications

Full-thickness skin graft

A scar is an inevitable result at a full-thickness skin graft donor site. Direct suture gives the best result, so that the graft should be removed from areas where there is spare skin, e.g. postauricular, preauricular, upper eyelid, supraclavicular or lower abdominal skin. When closure is not possible a split-thickness graft will be required.

Split-thickness skin graft

The donor site should be left with sufficient dermis and epithelial remnants for spontaneous epithelialization to occur. It must be kept clean and uncontaminated while healing takes place. Pain can be severe in the first two hours but usually subsides over the first 48 hours. An occlusive dressing such as Opsite helps the pain. The most important complication is delayed healing.

Predisposing factors to delayed healing

A thick split-skin graft gives a deeper donor site that heals more slowly (Fig. 3.7). The skin tends to be thin in older, especially female, patients giving rise to relatively deeper donor sites. Infection, particularly by β haemolytic steptococci, will cause

Figure 3.7
An unsightly donor-site scar resulting from a thick split-skin graft taken with a Padget dermatome ten years previously. This a particularly conspicuous site in a female patient and should be avoided if possible.

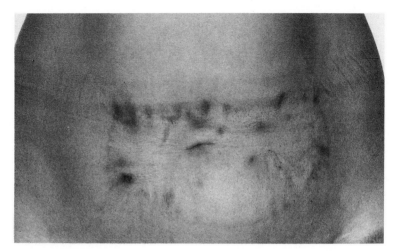

delay in healing. Trauma, when a donor site is disturbed frequently or knocked, can delay healing. The dressings should therefore be kept in place undisturbed for at least one week unless it becomes infected.

The donor site should be chosen away from the perineum, pressure areas or joint creases, so that maceration and trauma are avoided.

Prevention of delayed healing

1 Avoid a deep defect by careful selection of donor site and graft-knife setting. A donor site over a bony prominence will cause irregular graft thickness and should be avoided if possible.

2 Graft the donor defect if necessary. In elderly patients a little extra skin can be cut and applied to the donor site as a mesh graft to speed healing.

3 *Adequate dressing.* An occlusive dressing may speed healing but can predispose to infection. A fully absorbent dressing should be large enough to prevent breakthrough bleeding. If the dressing becomes wet, the outer layers should be removed and replaced with sterile dry dressings.

4 *Careful mobilization.* The early donor-site scar is vulnerable to increased hydrostatic pressure and elevation should continue until it is healed. Thereafter, a pressure dressing such as a tubigrip should be applied for several weeks, particularly in lower-limb donor sites. In out-patients it is preferable, all other considerations being equal, to take the graft from the upper limb to avoid interfering with patient mobility.

Late donor scar complications

The donor site may develop any complication of a scar (Fig. 3.8), including hypertrophic or keloid scar (Fig. 3.9), which will be discussed in Chapter 5. The donor scar tends to dry and crack and should be kept greased with moisturizing cream.

The scar will tend to be hypopigmented and vulnerable to sunlight (Fig. 3.10). For the first year, until the pigment returns the scar should be protected with clothing or a strong sunscreen cream. If the fresh donor scar is traumatized by sun, the subsequent return of pigment is often considerably delayed.

Graft Failure

Diagnosis
The graft is white or translucent when first applied but becomes pink as it is revascularized, usually starting within 48 hours. A thick, partial-thickness or full-thickness skin graft will stay white longer, possibly up to a week.

Signs of failure
● A persistently white graft.
● A graft remaining loose on its recipient bed.

Figure 3.8
The textural pattern in this well-healed, rather atrophic donor scar may be caused by the pattern of weave in the dressing gauze (a). It is quite obvious when the skin is not under tension (b).

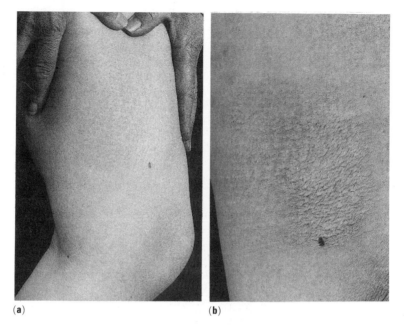

(a) (b)

Figure 3.8 The textural pattern in this well-healed, rather atrophic donor scar may be caused by the pattern of weave in the dressing gauze (a). It is quite obvious when the skin is not under tension (b).

- A black, dry graft is dead.
- In the presence of a haematoma, a dark or blue graft may be merely bruised but viable. Slow take may occur.

Predisposing factors

Graft take depends on close immobile contact between graft and bed, allowing it to pick up a sufficient blood supply before death from ischaemia occurs. The initial adhesion is by surface tension with fibrin deposition for the first few hours, followed by vascularization starting at 24–48 hours. Firm union with collagen formation begins after a few days (Fig. 3.1). Anything that prevents the adhesion is a cause of graft failure.

Haematoma or seroma between the graft and its bed acts primarily as a mechanical barrier to vascularization. An expanding haematoma will strip off graft that has already been adherent. Haematoma, left undrained, will act as a focus for infection.

Movement at any stage within the first seven days is a common cause of graft failure by preventing adhesion of the graft to its bed.

Infection with pus, under the graft acts as a mechanical barrier to take. Contamination by most of the common skin flora will not interfere with graft take. *Steptococcus pyogenes* is an absolute contraindication to any skin graft procedure. The graft may be completely destroyed and liquified. *Pseudomonas pyocyaneas* has similar but less marked effects.

Figure 3.9
Hypertrophic donor
scar on thigh at 6
months (a) and two
years (b) after skin
graft.

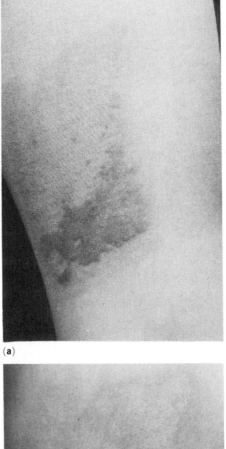

(**a**)

(**b**)

Figure 3.10
A forearm donor site showing hypopigmentation. Early exposure to sun can cause blistering and exacerbate hypopigmentation of a donor site. The graft seen on the flexor aspect of wrist has an exceptionally good colour match, because it is taken from an anatomically similar site.

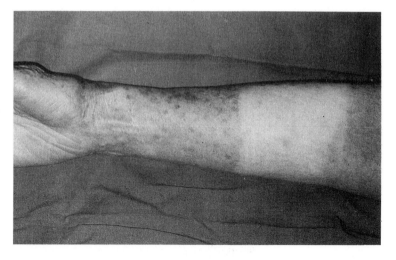

Tissue interposition forms a mechanical barrier to revascularization. Placing the graft upside down brings an impervious keratin layer against the bed preventing take. If the graft is lifted off its bed repeatedly by seroma or haematoma, epithelial elements may begin to cover the graft's deep surface preventing adhesion. In the full thickness graft, fat remnants in the deep surface can act as a barrier.

Inadequate bed. Avascular tissue in the bed such as exposed bone, cartilage or tendon will prevent take.

Dead graft. When a graft has been stored badly and allowed to dry out or heat up it will die. Storage longer than three weeks in the domestic refrigerator is very likely to give rise to a non viable graft.

Prevention—adequate preparation of the recipient bed
1 *The clean surgical wound.* Complete haemostasis is the key to the good graft take and can be achieved in several ways.
   (a) Arrest of large bleeding points by ligature or bipolar coagulation.
   (b) Small oozing vessels can be stopped by firm pressure from saline gauze pack applied for a few minutes. Additional measures include adrenaline saline soaks 1 part in 500,000, topical thrombin or warm packs.
   (c) If adequate haemostasis cannot be obtained, consideration should be given to a delayed application of the graft. The wound is dressed with a firm occlusive dressing to prevent desiccation of the bed and the graft should, ideally, be applied within 48 hours.
2 *The chronic granulating wound.* Clean, flat, healthy granulation

tissue over the wound bed is the aim. Fleshy, proud granulation tissue can be subdued by firm pressure dressings or removed by curettage at operation prior to the application of the graft. The granulations tend to bleed profusely and good haemostasis is essential.

Routine bacteriological swabs should be taken to detect pathogenic organisms, and infection should be treated, as necessary, by local dressings or by appropriate systemic antibiotics.

Slough must be removed by:

(a) surgical debridement, which can be perfomed by scalpel, without pain, during a wound dressing without anaesthetic;

(b) repeated dressings using antiseptic or enzymatic agents;

(c) absorbent preparations that soak up and remove debris from a wound—these may be useful but are of little help in the presence of large volumes of slough.

Accurate application of the graft Intimate contact with the recipient bed without differential movement is essential. There are two basic methods of achieving this.

1 *Pressure dressing techniques.* A full-thickness graft must be sutured edge-to-edge to the skin margin of a defect but a split-thickness graft can be overlapped (Figs. 3.4, 3.11). A pressure dressing is then applied.

(a) A bolus dressing (synonym Stent or tie-over dressing) of wool, foam or shaped material such as acrylic is tied over the graft using the long ends of the marginal sutures (Fig. 3.11). A further padded dressing can be applied at the periphery of this dressing and the whole is covered by an outer layer of crepe or elastoplast. Alternatively, the tie-over bolus can be exposed. This method is helpful on concave or irregular surfaces or in mobile areas and is preferable for full thickness skin grafts. It is usually left in place for 7 days.

(b) On convex surfaces, pressure can be applied by a conforming padded dressing without the need for a tie-over. An inner non-adherent layer of tulle gras or similar material is essential to aid removal of the dressing without disturbing the graft from its bed. Near a joint, a splint should be applied to immobilize the part.

2 Exposed grafting. Pressure is not essential for graft take and in some areas the tie-over can cause problems by friction and exertion of irregular pressure or pulling. Exposed grafting is especially suitable for split-skin grafting but is *contra-indicated* under the following circumstances.

(a) *If the patient is unable to cooperate.* Young, old or confused patients may interfere with the graft.

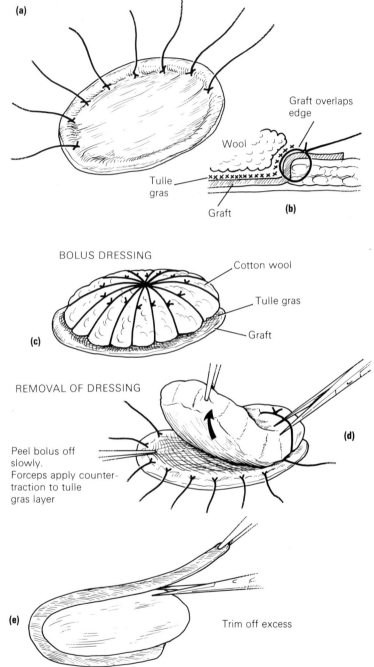

Figure 3.11
The technique for applying a split skin graft using a tie-over dressing. Note the graft must overlap the wound defect (a), (b) to prevent it retracting and exposing the wound margin.

(a)

(b) Graft overlaps edge
Wool
Tulle gras
Graft

BOLUS DRESSING
Cotton wool
Tulle gras
Graft
(c)

REMOVAL OF DRESSING
Peel bolus off slowly.
Forceps apply counter-traction to tulle gras layer
(d)

(e)
Trim off excess

(b) *Circumferential grafting.* It is impossible to avoid friction if a graft is exposed on a surface the patient has to lie on.

(c) *If experienced staff are not available for postoperative care.* The exposed graft has a greater tendency to form haematomas and is therefore best performed in a specialist unit where the nurses are capable of dealing with this problem.

(d) Exposed grafting is not suitable for out-patient care.

(e) To avoid the excessive mobility of the restless patient waking from an anaesthetic, and save operation time the exposed graft can be applied as a delayed procedure when stored skin is used. No fixation is usually required, as the skin sticks firmly by surface tension to the moist recipient site.

(f) Dependancy of the graft must be avoided if it is exposed.

Good postoperative care   Neglect of this vital facet of grafting technique can cause delayed healing or loss of the graft and also lead to later loss of a graft even if it has taken well initially.

1 If the graft is dressed, a decision is needed about the first change of dressing. The precise timing is not usually of crucial importance, but the custom has grown to inspect at weekly intervals. This is usually determined by the weekly operating session or out-patient clinic. It is important to inspect a graft early if problems such as infection or haematoma are suspected. If the dressing is adherent, there is little point in forcibly removing it, possibly disturbing the graft, and it can be left on longer than a week.

2 Exposed grafts must be carefully inspected at regular intervals for haematoma or seroma formation. Accumulations must be expressed and removed at the edge of the graft or released directly by snipping a small hole in the graft. This process must be carried out every few hours at first, day and night. After 48 hours, when the graft is pinking up, less attention is required.

3 Mobilization must be gradual. After 5–7 days, once the graft has taken, increase of activity is allowed. However, the graft is still vulnerable to trauma and increased hydrostatic pressure can lead to expanding haematoma and graft failure. Before dependancy is allowed, a supporting pressure dressing must be applied. If the recipient site is relatively avascular and take is expected to be slow, Buerger's exercises of graduated dependancy can be used initially before full dependancy. On a weight-bearing area, dependancy with partial weight bearing should be used at first.

A graft crossing a joint should be splinted to stop shear forces disturbing the graft and mobilisation must be carefully supervised. If there is a tendency to contract across a joint, a splint must be applied and worn for up to six months; see Chapter 5.

4 Hygienic care of the graft is most important. The early graft tends to desquamate excessively for a few weeks owing to the lack of sebum production. Scabs can develop that lead to infection and pressure. It is essential that they are removed and the graft is cleaned. In favourable circumstances, soap-and-water washes can be allowed early after graft take, i.e. about 10–14 days after graft application. Lubrication should be applied regularly by massage with a moisturizing cream.

Treatment of graft failure

1 Soft tissue infection should be treated by the appropriate antibiotic, given systemically, to try to boost graft survival.
2 *Slow take with incipient failure.* Continued pressure dressing and rest and elevation may allow a take to proceed, particularly if there is some capillary refill or slight blistering.
3 Haematoma or seroma must be removed as soon as it is detected. Recurrent haematoma can be a difficult problem and, if necessary, a large incision should be made to allow the graft to redrape and adhere. A small new graft may then be required at this site.
4 Small insignificant areas of complete failure can be left to form a dry scab and will epithelialize from the margins.
5 Large areas of failed graft should be removed, allowing the defect to be prepared in time to use any stored skin. This avoids the need for a fresh donor site.

Tactics to improve the skin graft take

The search for drugs and dressings that will improve graft take has been as elusive as the search for the philosopher's stone. However, there are manoeuvres that can enhance graft take.

Biological dressings   These probably work by ensuring more efficient preparation of the recipient bed, being occlusive and possibly bacteriocidal, although their efficacy has been over-emphasized. Amnion may have a special effect in increasing vascularization.

Delay   Delay may be effective in speeding healing by its action on the graft and the bed.

1 One method is to replace the graft on its donor site for 24 hours. When it is applied to the recipient site, such a graft gives an impetus to the capillary buds in the wound bed immediately after transplantation.
2 If a graft is placed on a bed where healing has progressed to the proliferative phase, the initial ischaemic phase of the graft is greatly reduced. This is similar to the more rapid healing of resutured wounds known as acceleration of healing.
3 Delayed graft application helps to eliminate haematoma formation.

Cooling The metabolic activity of a graft is decreased by cooling and it is then able to withstand the initial ischaemic phase more easily. This may explain why exposed grafts can give more satisfactory results.

Thinner grafts Thin grafts take more easily than thick split-skin grafts, full-thickness grafts or composite grafts. Thin grafts may not perform well in the long term but can be used as a temporary cover to be replaced later by direct closure, a thicker overgraft or flap repair.

Mesh or patch grafting If there is likely to be slow healing or an oozing surface, skin grafts will take more easily if they are applied as small strips or patches (postage-stamp grafts). This has the added advantage of increasing the area of cover but the cosmetic result is worse.

 Mesh grafts are made by passing the graft through a machine that makes longitudinal parallel serrations allowing the graft to expand like a string vest. Blood, serum and pus can ooze out freely and the graft will conform easily to irregular surfaces. The cut edges of the mesh also increase the number of exposed vessels for anastomosis. The interstices of the mesh heal rapidly by epithelialization from the adjacent graft margins (Fig. 3.12). The cosmetic result may be less satisfactory but, when rapid healing is required, it allows more reliable take in difficult areas.

Expanding grafts to cover large areas

If the area of skin loss is very large, e.g. in a big burn, there may not be sufficient donor sites available to provide conventional skin grafts. Several methods are available to augment skin graft availability.

Figure 3.12
Application of mesh grafts. When the graft bed is moist, as in this excised burn (a), mesh grafts allow serum and blood to ooze out (b) and bleeding points can still be treated through the interstices of the mesh (c). The gaps in the mesh epithelialize rapidly (d), as seen here at three weeks.

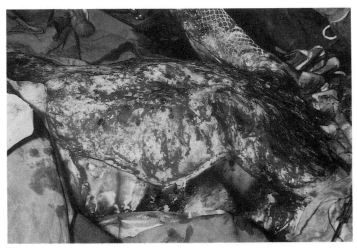

(a)

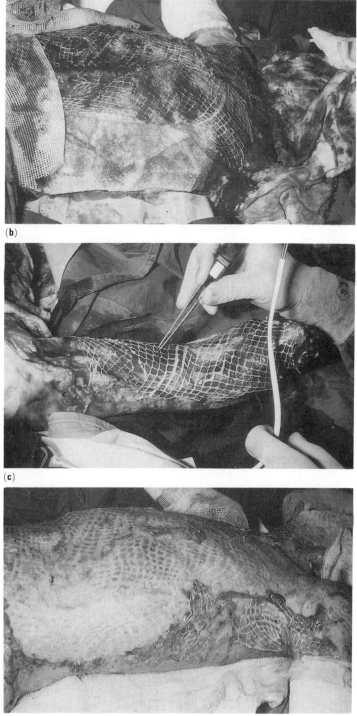

(b)

(c)

(d)

1 By the use of an electric dermatome, skin can be cut from virtually any part of the body. The shaved scalp is a very useful source of grafts. It heals rapidly if thin grafts are taken and repeated crops of graft can be taken at frequent intervals.
2 Mesh, strip or patch grafts will cover a larger area (Fig. 3.12).
3 When rapid skin grafting is required for a very ill patient, allograft sheets can be taken from related or unrelated donors and used to resurface large areas. Small patches of autograft, if available, can be seeded into holes in the grafts or between sheets. As the allograft is rejected these seeds spread out to cover the wound.

Complications of allografts

Rejection is a common complication when a skin graft is used from a donor, whether related or unrelated. Cross-matching is possible but the antigenicity of skin is high and rejection is likely to occur. However, in some severely ill patients, allografts will survive for long periods, for example in large burns, or if the patient is immunocompromised.

The most serious complication of an allograft is the risk of transmission of infection, notably HIV virus but also syphilis and hepatitis. An allograft donor must therefore be screened very carefully for these diseases and for malignant disease that could also, theoretically, be present in the graft and therefore be transplanted. The risks are potentially fatal and therefore the use of allografts must be reserved only for life-saving situations where there is no alternative.

4 Tissue-culture techniques are experimental at present, but epithelial sheets have been used successfully to graft burns. The main problem with this method is the time needed to grow sheets and their poor cosmetic appearance.

Other Skin Grafts

Composite grafts
These are full-thickness grafts including the underlying fat or cartilage (Fig. 3.13). The take is extremely slow and precarious, and very small or narrow grafts are inserted to ensure take. Great care must be paid to meticulous haemostasis and it is unlikely that the blood supply will be sufficient if any part of the graft is more than a few millimetres from the recipient bed. Cooling may help the survival.

Hair transplants
Punch grafts of hair are small composite grafts. It is essential that these grafts contain sufficient depth of subcutaneous tissue to include the hair follicles and they must be cut at an angle parallel to the shafts of the hairs (Figs 3.13, 3.14).

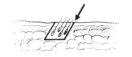

Punch graft of hair, cut parallel to hairs and include hair follicles

Figure 3.13
Composite skin grafts. Note that only relatively small pieces of tissue will take in this way. Hair grafts must be cut parallel to the hair follicle to include the entire hair shaft and bulb if they are to grow hairs.

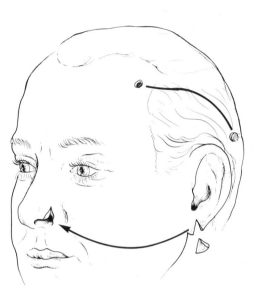

Figure 3.14
These hair grafts contain only one or two hairs in each punch because they were cut across the grain of the hair follicles.

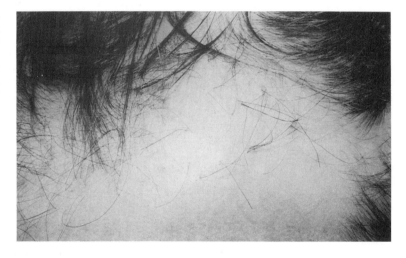

Pinch grafts

Small pieces of skin snipped off with scissors or scalpel have been used in the past to graft difficult areas. They are easily dislodged before they are healed and are vulnerable to desiccation. Regular gentle irrigation with isotonic saline is needed for several days. The donor-site scarring is very unsightly (Fig. 3.15).

Figure 3.15
Pinch graft donor
scars have a
characteristically
unsightly appearance.

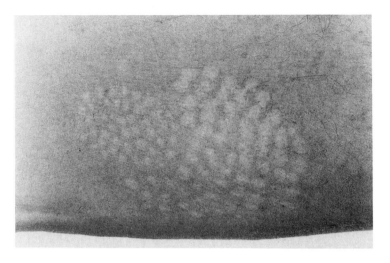

Dermis or dermal fat grafts

Skin grafts free of epithelial elements can be used subcutaneously to build up defects of soft tissue. They must be in thin sheets if they are to take effectively. It is preferable to insert two thin dermal fat grafts on separate occasions than to use a thick graft. The take of the fat is poor. Near the surface, the dermis should be placed outermost for the best cosmetic result. Complications include absorption of the fat, fat necrosis or late calcification (Fig. 3.16).

Late Complication of Skin Grafts

General unsightly appearance

Skin graft cover of a defect is never as good as the original skin even if the take has been totally successful (Fig. 3.17). Dissatisfaction with the appearance is largely a matter of patient expectation. If a realistic prospect is discussed with the patient prior to surgery and adequate informed consent is obtained, problems are unlikely. Measures to minimize the cosmetic defect include the following:

1 Use the anatomically nearest donor site that is possible. For example, when a graft is required on the face, pre- or post-auricular skin will give a better result than groin or abdominal skin.
2 Large sheets are preferable to mesh or patch grafts.
3 Apply grafts in anatomical units, see Chapter 11 (Fig. 5.18).
4 Thicker grafts give better results and full-thickness skin grafts normally look better than split-thickness grafts (Fig. 3.18).
5 Contour defects caused by lack of subcutaneous fat can be camouflaged by a prosthesis or treated by flap repair in carefully selected cases.

Figure 3.16
Late calcification in a dermal fat graft used for breast augmentation. Over the passage of twenty years this graft atrophied and shrank in size to leave this calcified nubbin. The X-ray also shows that a repeat augmentation using a silicone implant has been performed.

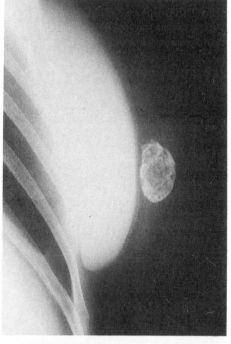

Figure 3.17
This split-skin graft applied to the neck to treat a burn took exceptionally well. The graft was put on when the patient was a child and looked very good initially, but on his reaching puberty it became more obvious. The hairless graft with its clearly defined margin stands out in contrast to the beard skin. The colour changes associated with exposure to sun make the difference more obvious.

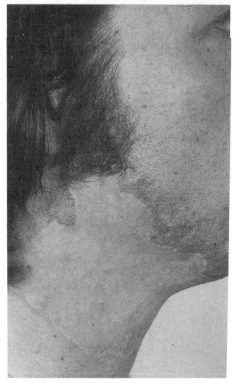

Marginal scar

A scar at the edge of a graft is inevitable. These scars can become hypertrophic or keloid (see Chapter 5). Measures must be taken to minimize the effects of scars, especially if the patient is a known hypertrophic scar former. The defect should be planned, where possible, to leave marginal scars parallel to skin tension lines. Indentations or lateral gussets to break up linear scars will help healing. When strips of graft are used, they should be placed spirally or obliquely, and transversely at a joint crease line.

Contraction

An open wound left to heal by epithelialization will contract. Split-thickness skin grafts diminish this tendency to contract. The thicker the graft the more effective it is. Contraction can bunch the graft into ridges or nodules and also distort the adjacent tissues, giving an unsightly appearance as well as a functional disability. A full-thickness skin graft is less likely to contract, but can do so (Fig. 3.19).

Application of splints and pressure dressings helps to prevent contraction. The process is maximal at two months and continues for up to six months. Treatment will be needed at least

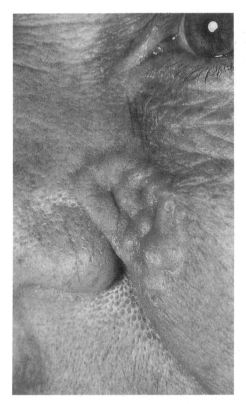

Figure 3.19
This severe hypertrophic reaction with contraction of a post-auricular full-thickness skin graft is unusual particularly in an elderly patient. The thickening slowly subsided over the following two years to leave an acceptable result.

that long. Once the graft is stabilized, further contraction is unlikely, but growth is limited in young patients and further tightness may develop at growth spurts such as that at puberty.

Durability

The functional performance of a graft is limited by its structure. Split-thickness grafts are deficient in dermis, including sebaceous and sweat glands, and have little sensation initially. They tend to be dry and crack and develop hyperkeratoses, particularly when subjected to pressure or friction. With time the graft can thicken and become more robust, but it will have to be protected initially by suitable padding and support.

Sensation is absent for the first few weeks but if there is sensation in the graft bed it will recover to some extent. The sensory return is better in thicker or full thickness grafts. If the graft bed is insensitive, no recovery of protective sensation is possible, and special care will have to be taken to see that the graft is not damaged.

In the long term the performance of a graft is greatly dependent on the quality of the recipient site. If there is a good soft-tissue base with sensation, the graft will stand up well to wear and tear. If the graft is placed over dense adherent scar tissues, it is unlikely ever to perform well and flap repair should be considered. Innervated local flaps give the best functional and cosmetic results.

Colour change

Colour change in a graft arises either from keratin abnormalities or abnormal melanin deposition.

Hyperkeratosis results from the dryness of the graft and surface friction. It is particularly common in skin grafts on the palm and sole, giving a dirty, unwashed appearance. It cannot be wholly prevented but grease massage, simple washing and pumice-stone abrasion helps.

Melanin abnormalities occur because there is a tendency for all skin grafts to hyperpigment and the most plentiful donor sites, e.g. the thighs, have darker skin than the rest of the body (Fig. 3.20). Early exposure to sun accentuates the hyperpigmentation.

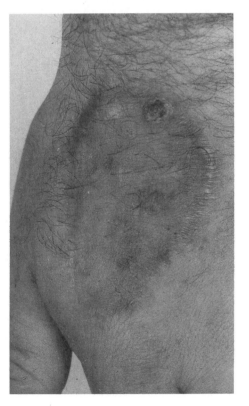

Figure 3.20 Hyperpigmentation in a split-thickness skin graft taken from the thigh and applied to a burn on the back of the hand. Note that exposure to the sun has given rise to markedly increased pigmentation as well as blistering and redness of the marginal scar several years after the graft was applied.

Prevention

1 On the face, use a local donor site, e.g. pre- or post-auricular skin. These grafts will tend to be red at first.

2 In conspicuous areas such as the face and neck, avoid thin split-skin grafts because they tend to hyperpigment more than thicker grafts.

3 A second skin graft, taken from a donor site from which a split-skin graft has already been harvested, will sometimes give a paler colour but it is difficult to control and may end up too pale.

4 Avoid early exposure to sun by clothing or sun-screen cover creams for at least six months after grafting. Once the graft is hyperpigmented, it will take many years to fade even if subsequent exposure to sun is avoided.

5 Persistent hyperpigmentation can be bleached using hydro-quinone creams or disguised with makeup. A hypopigmented area can be tattooed an appropriate colour.

6 When pigmented grafts are needed, as in nipple reconstruction, the graft should be taken from a pigmented donor site e.g. upper inner thigh.

Abnormal hair

Soft tissue or skeletal injury tends to induce abnormal growth of coarse, dark hairs. Grafts taken from hairy donor sites will grow hair if they are thick split-thickness or full-thickness grafts. If hair is not wanted, a hairless donor site must be selected. Particular care should be taken in grafting children, as a non-hair-bearing site may change to hairy and hairs will grow in the graft at puberty. For example, a full-thickness groin skin graft must be taken far enough laterally to avoid pubic hair follicles.

Complications of Cartilage Grafts

Predisposing factors

A cartilage graft, unlike other free grafts does not require revascularization, since cartilage gets its nutrition by diffusion of fluid from the surrounding tissue. Nevertheless, a good vascular supply is required in the graft bed. Any factor, such as infection, haematoma or foreign material, that acts as a barrier will prevent graft take. Exposed cartilage devoid of soft-tissue cover will dry out and may be absorbed, or will slough, particularly if infection sets in.

Allograft tissue, of any type, carries grave risks of transmission of infection such as HIV, slow viruses or hepatitis and should not be used. Treatment by gamma irradiation designed to prevent transfer of infection alters the nature of the cartilage and it may be absorbed or calcify even if the initial take is good.

The internal anatomical structure of cartilage makes it a difficult substance to shape. There is a tendency for struts to deform and bend unless the graft is carefully selected and cut symmetrically from the donor site.

The donor site can be very disfiguring when rib cartilages are used, leaving scars or contour deformities. Sub-perichondrial dissection is best performed to avoid pneumothorax. If a thin sheet of cartilage is required, the conchal hollow of the ear is a good source of material.

Prevention of complications
Careful technique, ensuring sterility and meticulous haemostasis of the recipient pocket is essential. Cartilage grafts take better if the perichondrium is removed. The graft must be handled carefully with non-toothed instruments to avoid splits that might cause distortion (Fig. 3.21). The wound must be closed carefully, without tension, to prevent the risk of extrusion. If there is excessive tension, either the pocket must be enlarged or the graft reduced in size. A snug fit is desirable to prevent movement of the graft. Any surplus cartilage can be stored in the abdominal subcutaneous fat through a small stab incision to be used later if necessary. This manoeuvre may avoid the need for a second donor site.

Management
Any sizable haematoma must be released and infection treated with antibiotics if graft loss is to be avoided. Exposed cartilage must be trimmed back to healthy graft and covered with viable skin. Padded protective dressings can be used to prevent further trauma.

Complications of Bone Grafts

Predisposing factors
The graft must be held in intimate contact with bone. Cortical bone does not take easily in any circumstances. Cancellous bone and marrow take better, but not in the presence of infection. Exposure of the graft or excessive mobility interfere with healing. All bone donor sites, except the skull, will leave visible scars that may be tethered. The bone defect may also be visible as a contour defect and there may be stress pain or even stress fracture owing to weakening of the donor bone.

Prevention
The bone must be carefully handled to avoid contamination and kept moist. Prophylactic antibiotics should be considered if there is any possibility that the operation site is contaminated or when the recipient site has been subjected to irradiation. The graft must be placed in close contact with bone in the recipient site and covered by viable soft tissue. A donor scar can be avoided in some cases by using Kiel bone graft—a xenograft of

Figure 3.21
A cartilage graft taken from the nasal septum. Note that it is straight (a). If the cartilage is damaged on one side it will bend in the opposite direction causing a convex curve. This property is exploited by cross-hatching this graft with part thickness knife cuts (b) to create a curve (c) as it is to be used in an eyelid reconstruction to substitute for the tarsal plate.

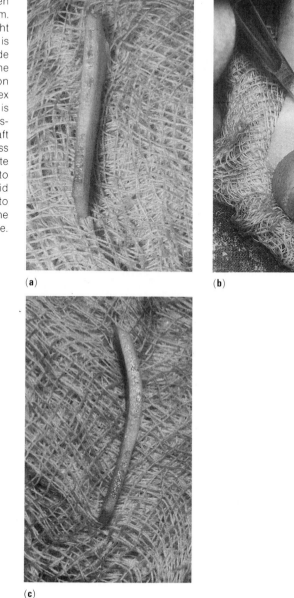

(a)

(b)

(c)

antigen-free calf bone that acts as a matrix for the host osteocytes to colonize.

When bone grafts are used to fill in a contour defect, the amount of bone inserted should be strictly limited in volume to give an accurate correction. Excess bone does not usually remodel.

Management

If the graft is to be saved, infection must be diagnosed early and treated vigorously by antibiotics and drainage of pus when necessary. Any exposed bone should be covered by soft tissue to prevent desiccation and sequestrum formation. Once sequestrum has formed, it should be allowed to separate spontaneously or encouraged to do so by curettage. If there is non-union, prolonged splintage may help or the bone ends can be freshened and re-approximated or treated by further bone grafting as necessary.

Persisting controversies
- Prevention of contraction in free skin grafts.
- The ideal dressing for split skin graft donor sites.
- Control of pigmentation in skin grafts.
- The use of chemotherapeutic agents to increase long-term skin allograft survival.

Further reading

McGregor, I.A. (1980) *Fundamental Techniques of Plastic Surgery.* Edinburgh: Churchill Livingstone.

Grabb, W.C. & Smith, J.W. (Eds) (1980) *Plastic Surgery: A Concise Guide to Clinical Practice.* Boston: Little Brown.

Barron, J.N. & Saad, M.N. (Eds) (1980) *Operative Plastic and Reconstructive Surgery.* Edinburgh: Churchill Livingstone.

Barclay, T.L. & Kernahan, D.A. (Eds) (1986) *Plastic Surgery.* London: Butterworths.

Walker, W.F. (Ed) (1986) *A Colour Atlas of Minor Surgery.* London: Wolfe.

4 Complications of Flaps

A skin flap is designed and transferred so that there is always attachment at one side to carry the nutrient blood supply. The flap has greater versatility than a graft, as it can be placed over an avascular area, and the quality of transferred tissue is better, as it contains all the elements of skin (Fig. 3.2). A flap procedure is much more vulnerable to planning and technical errors and the penalty for failure is greater. If a flap necroses, it fails to achieve its objective, re-establishing the defect. There is also an equivalent-sized donor defect to repair (Fig. 4.1).

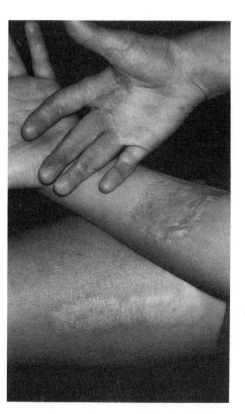

Figure 4.1
A cross-arm flap repair of the right middle and ring fingers. Note the severe depressed donor scar on the left forearm which has in turn been covered by a split-thickness skin graft taken from the left thigh, also leaving a scar.

General Complications

Predisposing factors
Most of the factors detailed in Chapter 2 (on wound healing) are relevant to flap procedures.

- In emergency patients, with severe associated injuries, it may be prudent to postpone definitive flap repair. Flap surgery is rarely life-saving and should be performed when the patient is in a good stable condition.
- The wound can be kept moist and clean by an occlusive dressing or a temporary split-skin graft. The operating time is thus kept to a minimum.
- In the presence of shock with poor tissue perfusion, it is difficult to assess the blood supply of a potential donor site.

Surgical technique   Flap repair is demanding of experience and technical skills in assessing defects, planning methods of repair and performing the surgery. The surgeon must be familiar not only with the technique being used but with alternative methods and salvage procedures. If in doubt, the inexperienced operator should be prepared to seek help and advice. Gentle handling of all tissues to avoid further damage to a flap is essential.

Timing of surgery   In the non-emergency patient with a clean surgical defect, the ideal time for a flap is for immediate or delayed primary repair before the wound becomes contaminated and oedematous.

After severe trauma, the surrounding tissues become bruised and swollen and it is difficult to assess tissue viability. Local flaps should be used with extreme caution in these circumstances. Immediate free microvascular flaps may also be contraindicated after injury of a crushing or avulsion type, as the local vessels can be damaged well beyond the obvious site of injury.

A delay of up to 10 days allows oedema to settle, infection to be treated and ischaemia to declare itself.

Ischaemia   The prime cause of flap necrosis is ischaemia arising from two main synergistic factors: excessive tissue tension and deficient blood supply.

Poor planning with an inadequate size of flap causes excessive tension. Careless design may compromise the blood supply.

Haematoma stretches the flap, increasing tension, decreasing the blood supply and may lead to necrosis. The haematoma can act as a foreign body in the wound giving a focus for infection or lifting the flap off its bed.

Infection, chronic or acute in a wound is a contra-indication to flap repair.

- Chronic infection gives rise to stiffness and impairs mobilization of the flap. Even if flap necrosis does not occur, the increased oedema and fibrosis marr the final result and rehabilitation will be slower.
- Acute inflammation developing after flap transfer can cause wound breakdown or loss of a flap. The excessive demands of inflammation may tip the balance against viability in a flap when the blood supply is marginal.

Local X-irradiation in a donor site causes ischaemia by damaging small vessels and excessive fibrosis develops, making flap movement difficult. These changes are worst after a few weeks and never return to normal. The best time for flap surgery is either immediately before or after radiotherapy, or delayed as long as possible. If feasible, all irradiated skin should be removed when the defect is being established and X-irradiated skin should not be incorporated in the flap.

Prevention of complications
Prophylaxis depends on accurate identification of risk factors, their treatment or avoidance.

Indications   *Is a flap necessary?*
If the defect is small and not causing significant symptoms, the need for flap repair should be reconsidered. A trial period of conservative management may suffice. A split-thickness skin graft applied as a temporary dressing to clean the wound may take and provide adequate cover. In former days, when delay of flaps to fashion tube pedicles was commonly practised, the defect sometimes healed spontaneously and the flap was not required.

Is a flap advisable?
At the time of acute injury, primary local flap repair should be used with caution. Distant or microvascular flaps will be more reliable, but their emergency use should be very carefully considered.

When a flap is to be used to repair a defect following excision of a malignant tumour, it is vital to perform adequate clearance, particularly in depth, as a flap might conceal a recurrence. If there is any doubt about excision, a split-skin graft should be applied, replacing it with a flap later.

Which flap?
Local flaps, if available, are simplest and usually give the best skin match. Distant flaps involve more extensive multiple procedures, increasing the likelihood of complications. Free microvascular flaps are extremely versatile allowing one-stage transfer, but the operating time is prolonged and the penalty for failure may be complete loss of the flap. All other considerations

being equal, the aim should be to keep any repair as simple as possible.

The recently developed fascio-cutaneous and musculo-cutaneous flaps have increased the reliability and availability of local flaps. An alternative is to cover the defect with a muscle or fascia flap and place a split-thickness skin graft on top.

Planning The object is to provide a viable flap of skin sufficient in size and quality to cover the defect. The dilemma is that the true extent of the defect may not be fully revealed until after the flap has been made at the time of surgery. A tumour may be more extensive than expected. When a contracted, scarred area is excised, the defect may expand dramatically, making the planned flap cover impossible. The basic plan must therefore include alternative strategies that must be considered in advance so that informed consent can be obtained from the patient. At operation, it is best to prepare the surgical defect first, so that the design can be checked before the flap is raised.

The quality of the available donor sites also determines flap use on the basis of such factors as colour, texture and pliability of the skin, presence or absence of hair, and quantity of subcutaneous fat.

Prevention of ischaemia

Design the flap with adequate blood supply The shape and size of a viable flap is constrained by the anatomy of its blood supply. The nature of the nutrient vascular supply forms a convenient classification of skin flaps.

Random pattern flap

The random pattern flap is the basic traditional skin flap and has no specifically known or identifiable main arterial or venous blood supply. There is a severe restriction of size for these flaps and in practice it has been found that the length must not exceed the size of the base of the flap, i.e. a one-to-one ratio must be observed (Fig. 4.2a). The relative shortness of these flaps makes them very difficult to transpose into a defect. Longer random flaps are possible in the head and neck region because of the better blood supply but, in general, if longer flaps are needed a delay procedure will have to be employed or the design must be altered to one of the safer, more reliable axial pattern, fascio-cutaneous or musculo-cutaneous flaps.

Venous drainage is as important as arterial inflow. On a limb where the venous system has valves, a proximally based flap is much safer than a distally based flap.

Axial pattern flap

The blood supply to the axial pattern skin flap arises from an anatomically known and identifiable arterio-venous system. The flap must therefore be designed and raised containing this blood supply (Fig. 4.2b). If the artery is a large one it can be checked

Figure 4.2
(a) When a random pattern skin flap is raised, length and breadth must be of an equal size. (b) An axial pattern flap contains an arteriovenous system of blood supply and longer flaps can be used. (c) Provided that the arteriovenous supply is preserved the flap can be raised as an island flap. (d) A free flap can be transferred by joining the blood supply to the recipient site by microvascular anastomosis.

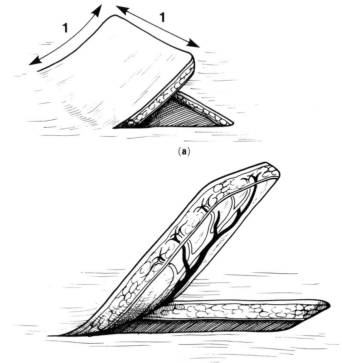

(**a**)

(**b**)

(**c**)

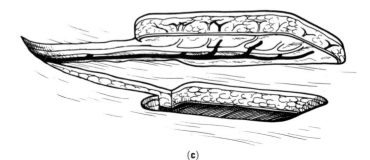

(**d**)

pre-operatively by palpation or a Doppler probe. Arteriography is not usually recommended.

As long as the supplying vessels are not divided, the flap can be raised as an island or it can be used as a free flap, when the vessels are divided and anastomosed to the recipient site by microvascular repair (Fig. 4.2c, d).

The possible length of these flaps depends on the size of the supplying vessels and varies with the site of the flap. In favourable circumstances a random 1:1 ratio flap can be added on to an axial flap to increase the length.

Fascio-cutaneous flap

When a skin flap is raised incorporating the underlying deep fascia, the blood supply is enhanced by a rich plexus of vessels and longer flaps can be designed (Fig. 4.4c).

Musculo-cutaneous flap

In certain areas of the body the skin derives its blood supply from the underlying muscle, so that a skin flap raised in continuity with the muscle will have an enhanced blood supply and longer or island flaps can be raised. They can also be transferred as free flaps by microvascular anastomosis.

Flap delay   When blood supply is thought to be inadequate, it can usually be enhanced by the use of a delay procedure (Fig. 4.3). The principal action of a delay is to preserve the vessels on which the flap will be based for its transfer and serially divide the supplying vessels on the other three sides and beneath the flap. There are several disadvantages to delay.

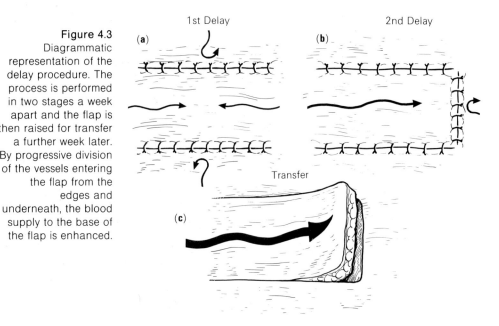

Figure 4.3
Diagrammatic representation of the delay procedure. The process is performed in two stages a week apart and the flap is then raised for transfer a further week later. By progressive division of the vessels entering the flap from the edges and underneath, the blood supply to the base of the flap is enhanced.

1 It converts the operation into a multi-stage one with a potential incidence of complications at each stage.

2 Infection or haematoma, if it occurs, will make the flap stiff and oedematous.

3 A delayed flap can develop fibrosis that may limit its mobility and pliability.

4 The flap may not have sufficient blood supply even after the delay and necrosis may result. Delay will not rescue a badly designed flap (Fig. 4.4).

Tube pedicle flap. The preparation of a tubed flap involves a series of delay operations to orientate the blood supply along the length of the flap. All the complications of flap delay are possible. It can be difficult to determine which is the dominant end of the pedicle. Before one end is detached ready for transfer, a further delay operation by partial division is advisable.

Tissue expansion. One effect of tissue expansion is to delay the flap very effectively.

Avoid tension Good planning is the first essential in preventing tension. The flap must be big enough to cover the defect with a little spare, to allow for slight expansion with oedema and swelling that inevitably occurs as a result of the trauma of surgery.

Avoid kinking and twisting The design should allow the flap to turn into position without undue tension or twisting. Any torsion or acute folding can interfere with the blood supply.

Do not rely on diagrams All surfaces of the body are curved. A flap must not be designed by direct transfer of a two-dimensional plan from a book. Any proposed flap must be designed so that allowance is made for the third dimension.

The best way is to plan and rehearse the procedure preoperatively using non-extensile material, such as jaconet or polythene sheet, as a template that can be kept and sterilized to be available at the time of operation. Once the defect has been established, the pattern can be used to check the design before the flap is raised.

Avoid vasoconstrictors If using local anaesthesia, adrenaline or noradrenaline infiltration should be avoided in skin where a flap is to be raised.

Surgical technique Accurate, gentle technique is essential in flap surgery. The tissue planes must be established on the basis of the design of flap being used and it is essential that dissection does not stray from the appropriate level. In axial flaps, the main vessels must be religously preserved and not stretched or separated from the flap. When a flap depends on its underlying attachments to muscle or fascia it is useful to place a few temporary tacking sutures to maintain the continuity, particularly if an island flap is being used.

Figure 4.4
Contrast the result
between these two
flaps. (a) The random
pattern flap to be used
to repair this wound of
the knee has been
delayed on two
occasions, but
underwent necrosis of
the tip shortly after
transfer (b). (c) A
wound of the knee
showing a similar
sized fascio-cutaneous
flap marked out for
transfer, without prior
delay. (d) The result
two weeks later shows
that the flap has
survived completely
because the blood
supply to a fascio-
cutaneous flap is
superior.

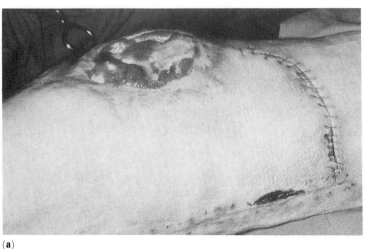

(a)

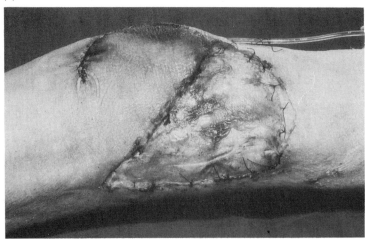

(b)

Fat patients are not ideal candidates for flap surgery and no attempt should be made to thin the main body of a flap at the first stage, for fear of interfering with the blood supply.

Haematoma must be prevented by careful haemostasis and drainage under the flap. Closed suction drainage is the most efficient method. If possible the wound should be sutured and closed completely to minimize wound infection risks.

Postoperative care   Specialist postoperative nursing care should help to minimize flap complications. External pressure from tight dressings or the patient's lying on the flap must be prevented. The most crucial period is the first few days and nights. If the patient's posture is allowed to move so that the flap is kinked, necrosis can occur (Fig. 4.5a).

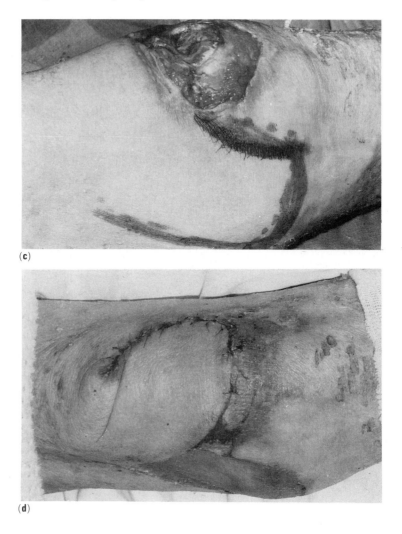

(c)

(d)

Flap Necrosis

All flap procedures have a definite but variable incidence of necrosis. Eventually, if enough flaps are performed, necrosis is inevitable on occasion. The incidence depends on the region of the body and the type of flap. The blood supply is better and flap necrosis is less in the head and neck region.

Random pattern flaps such as a cross-leg flap may have patchy peripheral necrosis of small areas in up to 30% of flaps, but this is sufficient to cause failure in fewer than 10% of all flaps. Axial pattern flaps, on the other hand, have a better blood supply and develop less minor necrosis, but when the blood supply is compromised any necrosis usually involves a larger area of the

Figure 4.5
Note the distribution of flap necrosis in this axial-pattern groin flap which had become kinked when the fixation slipped on the second postoperative night (a). Blisters should not be deroofed unless infection occurs under them, as the flap skin cannot cope with the added stress of dehydration. The black area where a blister was deroofed is the only part of the flap to go on to full-thickness skin necrosis. (b) Three weeks after being raised, the flap is clamped with a soft bowel clamp to test the circulation. The absence of colour change signifies that the pedicle can be safely divided. (c) The flap, fully healed four weeks later.

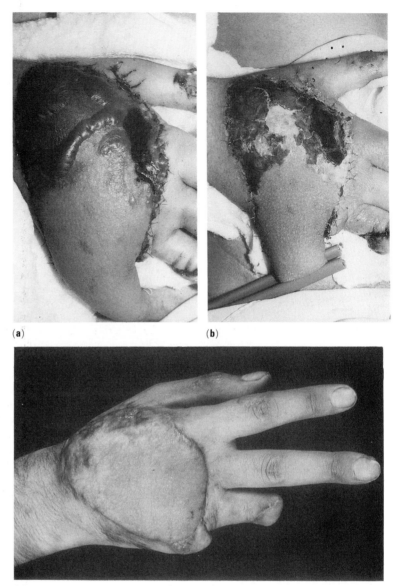

(a)   (b)

(c)

distal flap (Fig. 4.5a). The necrosis rate in axial pattern flaps such as delto-pectoral or groin flaps is approximately 10%. The viability of a flap may be in doubt from the moment it is raised; or ischaemia can develop at a later stage during transfer and in the postoperative period. It is vital to diagnose potential ischaemia as soon as it develops if any help is to be given to an ailing flap to prevent it proceeding to frank necrosis. The flap should be monitored continuously if possible, and it should not be totally covered by dressings.

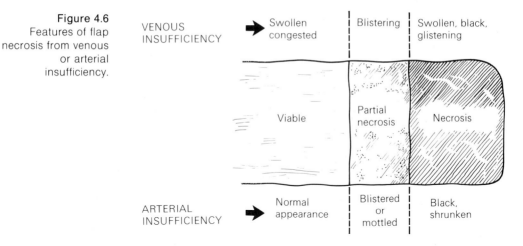

Figure 4.6
Features of flap
necrosis from venous
or arterial
insufficiency.

Incipient necrosis

Diagnosis The skin of a healthy flap is similar in colour and texture to the donor skin. It blanches easily on compression with brisk return of capillary flow. When first raised there should be bleeding from the periphery of the flap. Venous insufficiency will cause a deep cynanosed colour but, if arterial inflow is poor, the flap will be pale with little or no capillary return after pressure. The fluorescein dye test is a good indicator of viability of a flap if there is any doubt when it is raised. It cannot be used repeatedly as a continuous monitor, because the tissue stains.

If venous ischaemia persists, the tip of the flap will become progressively darker and colder. There may be blistering in the proximial part of this area. In arterial insufficiency, the flaps will become mottled and the tissue will lose its normal tone, gradually becoming shrunken, black and necrosed (Fig. 4.6).

Management All reversible factors should be sought out and corrected as soon as possible.

1 If the flap appears non-viable when first raised, transfer can be abandoned and it should be returned to its bed. This then becomes a delay operation and the flap will sometimes recover. Alternatively, the flap can be applied to the defect in the hope that enough will survive to allow it to be advanced later. Such decisions require experience and the junior surgeon should ask for help and advice if necessary.

On rare occasions, if the blood supply is damaged by a technical error, e.g. if the vascular supply of an axial flap has been divided, microvascular repair may be possible. Venous insufficiency can sometimes be relieved by additional venous microvascular anastomosis at the margin of a flap—known as microvascular augmentation.

2 Excessive tissue tension can be eased by releasing sutures
until the circulation has improved. It may then be possible to
resuture the wound at a later date, or a split-thickness skin
graft can be applied to the marginal defect. Haematoma must
be released and drained (Fig..4.7).

Figure 4.7
(a) The haematoma
under this flap
developed late at 10
days when the patient
yawned. (b) It should
be aspirated or
drained to prevent
delayed healing and
possible infection.

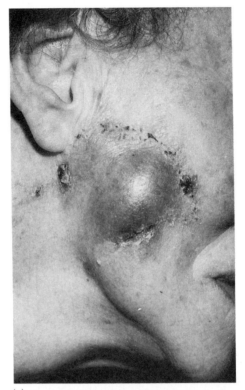

(a)

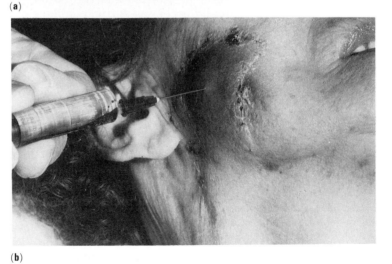

(b)

3 Infection must be treated by releasing and draining any pus. Systemic antibiotics should be used to treat soft-tissue infection.

4 Kinks and creasing caused by tension or shearing forces must be prevented and relieved. This is particularly likely in distant flaps where a crossed position is employed, e.g. cross-leg flap. The fixation must be checked and corrected as necessary. External pressure from dressings, tapes or fixation apparatus must be relieved.

5 Posture of the patient can sometimes be used to aid the circulation by gravity. An oedematous flap with impaired venous drainage can be elevated or a flap with arterial insufficiency can be lowered.

Resuscitation of the ailing flap

Once signs of ischaemia have become developed, it is usually too late to prevent necrosis, but several measures have been tried.

Cool the flap. Keeping the flap exposed and cool will decrease the metabolic requirement. At the same time, warming the patient may increase tissue perfusion (reflex heating).

Massage. Gentle rolling pressure on the flap from tip to base may aid venous return.

Hyperbaric oxygen. Intermittent increase in oxygen tension by hyperbaric oxygen treatment may give rise to enhanced tissue survival. In practice, treatment is difficult to organize and a special hyperbaric chamber is required.

Vasodilators. Alpha-blocking drugs may be useful in theory but the clinical results are disappointing. An alcohol infusion, intravenously, is an effective peripheral vasodilator but it is not so effective in a compromised flap.

Dextran. Low-molecular-weight dextran, by decreasing blood viscosity, helps tissue perfusion.

Anti-oedema treatment. Drugs such as Chymar that decrease oedema may reduce tissue tension and help the circulation. Diuretics have no beneficial effect. Intermittent positive-pressure compression treatment may help viability by increasing venous return and decreasing oedema, but this method must not be used if infection is present as it can be spread.

Stop smoking. Cigarette smoking is a potent vasoconstrictor and should not be allowed if the viability of a flap is marginal.

Leeches. The use of medicinal leeches has had a renaissance recently. They are useful in decreasing congestion in a swollen flap by sucking out blood, but they also release anticoagulants into the tissues that promote blood flow and cause the wound to ooze for several hours, relieving venous congestion. A major complication of leech therapy, in the presence of arterial insufficiency is infection by *Aeromonas hydrophila* and leeches should be used with caution in such cases.

Established necrosis

Diagnosis   Flap necrosis presents in several patterns.

- Superficial skin loss with blistering, which should heal spontaneously.
- Full-thickness skin necrosis including subcutaneous tissues.
- Full-thickness skin necrosis with preservation of some subcutaneous tissue. This is more likely to occur in fasciocutaneous or musculo-cutaneous flaps.
- Loss of subcutaneous fat with preservation of the overlying skin. This may present late, with fat necrosis and oozing of liquid fat from the wound.

Management   The precise treatment depends on the nature and extent of the necrosis. If the loss is small and does not compromise vital structures, spontaneous separation of the eschar can be awaited (Fig. 4.6). The resultant wound may heal spontaneously or require a small graft.

Alternatively, the necrotic tissue can be excised and the defect repaired surgically. The flap can sometimes be elevated and readvanced, but a small additional local flap may be required. If vital structures are exposed or compromised, it will be necessary to perform an alternative flap repair.

Donor-site Complications

Prevention
A scar is inevitable, but the degree of deformity must be kept to a minimum. The donor site should be selected so that the scar is favourably placed and vital structures are not put at risk. It is essential that an avascular base is not exposed during elevation of the flaps if direct closure of the donor site is not possible. Otherwise, a second flap repair will be necessary to close the donor defect! A planned bilobed or trilobed flap can overcome this problem. Care must be exercised during elevation of a flap to ensure that adjacent structures are not damaged.

Direct closure of the donor defect gives best results but, if there is excessive tension, a split skin graft will be required. This skin graft may be excised later by serial excision or with the aid of tissue expansion.

Management
See Chapter 5 on the treatment of scars.

Late Complication of Flaps

Patient dissatisfaction   As in all reconstructive procedures, the result may be technically excellent and yet the patient may not be satisfied. The commonest cause is excessive expectation on the part of the patient coupled with inadequate pre-operative assessment and counselling.

Marginal scar   The marginal scar is subject to all the complications of scars. Careful planning will keep complications to a minimum. The best results will be obtained if flaps are planned to replace whole aesthetic units, putting marginal scars in neutral areas (see Chapter 5) (Fig. 4.8).

Poor tissue match   A flap retains the properties of the donor site. For the closest possible match, a skin flap should be derived from local skin of the same anatomical type. For example, load-bearing areas

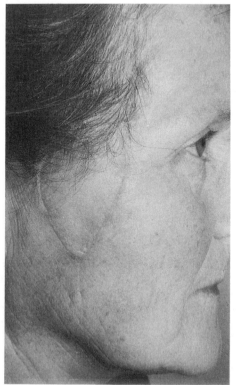

Figure 4.8
An unsightly donor scar from an advancement subcutaneous island flap. If the flap had been advanced obliquely from the pre-auricular area the donor scar would have been less conspicuous, as a large part of it would have merged into the pre-auricular skin creases.

should be replaced with load-bearing skin. Distant flaps will usually be more conspicuously different.

Fat If the donor site is fat or from an area such as the abdomen that is subject to fat deposition later, the flap will be fatter than the surrounding skin. Prevention is achieved by selecting the donor site in a thin area. Excess fat can be removed later by trimming under direct vision or by suction lipectomy. An alternative is to use the crane-flap method, whereby the flap is applied for about a week. It is then returned to its donor site leaving the viable deeper layer attached to the base of the defect. This subcutaneous fat is then covered with a split skin graft.

Hair The donor site must be selected to give the appropriate repair (Fig. 4.9). If a non-hair-bearing flap is required, it must be

Figure 4.9
Hair growth can be a problem by its absence or presence. (a) A non-hair-bearing naso-labial flap is fairly conspicuous on the upper lip of this elderly female patient. (b) This reversed dermis flap from a hairy chest has developed hair growth on the finger tip.

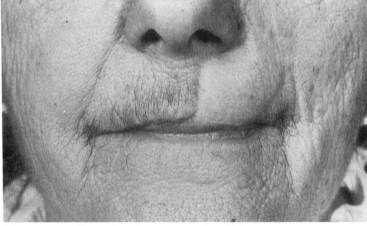

(a)

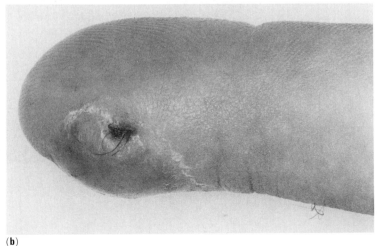

(b)

selected accordingly. It is important in children to avoid areas that will become hairy at puberty. When a hair-bearing flap is required, areas subject to male-pattern baldness should be avoided. Inappropriate hair growth can be removed by electrolysis, but radiotherapy should be reserved for severe or persistent cases.

Colour Distant flaps can be very different in colour. For example trunk flaps transferred to the face will be very pale compared with the surrounding skin. In avoiding this problem, local flaps give the best results (Fig. 4.10).

Treatment by skin camouflage cosmetics is sometimes effective. If a darker flap is required, it may be possible to shave the skin to remove the outer layers and cover it with a split-thickness skin graft taken from a darker area. However, this negates many of the properties of the flap and the colour of the graft is very difficult to control.

Sensation Unless a flap is designed to contain a nerve supply, the return of sensation to a flap is very slow, taking up to two years. The quality of return depends on the nerve supply of the recipient

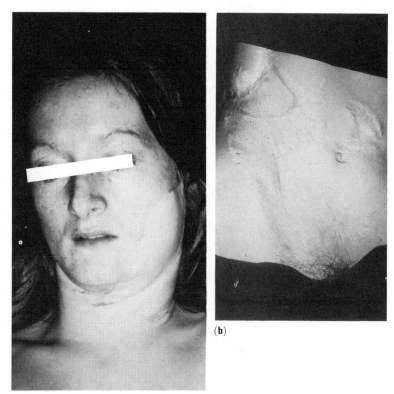

Figure 4.10
(a) A pale flap resulting from the transfer of abdominal skin to the face by tube-pedicle flap. (b) A flap donor site is usually very conspicuous on the abdomen because of the absence of subcutaneous fat.

(b)

(a)

site. In favourable cases the return of sensation will eventually be comparable to the recipient site and may be better than the sensation in the donor area.

Until protective sensation returns, the skin flap must be carefully protected from trauma, particularly on weight-bearing areas. The fat in the flap may atrophy or trophic areas may develop if precautions are not taken. A method of prevention is to use sensate flaps, if possible, on weight-bearing areas (Fig. 4.11).

Contracture   True contracture in a flap is very rare with the exception of the marginal scar. The flap may slip or retract with the passage of time, a problem particularly troublesome in a musculo-cutaneous flap that is still innervated (Fig. 4.12). The motor nerve branch to the muscle can be divided. Fat, bulky flaps are

Figure 4.11
The effect of using a sensate flap. (a) An ischial pressure sore in a paraplegic patient with an L.3 lesion. (b) When a tensor fascia lata flap containing sensation from the lateral cutaneous nerve of the thigh was applied, the patient had to shift his weight off the flap because it became uncomfortable, but unfortunately the insensate opposite side then developed a pressure sore and a similar flap was required there.

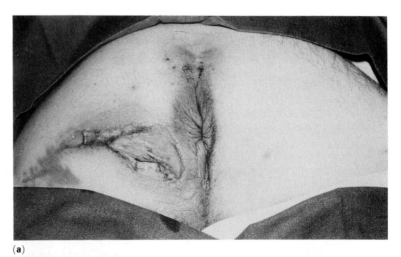

(a)

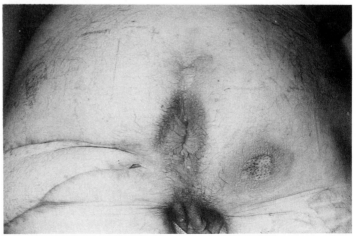

(b)

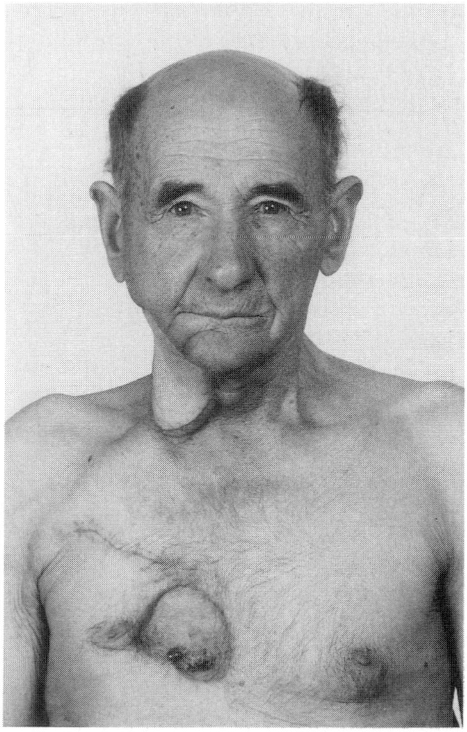

Figure 4.12
Pectoralis major
musculo-cutaneous
flap containing
innervated muscle.
Note that the flap has
slipped down under
the influence of gravity
and muscle
contraction four weeks
after it was raised.

Figure 4.12
Pectoralis major
musculo-cutaneous
flap containing
innervated muscle.
Note that the flap has
slipped down under
the influence of gravity
and muscle
contraction four weeks
after it was raised.

vulnerable to the pull of gravity and thinning may make the flap more stable.

The reversed dermis flap, placing the de-epithialized dermis on the base of the defect gives better adhesion and may prevent slippage.

Small flaps, especially circular ones, are more liable to contract and thicken causing a 'pin-cushion' effect. This usually subsides spontaneously, but can be helped with massage or pressure treatment.

Complications of Specific Flaps

Local flaps Flaps using local skin give very satisfactory tissue match for a defect. The enormous variety of named local flaps easily confuses the inexperienced surgeon. A detailed description of the various types of flap is beyond the scope of this book but the basic principles will be outlined and should help to guide the newcomer to flap surgery through the potential minefield of complications. There are three basic types of flap classified by the direction in which their axis moves (Fig. 4.13).

1 *Advancement flap.* Movement is in the direction of the straight flap axis.

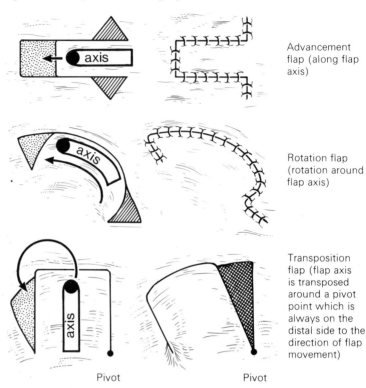

Advancement
flap (along flap
axis)

Rotation flap
(rotation around
flap axis)

Transposition
flap (flap axis
is transposed
around a pivot
point which is
always on the
distal side to the
direction of flap
movement)

Pivot   Pivot

2 *Rotation flap.* Movement is rotatory around a curved axis.
3 *Transposition flap.* The flap is raised and transferred into a
   new site hinged at its base.

All three can be used as local flaps. All distant flaps are
transposition flaps. In practice, many flaps are moved in a
combination of rotation and advancement.

Prevention of complications

Flap selection The random-pattern local skin flap is limited by the need to
observe the 1:1 length-to-breadth ratio, particularly in areas of
the body where the skin is tight and inflexible. Such flaps are
best avoided in the lower limb, where fascio-cutaneous or
musculo-cutaneous flaps are more reliable and move more easily
because of their greater length.

   In the trunk and upper limb, local flaps are more satisfactory
because the skin is usually softer and more flexible. In the head
and neck region, the better blood supply and softer skin makes
local flap repair much more feasible and several axial pattern
flaps are available.

   If the defect to be repaired is the result of trauma, it is very
important to beware of damage to the local skin and local flaps
must be used with caution.

Flap design   Accurate planning is the key to obtaining a healthy flap that will cover the defect.

1 The defect must be defined in size and shape. The margins of the defect should preferably be free of scars and allowance should be made for excision of doubtful marginal tissue. This will increase the actual size of the defect.
2 The flap is then planned to make the most efficient use of local skin, keeping flap size and the distance to be moved as small as possible. The direction of skin laxity in the donor site determines the flap availability.
3 The flap must avoid local vital structures such as eyelid and nose, and a flap must be based on a neutral area of the face.
4 Direct advancement flaps are best used for circular or square defects when excess tissue is required in the same axis as the direction of flap movement.
5 Bipedicle skin flaps must be used with great caution. They need to be longer than the defect to be closed if they are to move into position and are only reliable on the scalp. Fasciocutaneous bipedicle flaps are safer on the limbs.
6 Rotation flaps are most useful if there is a diffuse excess of skin. A flap made four times broader than the defect it has to cover can usually be rotated into its new site and sutured directly without undue tension and without causing a secondary defect. Smaller flaps will not rotate so easily and a back cut may be required. This should be done with caution, as a back cut will interfere with the blood supply.
7 A local transposition flap moves into its new site by angulation around a pivot point. The flap must be longer than the defect because its pivot point (Fig. 4.13c), is always on the opposite side of the flap to the defect (Fig. 4.14). The whole flap must be elevated to allow it to transpose.

Avoiding a dog ear   Triangulation of the defect is the classical method of avoiding a 'dog ear' (or standing cone) of excess tissue in rotation or transposition flaps. An alternative is to remove the excess once the flap is sutured into place. Either way, caution should be exercised to avoid interference with the blood supply of the flap. A relatively slight excess is acceptable, as it will tend to resolve spontaneously or can be revised at a later stage once the flap has settled into position.

Insufficient local skin

Prevention—tissue   If it is anticipated in advance that there is insufficient local skin
expansion   to cover the defect, and if the operation can be delayed, tissue expansion may be possible. The tissue expander must be inserted in the correct plane of cleavage under the potential flap. It is expanded slowly over several weeks. The expanded skin is then elevated and used as a local flap to cover the defect after the

Figure 4.14
A local transposition flap on the calf to repair an area of radionecrosis. An arc of rotation on the same side as the defect (a) gives the false impression that the flap is excessively large. (b) The arc of rotation from the true axis shows that the flap is only just large enough. (c, d) The donor defect is covered with a split-thickness skin graft.

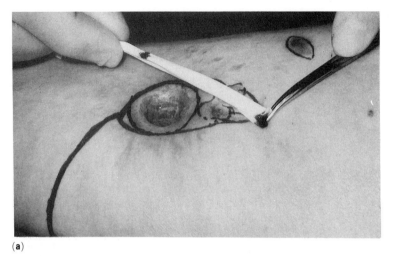

(a)

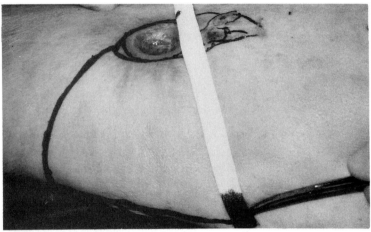

(b)

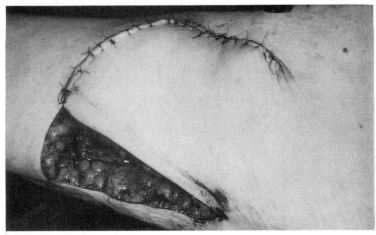

(c)

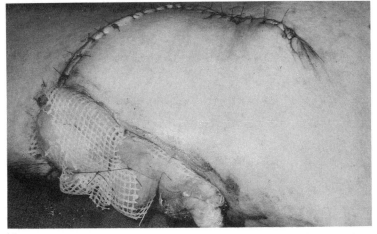

(**d**)

expander is removed. Tissue expansion is particularly useful in the scalp, to enlarge hair-bearing donor sites.

Complications of tissue expansion include infection and extrusion of the expander (Fig. 4.15), or skin necrosis if the expansion is carried out too quickly.

Figure 4.15
Exposure of a tissue expander. The expansion was continued rapidly and the flap was advanced to repair the eyelid.

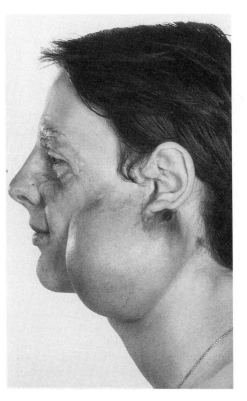

Management Once the defect is made, it may be too big for the planned local flap. There are several strategies available.

1 Abandon the flap repair and dress the wound while alternatives are discussed with the patient.
2 Apply a skin graft or use a distant or free microvascular flap as appropriate.
3 If the flap has already been raised, transfer it but add a marginal graft or additional flap to relieve tension.
4 Avoid the extensive use of back cuts to allow flap advancement, as this may compromise the blood supply. If necessary, suture the flap part way into position under slight tension. Creep is a property of skin that allows it to become accustomed to and adapt its shape to a new position. If it does not relax sufficiently, within twenty minutes or so, leave it sutured where it is and consider further advancement at a later date.
5 It may be possible to expand a flap donor site at the time of operation by inflating an expansion device under it—this is called instant expansion. Inflation is for three minutes at a time to blanch the skin, followed by deflation. This cycle is repeated three times.

Distant flaps There are two main types of distant flap:

1 direct (bridge) flap;
2 tube pedicle flap.

Direct flaps
A direct-transposition random-pattern flap is extremely limited by its short length-to-breadth ratio. Longer, axial-pattern, fascio-cutaneous or musculo-cutaneous flaps allow a longer bridge segment so that easier flap transfer can be achieved with fewer problems of tension and kinking. The most commonly used bridge flap today is the cross-finger flap. The basic principles apply equally to cross-arm and cross-leg flaps, or abdominal and groin flaps used for hand repair.

Prevention of complications

Planning A comfortable relaxed position of donor and recipient site should be planned to avoid unwanted stretching of joints. If possible, the limbs or digits should be placed side by side to allow mobility in tandem, so as to prevent stiffness. The flap must drape easily across the bridge to eliminate kinking and twisting. In a cross-finger flap, the donor site is preferably sited on the dorsum of the finger, so that, if the volar aspect is to be covered, a reverse dermis flap sits more easily.

Surgical procedure   The defect should be prepared first, removing all tissue that is scarred or of doubtful viability at the margin to give a good vascular inset for the flap. This is because, unlike a local flap, the bridge segment will be divided and the flap will depend for its survival on the adequacy of the blood supply from its base or periphery. If the base is avascular, all the vascular anastomoses will be at the periphery. The quality of inset can be improved by de-epithelializing the edge of the flap, or, with a fasciocutaneous flap, cutting a wider margin of fascia and inserting this rim under the edge of the defect. The tissues must be handled gently and kept moist at all times to prevent further devitalization of the defect or the flap.

Once the defect has been prepared, the design must be checked before the flap is raised. The flap is then elevated and the donor site sutured or covered with a split-skin graft, which is also applied to the bridge segment to eliminate raw surfaces and prevent infection. Depending on the flap being used, it may be more convenient to suture the flap in place or to arrange the fixation first.

Fixation   This may have to be rigid in cross-limb flaps but if there is a generous lax bridge more mobility can be allowed in order to prevent joint stiffness. In cross-finger flaps a band of sticking plaster is often sufficient. Cross-leg flaps should be avoided in older patients as there is a risk of permanent joint stiffness and deep-vein thrombosis.

Division   The timing of division of a bridge flap is crucial. The flap must have picked up sufficient blood supply from the recipient site or it will suffer ischaemia and necrosis. Many factors affect the timing.

1 *Site*. In relatively avascular areas such as the lower limb, the recommended time is three weeks after attachment. Arm and finger flaps can be divided earlier, at two weeks and ten days, respectively.

2 Complication at the attachment site such as infection and separation or mobility of the flap from the bed make a longer wait essential.

3 *Area attached*. If the whole flap is attached and no part of the bridge segment is required, earlier division is permissible, but if the bridge segment is required to cover the defect, a longer wait is necessary and a delay procedure may be advisable.

4 The reversed dermis flap picks up a more robust blood supply and can be divided relatively early, at about one week.

5 If there is a dominant vessel in the base of the flap, pick up of blood supply from its bed will be slow and a delay procedure is therefore advisable in axial pattern or musculo-cutaneous flaps.

6 *The crane flap*. When a thin layer of cover is needed, the flap

can be elevated after a week, leaving the viable deep layer that has picked up an adequate blood supply to support a split-skin graft. The flap is returned to the donor site, minimizing the donor scar.

Tests of blood supply   If there is any doubt about the flap's vascular supply from its bed, the viability can be gauged in various ways.

1 Clamping the bridge with a soft bowel clamp applied across the bridge. The behaviour of the flap blood supply can then be judged by any change in colour. If it is unchanged, then the flap is viable. A second check involves the amount of reactive hyperaemia when the clamp is released. If it is absent, the flap has a good attachment.

   Care is essential in using this technique because of the absent sensation. The clamp must not be left on for long periods or clamped very tightly, as the flap may be damaged severely.

2 A dye such as fluorescein, atropine injection or radioactive markers can be used in conjunction with a clamp on the flap bridge or tourniquet on the donor limb to assess the circulation.

Delay before attachment   This is a means of augmenting the blood supply from the bed. It is advisable in axial flaps that the vascular supply be divided one week before the skin bridge is divided. Clamping the bridge for progressively longer periods can be used as a physiological delay.

At division, if a significant part of the bridge is to be used to cover the recipient site, it is advisable to dress it and delay the formal inset of the flap for a few days.

Tube pedicle flaps

The classical tube pedicle flap is in effect a delayed random-pattern bipedicle flap that is tubed. This encourages the blood supply to run in a linear fashion. After a period of three weeks or so, one end is divided after a delay procedure. The raised end can then be applied to the recipient defect. This is a difficult multistage procedure with numerous pitfalls and potential complications; it is rarely used today and is not recommended to the novice. The experienced plastic surgeon uses it only for special indications such as penile reconstruction. A tubed axial-pattern flap such as a groin flap or musculo-cutaneous thigh flap is then used for preference because of the more reliable blood supply, which enables it to be raised and tubed in one stage without prior delay procedure.

Free flaps

The increasingly skilful use of microsurgical techniques has allowed free microvascular flap transfer to develop and flourish in the last decade. The methods are extremely versatile and have largely replaced other forms of distant flap transfer. The gains are great but the penalties of failure are also considerable. If one of these flaps fails, failure is usually complete (see Chapter 6).

Persisting controversies

- How to resuscitate an ailing flap?
- Is the delay procedure helpful or counterproductive?
- Are free flaps over-used?

Further reading

McGregor, I.A. (1980) *Fundamental Techniques of Plastic Surgery.* Edinburgh: Churchill Livingstone.

Grabb, W.C. & Smith, J.W. (Eds) (1980) *Plastic Surgery: A Concise Guide to Clinical Practice.* Boston: Little Brown.

Barron, J.N. & Saad, M.N. (Eds) (1980) *Operative Plastic and Reconstructive Surgery.* Edinburgh: Churchill Livingstone.

Barclay, T.L. & Kernahan, D.A. (Eds) (1986) *Plastic Surgery.* London: Butterworths.

5 Complications of Scars

A scar is the visible result of normal healing. Any injury to the skin that extends into the papillary dermis or deeper, whether traumatic, surgically induced or the result of other morbid process, will form a permanent scar. Most patients expect and understand that an operation will result in a scar but the quality of the scar may not be acceptable in certain circumstances. There may be an identifiable defect in wound healing that makes the scar unsightly or functionally unsatisfactory. Unrealistic expectation by the patient is a potent cause of disappointment and satisfactory results may be questioned.

Normal scar formation
Scar formation is a function of the wound-healing capacity of the skin. The wound-healing process starts with a phase of haemostasis when fibrin is laid down to fill the wound defect and a phase of inflammation with exudation into the wound of plasma proteins and invasion by polymorphonuclear leucocytes and later lymphocytes and monocytes. After three or four days there is a sudden change to a proliferative phase of cellular mitosis with new collagen deposition—fibrosis. From day five the tensile strength of the incision rises quickly as new collagen fibres are laid down and the process continues up to three weeks after injury. At this stage the scar is a depressed pink line, but gradually begins to swell slightly to form a pink or red indurated scar (Fig. 2.15c). This process of proliferation in hypertrophic scar formation lasts six months to two years. Finally by a process of maturation, vascularity decreases, the excess collagen disappears and the scar becomes paler, flatter and softer (Figs. 2.15a, 5.7a–c).

The visible scar is an inevitable result of this wound-healing process and, while there is a large range of measures available to try to improve scars, there is no known way at present to remove a scar completely without trace: 'Once a scar, always a scar'. All patients should be counselled thoroughly pre-operatively and during the postoperative period to expect and understand that after an initial good phase the wound may thicken and become red and unsightly during the proliferative phase. Although the scar may improve by maturation with the passage of time, it will never completely disappear.

The plastic surgeon and scar formation

The plastic surgeon starts at a disadvantage in treating scars. The patient may arrive with glowing recommendations from the referring clinician or may have totally unrealistic expectations that the plastic surgeon, using superior surgical skills, can remove the scars. This is palpably not true, although careful surgical technique and expertise can sometimes produce dramatic improvements. The most difficult task of all is to impress on an anxious patient that nothing need, nor should, be done surgically, in the early stages of wound healing and that maturation of the scar will give rise to gradual spontaneous improvement.

Unsatisfactory Scars

Predisposing factors

Impaired wound healing

Any of the general or local factors detailed in Chapter 2 that impair wound healing can cause an unsatisfactory scar. In particular, delayed healing may give rise to increased induration, oedema, tethering and irregular scar formation.

Mechanism of injury

The final appearance of a scar is more influenced by how it was inflicted than by how it was sutured. A contused, crushing injury with tissue loss or devitalized tissue will heal slowly with a more unsightly scar than a cleanly incised surgical wound. Deep or deep dermal burns leave intense scarring (Fig. 5.1). Explosions that cause multiple injuries with contamination of the wounds and ingrained dirt leave particularly unsightly scars.

Delayed scar maturation

Most scars undergo a maturation phase within six months. If the scar becomes progressively red, for up to two years, it is called a hypertrophic scar. Recurrent infection, retained foreign body or repeated trauma exacerbates the scar.

Age. Younger patients usually have a more prolonged proliferative phase in wound healing. Babies of less than six months and older adults have less tendency to form hypertrophic scars.

Tension. In a wound, tension predisposes to initial hypertrophic scar formation followed by an atrophic stretched scar.

Direction of the scar. This is the most important factor determining the result of scar formation. Generally, wounds parallel to natural crease lines and skin tension lines heal well and mature rapidly (Fig. 5.2); see Chapter 2. Longitudinal scars that cross joint creases tend to form thick, hypertrophic scars and contractures (Fig. 5.3).

Figure 5.1
The variable effect of mechanism of injury on scar appearance. The scattered white scars on the trunk are from small, deep, hot-metal burns—the patient is a welder. The hypertrophic scars on the right elbow are the result of a scald from a cup of coffee, which caused a deep dermal burn.

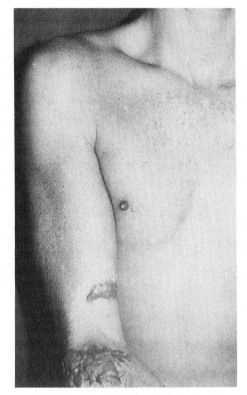

Figure 5.2
Scars placed in the natural skin crease lines shown on the face usually heal well. Alternatively, a scar placed in the hair line will be hidden.

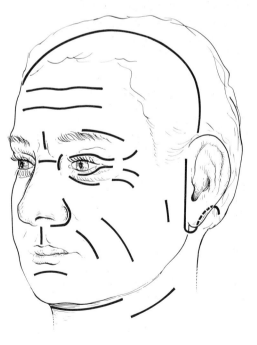

Figure 5.3
Severe hypertrophy
and contracture in a
scar crossing the
popliteal fossa (a). A
Z-plasty puts a
transverse scar across
the skin crease which
heals well, seen at 6
months in (b) and
1 year (c).

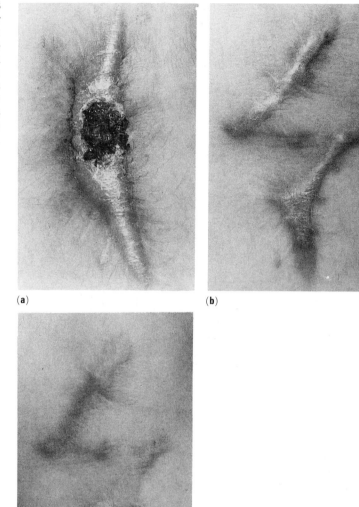

(a)

(b)

(c)

Site of the wound. Regional variations in hypertrophic scarring are not so marked as in keloid scarring. The face, neck and shoulder girdle areas tend to form hypertrophic scars, particularly over the sternum and deltoid.

Type of injury. Deep dermal (deep partial thickness) burns are particularly likely to cause unsightly hypertrophic scars (Fig. 5.1).

Skin type. The pink-skinned, red- or fair-haired person is more likely to develop red, raised scars.

Shape of the scar U- or V-shaped scars tend to become raised and unsightly, especially if the wound edges are shelved. As the scar contracts it will tend to bunch up the tissues causing a 'pin cushion' or 'trap-door' deformity. The smaller the flap, the greater the tendency for this to happen (Fig. 5.4).

Keloid A keloid scar is almost certainly a separate entity from hypertrophic scar. It is a progressive, sustained increase of scar formation lasting more than two years, frequently for tens of years, that tends to spread and involve the surrounding normal skin. It is much less common than hypertrophic scarring. Predisposing factors include the following:

Race. Keloid is more common in negroes but occurs in all races.

Previous history. Keloid tendency may be familial. A previous history of keloid in an individual means that there will be a greatly increased tendency for keloid to develop in subsequent wounds.

Type of injury. Recurrent trauma, infected wounds or burn wounds are particularly prone to develop keloid.

Site of wound. This is by far the most important factor in keloid formation. Even in a highly susceptible individual, not all scars behave in the same way. Some scars can become keloid, others may not. The presternal area is particularly at risk. (See Table 5.1.)

Prevention of the unsatisfactory scar
By recognizing and avoiding or treating predisposing factors it may be possible to minimize the development of unsightly or functionally unsatisfactory scars.

Planning Elective wounds or extensions of traumatic wounds should be kept as short as possible. Long, straight incisions should be avoided on the limb, particularly across joints, where the scar must be curved and angled to follow skin crease lines if possible.

Concealing the scar Try to conceal a scar by placing it in an inconspicuous place (Fig. 5.2). If a scar on the face crosses an aesthetic unit it will be more obvious. For example, if a lesion of the parotid is to be excised, a pre-auricular skin-crease scar will be less obvious than a direct incision across the cheek. A scar within or at the

Figure 5.4
Trap door scar from
an assault with a
bottle (a), treated by
partial excision and
Z-plasty (b), (c).

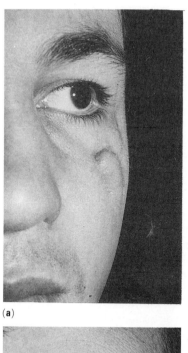

(a)

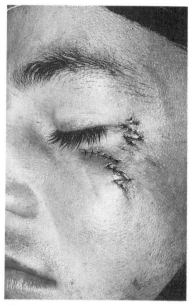

(b)

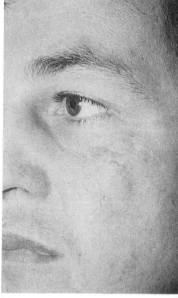

(c)

edge of hair-bearing skin is more difficult to see and a large
coronal incision of the scalp can give access to the whole frontal
area including the nose and orbits, leaving no visible scar.
Wherever possible, mucosal incisions for access to mandible or
maxilla and intranasal approaches for nasal surgery will conceal the scars and leave no external evidence of surgery. Scars

Table 5.1 Relative regional incidence of keloid scars.	
Presternal skin	1.0
Upper back	0.9
Beard area of face	0.8
Ear	0.8
Deltoid and preaxial upper limb	0.7
Front of chest lateral	0.6
Lower back	0.2
Abdomen	0.2
Lower limb	0.2
Post-axial upper limb	0.1
Central face	0.0

After Crockett D. J. (1964) *Brit. J. Plastic Surgery*, *17*, 245–253.

can also be planned so that they are concealed by clothing. If there is a choice of site for a scar, it is best to discuss the matter prior to surgery with the patient.

Plan for the future When making an elective incision, avoid compromising future surgical procedures. If the operation is part of a series, alternative methods of repair should be considered so that the incision does not, for example, sacrifice flap donor sites. In children, consider such factors as future hair and breast development. A scar near the nipple, for example, may damage the breast bud. In the female, it is better to place a scar some distance below rather than above the nipple. Scars grow, so as small a scar as possible is important in children. This applies equally to stitch marks (Fig. 2.19).

Surgical technique Most of the important technical points have been covered in Chapter 2. Trimming of skin wound edges should be kept to an absolute minimum. Dirt ingraining must be removed at the time of initial surgery or a tattooed scar will result. If necessary, dermabrasion must be used to remove all buried material (Fig. 2.8).

Sutures A large variety of suture materials is available, but in practice the correct placing of sutures and careful timing of suture removal are far more important than the relatively small differences between materials. Sutures should be fine and the tissue bites should be as small as possible so as to minimize stitch marks. Subcuticular repair with monofilament sutures will avoid suture marks altogether.

Avoid tension A wound under tension will tend to heal poorly with disruption. The sutures may cut out, causing stitch marks. When skin has been lost from a wound, it is often better to apply a graft to ensure early healing. The graft can be excised later and tissue-expansion techniques may be used to allow better repair with local skin.

Postoperative care Until wound tensile strength is maximal, at about six weeks, splinting of the wound can be very useful, particularly if the scar is on a mobile part of the body where repeated movement causes minute disruptions of the wound that increase fibrosis. If possible, the wound should be splinted, but extreme care should be taken that doing this does not compromise the eventual mobility of the underlying joint. After removal of the sutures, adhesive tapes kept on across the wound will help to relieve tension and decrease the tendency for the wound to separate. Correct timing of suture removal is important (see Chapter 2).

The new epidermal cover on a wound tends to be dry and to crack easily. Scabs should be removed as they loosen and general measures such as washing over the wound can usually be allowed after a few days if healing is proceeding well. A moisturizing cream should be applied to keep the skin supple and gentle massage may help to speed softening of the subcutaneous fibrosis.

Early application of therapeutic measures can be used prophylactically against such complications as hypertrophic scarring and contracture. Early pressure therapy and splinting will pay dividends.

Exposure to the environment A wound does not usually fully mature until at least one year after healing. During this time the scar is vulnerable to changes in temperature and will become blue, stiff and painful in cold weather, or red and itchy in hot conditions. Extremes of temperature should be avoided. Sunlight will damage a fresh scar by burning a hypopigmented scar or by making a pigmented scar become hyperpigmented. A fresh scar should therefore be protected from the sunlight for at least a year by appropriate clothing or high-factor sunscreen preparations.

Treatment of the unsatisfactory scar

Assessment The evaluation of a scar is partly subjective, and very careful pre-operative assessment must be made with the patient before scar revision is advised, planned or attempted. The patient's expectations and requirements must be fully understood. There may be pressures on the patient from relatives, friends and acquaintances, none of whom has any but the scantiest of knowledge about wound healing.

It is essential to establish a good rapport with the patient and, if necessary by repeated consultations, learn and explore the full background in order to determine the patient's wishes. At the same time the patient or his relatives should be gradually educated about the problems and possibilities of scar revision so that a realistic approach can be maintained. A careful balance must be struck between an over-optimistic approach by the surgeon or patient, when there may be disappointment as a result of exaggerated expectation, and on the other hand, pessimism from the surgeon that may deny the patient help when there is scope for some improvement.

If there is an objective defect that is amenable to treatment, such as a tattooed scar, and, if the surgeon's and patient's views coincide, the surgical result should be satisfactory. However, when there is still doubt about the true nature of the problem, a useful technique is to take colour print photographs of the scar and see the patient again after an interval. The wound can be reassessed and the photographs discussed with the patient. It may be helpful to recommend that the patient obtain a second opinion.

The patient's disfigurement as a result of an injury is a complex problem. It is important to evaluate and treat the patient as a whole, the mental state, the physical appearance, and rejection by the patient himself and by others. Surgery is only one part of the management, which should also include psychological assessment and support as necessary and disguise such as skin-camouflage techniques.

Conservative management
If the scar is newly healed and still undergoing a hypertrophic phase, evaluation should be delayed for at least a year after the time of the wound repair. Time is a great healer and many scars that are red, thick and unsightly will improve as maturation takes place. The patient should be seen at intervals so that the timing of scar revision can be planned. Frequently the improvement is so marked that surgery is not needed.

Early surgery in a hypertrophic scar is only indicated in certain circumstances as follows:

1 Contracture threatening other structures. For example, a cicatrical ectropian threatening the eye or a contracture affecting a joint should be corrected immediately.
2 If there is such gross malalignment or tattooing that scar revision is inevitable later, it is pointless delaying for long because the subsequent revision scar may undergo similar hypertrophic changes dating from the time of secondary surgery.

Additional measures
Conservative management should be active and is not a time of neglect. Suitable additional treatments include the following:

1 Grease massage to keep the scar moist and supple. Vitamin E application in the form of wheat germ oil softens scars.
2 Pressure therapy with elasticated garments or Tubigrip helps to prevent the tendency to hypertrophic scar formation.
3 Silicone gel sheets applied topically appear to relax and soften

scars. Pressure is not required for this effect. Contact sensitivity to the gel is a complication, and treatment must be stopped if this happens.

4 Splints, both static and lively, applied to a scarred limb help to prevent scar contracture. Passive splints worn at night and taken off for the patient to go to school or work are a compromise that may overcome patient non-compliance with wearing splints. Physiotherapy and exercises are useful additional measures.

5 Camouflage treatment is more difficult over a raised, knobbly wound but it is in the early stages after injury that most psychological help is required.

6 Sunscreen preparations should be applied whenever heavy exposure to sunlight is anticipated.

Scar Revision

There are five basic methods of scar revision (Fig. 5.5):

1 simple excision and resuture;
2 Z-plasty;
3 V to Y-plasty;
4 W-plasty;
5 release of contracture and graft or flap repair.

Simple scar revision

Indications   Most unsightly scars that are parallel to skin tension lines can usually be improved by simple fusiform scar revision (Fig. 5.5a).

1 Scars resulting from wounds healing by secondary intention are nearly always worth revising by this method.

2 Scars with large stitch marks, tattooed scars or small irregular scars are also suitable.

3 Tethered or depressed scars can frequently be improved. It is important not to re-explore the whole wound in depth, as the original conditions for tethering may be reproduced. The use of a buried dermis strip obtained from de-epithelialized scar and covered by lateral flaps is a useful technique to maintain correction of a depressed scar (Fig. 5.6).

4 Small trap-door scars can be excised and sutured directly—treating them like small skin lesions.

Contra-indications   It is important to realize that there can be no guarantee about wound healing after scar revision and if infection occurs the resulting scar may be worse. With all simple scar excisions, the scar will inevitably be slightly larger and therefore scar revision should only be undertaken if there is a positive indication to do something. Relatively inconspicuous scars should be left to mature further before a decision is made.

Figure 5.5
Basic methods of scar
revision. (a) Simple
excision and suture.
(b) Z-plasty. (c) Y to V-
plasty. (d) W-plasty.

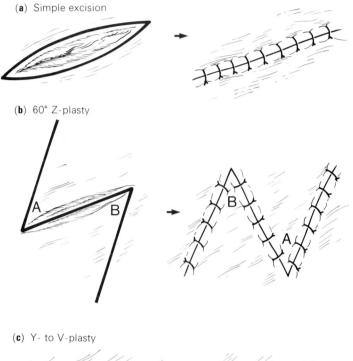

(**a**) Simple excision

(**b**) 60° Z-plasty

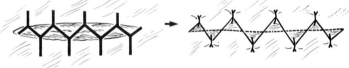

(**c**) Y- to V-plasty

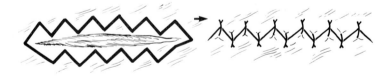

(**d**) W-plasty

1 Hypertrophic scars and widely spread scars will usually not respond favourably to simple scar revision. The hypertrophy and spreading will nearly always recur and the scar could easily become worse.

2 Keloid scars are an absolute contra-indication to simple scar revision. Recurrence is inevitable and the resulting scar will be worse.

Figure 5.6
Scar revision
incorporating a buried
dermis strip to correct
a tethered, depressed
scar.

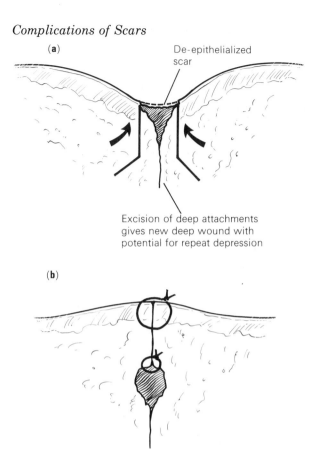

(a)

De-epithelialized
scar

Excision of deep attachments
gives new deep wound with
potential for repeat depression

(b)

Z-plasty

Indications

1 Tight or contracted linear or curved scars can be lengthened by Z-plasty, but only at the expense of lateral tension (Fig. 5.7).

2 If the line of a scar is not parallel to the skin tension lines, it can be adjusted so that the main limb of the scar comes to be in a skin tension line.

3 Long linear scars can be improved by serial small Z-plasties, which minimize the lateral tension.

4 Multiple small scars can sometimes be disguised by a camouflage effect using Z-plasties.

Contra-indications

The Z-plasty requires laxity of the skin laterally to allow the flaps to transpose. Diffuse areas of scarring cannot usually be helped by Z-plasty and scar release and grafting are required.

Linear hypertrophic scars can often be helped by Z-plasty, but there is a risk that all three limbs of the scar will become hypertrophic, so increasing the length of the scar. This must be discussed with the patient (Fig. 5.11a).

Figure 5.7
A hypertrophic scar causing nipple elevation treated by Z-plasty. (a) Severe hypertrophic scar from a scald in a 3-year-old child, proceeding to spontaneous resolution one year later (b). (c) At 14 years the scar has faded in appearance but is tight and distorts the breast on arm elevation. (d) A Z-plasty is planned, taking care not to include hair-bearing axillary skin in the flaps, and completed (e). One year later symmetry has been preserved (f), but continued follow up is required until growth is complete.

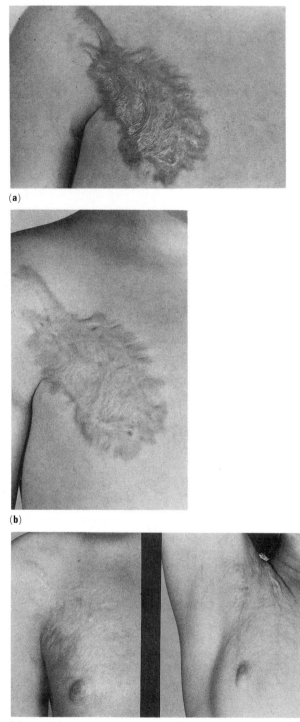

(a)

(b)

(c)

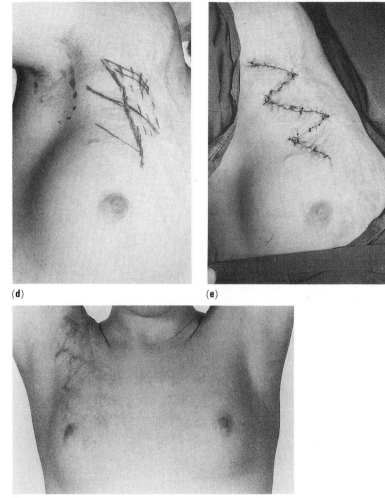

(d) (e)

(f)

On prominent plane surfaces, for example the cheek, a series of small Zs will be less noticeable, but larger Zs give better release when releasing a joint contracture.

Technique Z-plasty is a difficult procedure for the inexperienced surgeon to plan and execute. The following guidelines will help to minimize difficulties and errors (Fig. 5.8).

1 Plan the procedure. First mark the scar with ink, then mark the limbs of the Z-plasty.
2 Check the planning and marking before proceeding. If many trial ink marks have been made, erase the wrong ones with a Medi-swab to prevent confusion during surgery.
3 In each Z-plasty do not cut both flaps at first. Raise one flap,

Figure 5.8
A method to minimize
errors in Z-plasty. After
the flaps are marked
(a), only one is cut (b)
and the transposition
is checked (c), before
the second flap
is cut (d).

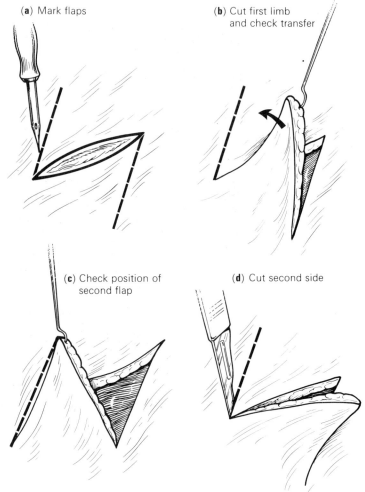

(**a**) Mark flaps

(**b**) Cut first limb
and check transfer

(**c**) Check position of
second flap

(**d**) Cut second side

check that it will transpose and remark a new flap if necessary before proceeding.

4 Flaps in scar tissue are very vulnerable to necrosis and must be cut vertically with a full complement of underlying subcutaneous tissue to preserve the blood supply. The flaps must not be widely undermined beyond their base.

5 Before suturing the flaps in the transposed position, check that all tight subcutaneous scarring in the wound has been released.

6 Ensure flaps are transposed into the new position (Fig. 5.9).

7 In tight scarred areas there may be so much tension that the wound cannot be closed. A skin graft must be inserted to relieve tension.

Figure 5.9
Failure to transpose a
Z-plasty, seen 6
months after surgery.
Three serial Z-plasties
were planned correctly
on the thigh of this
young female patient
to correct a ring
constriction. When
they were sutured, the
flaps of the posterior Z
were sutured back
where they came from
and the error was
discovered when the
dressing was removed.

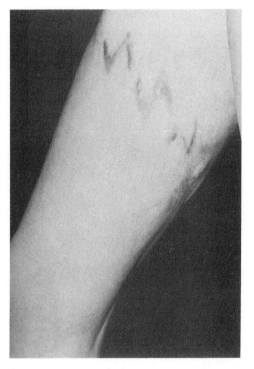

8 If the linear release is much greater than expected, so that the
flaps will not close in the intended position, extra parallel Zs
can be cut, but this must be done with great care. A 120° Z-
plasty can solve this problem in folds such as the thenar web
or axillary area.

9 In complex contractures a combination of scar revision and
asymmetrical Z-plasties can be used (Fig. 5.10).

V to Y-plasty

Indications   The V to Y-plasty has similar indications to Z-plasty. It is most
useful for releasing linear tightness. An advantage in severe
scarring from burns is that the flaps are not raised or transposed
and the chances of skin necrosis are decreased. The process can
be repeated after short time intervals in adjacent scars with less
risk of tissue necrosis.

Contra-indications   The method depends on lateral advancement of V flaps and
therefore loose skin is required on either side of the scar to be
released. It is thus not suitable in diffuse scarring without
bands.

Technique   A series of continuous V-shaped cuts must be made across the
whole thickness of the tight band. At the apex of each V a lateral

Figure 5.10
A severe contracture of the corner of the mouth (a) treated by a combination of scar excision and asymmetrical Z-plasties (b). If the flaps are cut at right angles to the skin surface with a generous amount of subcutaneous fat there will be minimal flap loss even though the flaps are cut in scar tissue; (c) 3 weeks postoperatively.

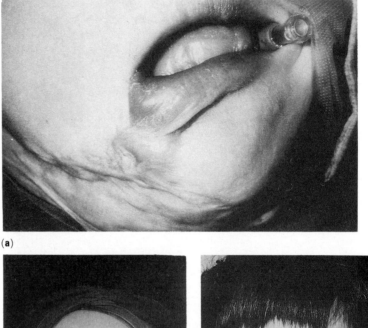

(a)

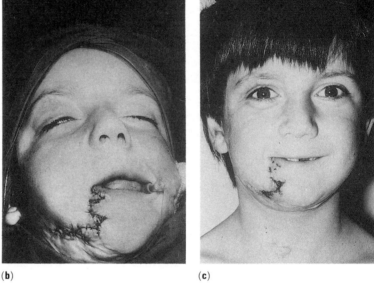

(b)   **(c)**

extension cut is made into the subcutaneous tissue. The release cut should be vertical with no undermining. The flaps are advanced, interdigitated and sutured in position (Figure 5.5c).

W-plasty

Indications   This technique is suitable for a limited number of linear scars, principally on the face and abdomen, that are not parellel to the skin tension lines. The scar is excised with an irregular pattern of normal skin to allow the wound to be closed in a zig-zag fashion.

Contra-indications The W-plasty technique is not suitable in areas of skin loss or contracture because it requires excision of normal tissue. It is contra-indicated for hypertrophic or keloid scars (Fig. 5.11).

If the limbs of the W are made too small, the series of trap door-scars that is formed can make the scar more conspicuous.

Release of scar contracture

Indications When there is extensive tissue damage or loss, with large areas of scarring, simple scar revision methods are not applicable. Once incision is made in the contracture, the wound gapes widely and flap or skin graft repair is needed.

Technique Transverse release of the scar is the most efficient way of releasing tension. The incision must be carried across the full

Figure 5.11
(a) Hypertrophic scar resulting from a Z-plasty. (b) If a W-plasty is performed, there is a risk that the scar will appear more obvious as it may itself develop a hypertrophic reaction.

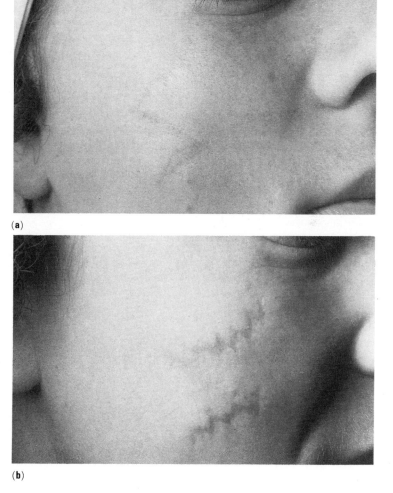

(a)

(b)

width and through the full thickness of scar into undamaged subcutaneous tissue. Scar is not usually excised. Often one release is not sufficient and two or more parallel releases are required. If a double release is used it is better to place the intervening bridge across the joint crease. Fishtail extension or trapezoid release gives even greater correction, allowing larger grafts to be inserted (Fig. 5.12).

Postoperative care   Even if there is a perfect take of the graft there will be a tendency to contract again. Prolonged splintage is required, particularly at night, for about six months (Fig. 5.13). Compression therapy can be used as a substitute during the day.

Hypertrophic Scar

Diagnosis   Hypertrophic scarring is severe thickening of a scar with a shiny red appearance (Fig. 5.7a). It is an exaggeration of the

Figure 5.12
Diagram of methods of scar release. (a) A simple transverse incision within the scar gives very poor release. (b) The incision must extend into unscarred skin for an adequate release. (c) Fish-tail incision to give wider release. (d) The double trapezoid flap method allows a much larger release.

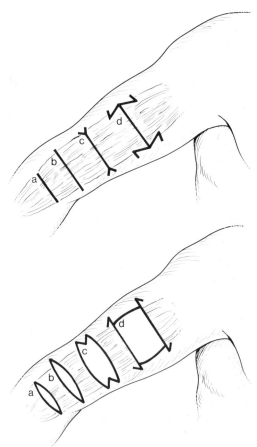

Figure 5.13
Release and skin graft of a neck contracture (a), after a flame burn. The transverse incision must be carried deeply through all scar tissue to allow full release. Note no tissue has been excised (b, c). A skin graft is applied and the result at 2 weeks is shown when the tie-over dressing was removed under general anaesthetic (d). In order to prevent contracture, a foam collar is worn continuously for 6 months (e). The result is a stable graft with full release maintained at 1 year (f).

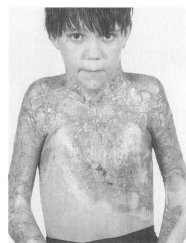

(a)

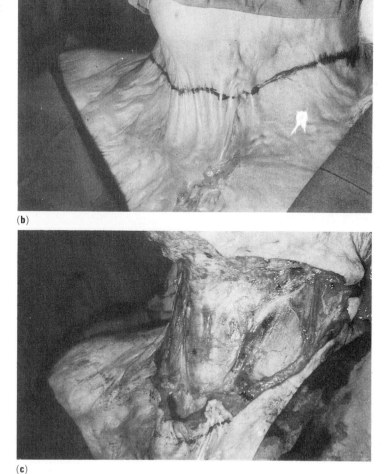

(b)

(c)

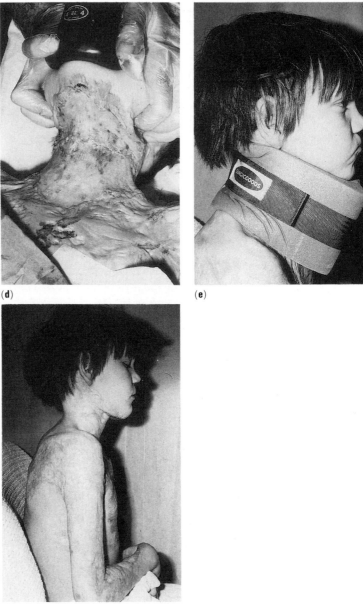

(d)

(e)

(f)

proliferative phase of healing and continues for at least six months and frequently as long as two years. It can sometimes develop so rapidly that it is mistaken for inflammation. It is accompanied by severe itching in the proliferative phase. The thick, plaque-like scar does not invade the normal surrounding skin but it causes severe cosmetic and functional disabilities.

Hypertrophic scarring may be a distinct entity from keloid scar or may be one end of a spectrum of scar pathology.

Predisposing factors The condition is more frequent in younger patients. It is particularly likely to occur in burn wounds of the intermediate thickness (deep dermal) variety (Fig. 5.1). Also, any wound that heals by secondary intention with the formation of granulation tissue is a potent predisposing factor.

Prevention All possible measures for gaining early primary healing without tension should be used. If a burn becomes infected or develops granulation tissue, grafts should be used as soon as possible to speed healing. Deep dermal burns should be shaved and grafted early.

Management *Conservative treatment* should be considered initially to await the spontaneous resolution that takes place by about two years (Fig. 5.7a, b). Antihistamine treatment and avoidance of hot baths and nylon clothing helps to relieve the itch in children.

Pressure applied by elasticated bandages such as Tubigrip or by custom-made pressure garments speeds maturation of the scar. Over a bony surface, acrylic pads using elastic traction give very localized pressure therapy. Treatment should continue for at least six months.

Steroids such as triamcinolone applied topically as Haelan tape or injected into the scar are an effective method of damping down hypertrophic scarring. It has to be repeated until the hypertrophic tendency has settled. Complications of steroid treatment include atrophy of subcutaneous tissues, depigmentation or telangiectasia.

Silicone gel applied by taping a suitably sized piece over the wound (without pressure) can give remarkable resolution of hypertrophic scar.

Surgical treatment is prone to high recurrence rates and simple excision and suture should be avoided. When the scar is interfering with function, various methods have been tried, including shaving and grafting, excision and grafting or flap repair. There is no doubt that flap repair gives the best results, but there is always a risk that the flap donor site will also become hypertrophic.

There is some evidence that early release of contractures, followed by grafting, allows more rapid resolution of hypertrophic scarring. Intralesional Z-plasty can give spontaneous resolution.

Keloid Scar

Diagnosis   Keloid scarring presents as a thick raised lump that starts off in a scar but can grow into the surrounding normal skin (Fig. 5.14). It is very important to suspect this diagnosis when presented with a fleshy intradermal skin tumour and a history of trauma, since excision is very likely to lead to a bigger and more unsightly lump. There may not be a history of trauma in susceptible individuals.

Prevention   The only way to prevent keloid is to avoid injury. Unfortunately, in susceptible individuals even the development of folliculitis is sufficient to spark off keloid formation. Spots should

Figure 5.14
(a, b, c) Progressive enlargement of a keloid scar over a period of seven years to become confluent by invading normal surrounding skin, in spite of triamcinolone injections. The process was finally halted by intrascar excision and grafting followed by superficial X-ray therapy (d).

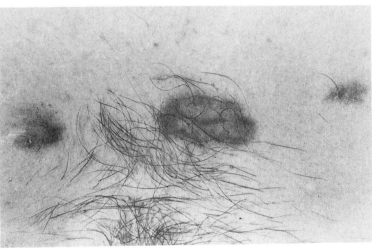

(**a**)

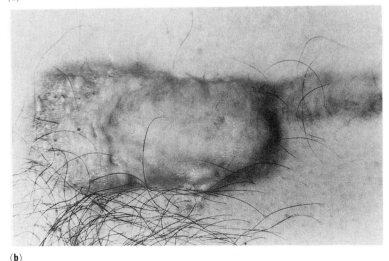

(**b**)

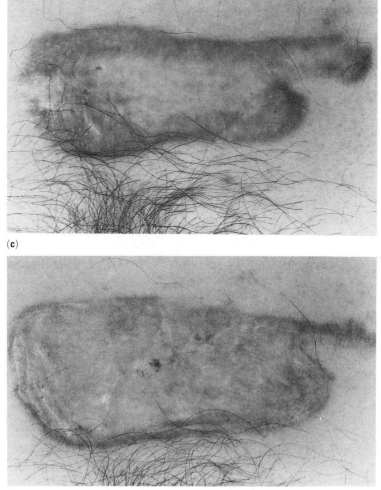

(c)

(d)

not be scratched or picked and even grazes should be carefully
looked after to avoid infection and to speed healing. There is an
unpredictability about keloid scars: some wounds in the same
area become keloid and others do not. Buried non-absorbable
sutures should be avoided so as to prevent a foreign-body
granulation reaction that may initiate keloid formation (Fig.
5.15).

Management   Keloid scars may remain active for many years, but if these scars
are asymptomatic it is prudent to leave them undisturbed rather
than risk making them worse.

Pressure therapy is sometimes effective but it has to be applied
for prolonged periods if it is to be successful.

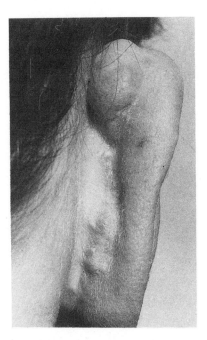

Steroid therapy is less successful than when used in hypertrophic scarring (Fig. 5.16).

Surgical treatment alone is very likely to result in exacerbation of keloid formation. If possible any surgery should keep within the confines of the keloid, and intralesional excision with or without Z-plasty or skin grafts may help. In addition, incorporation of triamcinalone directly into the wound on closure and immediate postoperative pressure may help, but results are disappointing and the recurrence rate is high.

Irradiation therapy is usually reserved for intractable cases. It must not be used in children or in women of childbearing age. When used as split therapy with radiotherapy on the day before and the day after surgery (Fig. 5.14d), it is successful in a proportion of cases (Fig. 5.17).

Treatment of Other Problem Scars

Multiple scars
Excision of scars that are closely parallel can remove several scars and replace them with one scar. Stellate scars can similarly sometimes be improved by excision and suture. If scarred areas are excised and grafted, the grafts should be applied to anatomical units to minimize the impact of the marginal scarring (Fig. 5.18).

Figure 5.16
The result of
triamcinolone
injections in a keloid
(a) is unpredictable
and in this case
caused necrosis and
exacerbation of the
symptoms of itch and
pain (b).

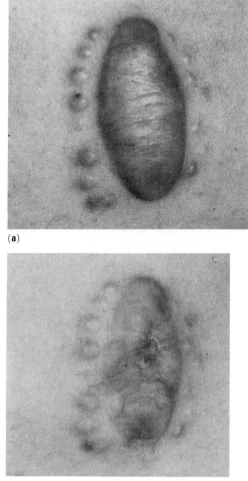

(a)

(b)

However, where there are large numbers of scars over a wide area, e.g. after suicidal gestures, excision is not feasible, but shaving with overgrafting gives quite good improvement. Careful selection is essential and if patients who form atrophic scars are chosen for treatment the graft is unlikely to produce hypertrophic scars.

Hyperkeratosis

Excessive thickening of the epidermal layers of the skin is a rare problem but when it occurs it can be painful and disabling. It usually occurs over weight-bearing areas. It is important to avoid placing scars on pressure areas. Shaving and over-grafting or flap repair to remove the marginal scar of a weight-bearing area may help.

Figure 5.17
(a) Treatment of a
keloid scar by excision
and postoperative
radiotherapy. (b)
Result 1 year later.

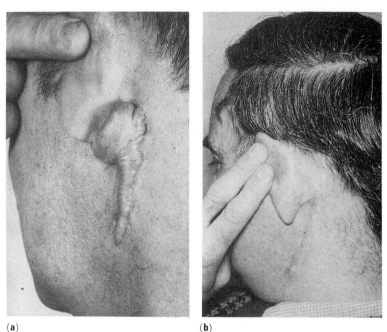

(a)　　　　　　　　(b)

Figure 5.18
This ungainly scarring
is the result of
applying small grafts
that do not cover the
complete aesthetic
unit.

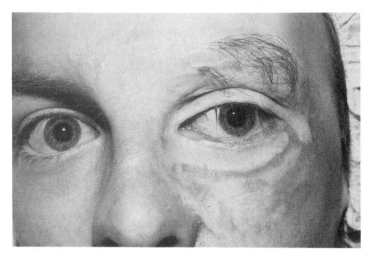

Raised scars

Bunching of tissue can be caused by contraction of a curved
scar, as in trapdoor scarring, or by lymphoedema in the subcutaneous tissue. Treatment consists of a combination of measures
to correct the causative factors. Scar revision by Z-plasty will
release the tightness and pressure therapy can prevent recurrence of the oedema (Fig. 5.4).

Pigmented scars

Tattooing of single scars is treated by scar revision. If a large area is involved with multiple tattoos, dermabrasion is the treatment of choice. If there are still a few areas of deep tattoo remaining, small excisions can be added (Fig. 5.19).

Hypopigmentation can occur after injury (Fig. 5.20). The pigment usually returns gradually and spontaneously if the original wound was superficial. In the meantime, the skin must be protected from sun, since repeated trauma causes blistering and further hypopigmentation. When the skin loss has been full thickness, it does not usually return. A pigment can be tattooed into the skin or dermabrasion and overgrafting with a very thin split-thickness graft can be tried. The degree of graft pigmentation is very difficult to control (see Chapter 3).

Hyperpigmentation may also occur after injuries to the skin. It is essential to screen wounds from the sun selectively to prevent hyperpigmentation. Another useful technique is to use skin bleach to lighten the dark patches.

Figure 5.19
Tattooed scar as a result of failure to clean and debride a dirt-ingrained scar adequately.

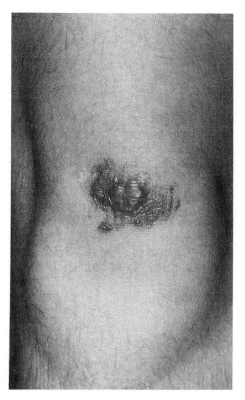

Figure 5.20
(a) This superficial
scald with blistering
caused a
hypopigmented area
(b) seen 3 weeks later.
(c) Six months later
the pigment had
almost completely
returned.

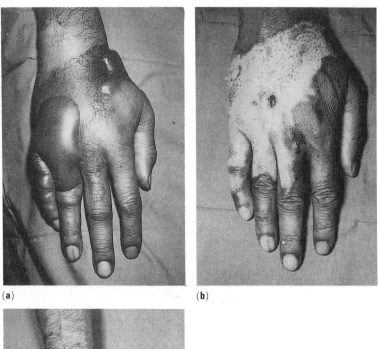

(a)   (b)

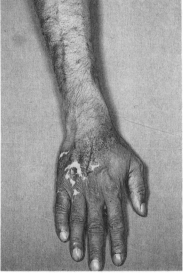

(c)

Painful scars

Most scars will be painful for a time after healing. The pain is worse in cold weather. Pain usually subsides after one or two years. A small minority of scars develop severe pain. The presence of any foreign body should be excluded. Sometimes the pain is due to nerve entrapment or neuroma. In the severe types of causalgia, help is required from a pain specialist.

When the scar is painful as a result of excessive pressure over an area with little padding, shaving and overgrafting or excision and flap repair will sometimes give relief.

Hair

Increased hairiness and the production of coarse darker hair after trauma can be a problem in some patients. Even a limb fracture in the absence of skin injury can give rise to excess hair production. Treatment is very difficult and shaving, plucking or electrolysis can be tried.

Any deep injury in a hair-bearing area that damages the hair follicle will cause a bald scar (Fig. 5.21). The only treatment possible is to graft in punch grafts of hair-bearing skin or to use a hair-bearing flap repair. Tissue expansion is particularly useful in these cases.

Figure 5.21
This deep hot fat burn in a hair-bearing area caused damage to the hair follicles and a consequent bald patch.

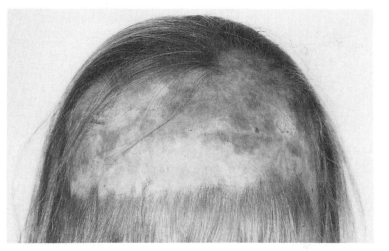

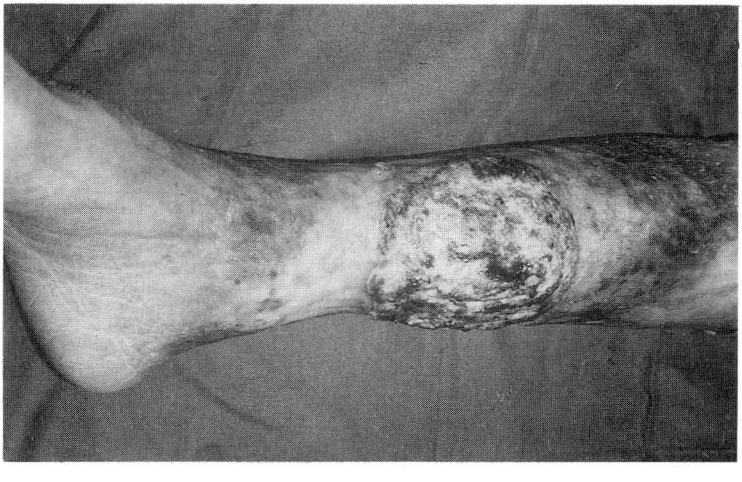

Figure 5.22
A Marjolin's ulcer that developed 30 years after a wound that caused a chronic discharging sinus.

Marjolin's ulcer

Malignant change can occur in unhealed wounds or unstable scars after a latent period of many years. Unstable areas subject to repeated trauma or breakdown should be treated by surgical repair if ulceration persists for longer than a few months of adequate conservative management (Fig. 5.22). When an unstable scar is being treated, consider sending a specimen of the wound margin for histopathological examination.

Persisting controversies
- Prevention of hypertrophic scar formation.
- Early surgery in hypertrophic scars.
- The treatment of keloid scars.
- The indications for surgical revision of scars.
- Control of pigment formation in scars.

Further reading

Borges, A.F. (Ed) (1977) Scar Revision. *Clinics in Plastic Surgery*. Philadelphia: Saunders.

6 Microsurgery

The technique of microsurgery has found many applications in different branches of surgery. Operating under magnification enables greater accuracy in dissection, better definition of fine structures and more accurate approximation of vessels and nerves in reconstructive procedures. The usual range of magnification used in practice varies from $2\frac{1}{2}$ times using loupes, to 40 times using a microscope. The greater the magnification, the more accentuated become the operator's movements, both voluntary and involuntary, and the more challenging and difficult becomes the surgery.

Improvements in optics have progressed with improvements in suture and needle manufacture so that sutures of 22 µm diameter (10-0), 18 µm diameter (11-0) and even smaller, are used in anastomosis of vessels down to less than a millimetre in diameter. Fine instruments are required for the use of these fine sutures, and it is important that the care of these is meticulous to avoid damage to the delicate points at the ends of the forceps, etc., which can jeopardize otherwise good technique.

Microsurgery is now widely practised in other branches of surgery, including neurosurgery, gynaecological surgery (for example in reversal of a tubal ligation procedure), in ENT surgery (middle ear work), etc. In this chapter, however, the discussion will centre around the use of the microscope in plastic and reconstructive surgery, which can broadly be divided into two categories—namely, emergency situations and elective surgery.

Emergency surgery
The use of the microscope has greatly improved the quality of repair of divided structures, nerves, vessels, etc.

Nerve injury   The repair of divided nerves requires care and precision to correctly identify corresponding fasciculi and execute their repair. This is particularly so in a mixed nerve (e.g. the median nerve at the wrist), containing both sensory and motor components. The better and more accurately the fasciculi are aligned, the better is the final result, though this is difficult to test experimentally. Methods of repair are

1 epineural;
2 perineural;
3 epiperineural (see Fig. 6.1).

Figure 6.1
Anatomy of nerve and
epiperineural repair.

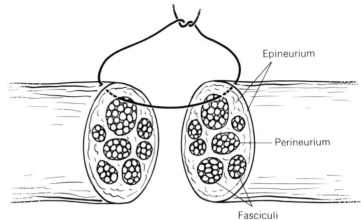

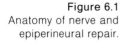

Figure 6.1
Anatomy of nerve and
epiperineural repair.

In an epineural repair, only the outer epineurium is sutured, usually with interrupted sutures of 8-0 to 10-0 depending on the size of the nerve. In a perineural repair, only the perineurium is approximated, but this is often thin and may not always hold the suture adequately. Using an epiperineural repair, the benefits of better fascicular alignment (as in a perineural repair) combined with the extra strength of the epineurium give the most satisfactory repair. Debate continues as to the correct timing of nerve repair—as a primary or secondary procedure. Generally speaking, in a clean-cut fresh wound, a primary repair should always be attempted. In crush injuries, avulsion injuries, and particularly when there is tissue loss, a secondary procedure may be indicated.

Vessel injury   Whereas limited magnification for repair of larger damaged vessels, e.g. the brachial artery, is helpful, repair of smaller vessels such as digital arteries and veins can only be carried out under magnification. A digit can survive on a single digital artery, but when both digital arteries are divided in the presence of an extensive skin laceration, repair of at least one digital artery is required if it is decided to preserve the digit. Replantation of a severed digit will likewise require repair of at least one digital artery and a vein, but preferably two veins. With greater numbers of these digital replantations being successfully carried out, a clearer picture of the long-term benefits of such lengthy procedures has emerged from various series published. In general, replantation of a severed thumb should always be attempted. Good results from replantation of severed single digits can also be achieved in children, but in adults this is usually not the case, particularly in zone II injuries, i.e. to the level of the DIP joint. Distal to this, although the operation is technically more difficult, good results can often be obtained. Replantation of multiple digits, hands and more proximally in the upper limb, again should be attempted. Replantation in the lower limb, however, seldom gives results as satisfactory, especially in adults. It is important to emphasize that, although this type of surgery is challenging and often very rewarding, it may not always be in the patient's ultimate interest to undergo prolonged surgery and a protracted period of rehabilitation. These patients should be referred to centres where specialized microsurgeons experienced in dealing with these problems are better qualified to make decisions about the advisability of particular procedures in particular injuries.

Duct injury The most common ducts injured seen in plastic surgery are the parotid and lacrimal ducts often transected in association with facial lacerations caused by sharp objects such as broken glass. Inaccurate repair can result in stenosis with recurrent infection in the parotid gland and epiphora in the eye. Parotid ducts can of course be simply ligated, but magnification must be used if repair is carried out. Lacrimal ducts must be repaired over a fine stent or thread and once again accurate apposition of the divided ends can only be achieved with magnification.

Elective surgery

Magnification with loupes is helpful in many aspects of plastic surgery such as fasciectomy in Dupytren's disease, cleft lip repair, etc. More particularly, microsurgery techniques are used in elective peripheral nerve surgery and free tissue transfer.

Elective peripheral nerve surgery In situations where primary nerve repair after division cannot be carried out, secondary nerve repair or nerve grafting procedures may be required. Several nerves have been used as donor grafts, the most commonly used being the sural nerve in the leg. Vascularized nerve grafts have also been used and although their full role and value have not been evaluated, they have proved valuable in situations where the bed on which the graft is to be placed is scarred or of limited vascularity. Nerve grafts are being used widely in the management of facial palsy, often being anastomosed to viable fascicles on the normal side and then routed across the face to the paralysed side to re-animate the denervated muscles there or used in conjunction with a vascularized muscle transfer.

Free tissue transfer Plastic surgery is involved in many situations in providing soft-tissue cover following trauma, elective excision of tissue, burns, etc. With a knowledge of vascular territories supplied by a particular artery and vein, flaps of tissue, together with this vascular supply, can be completely detached, transferred to the recipient site and revascularized by anastomosing the vessels into those in the recipient area. These flaps can be of simple skin and subcutaneous tissue only, or of compound design consisting of muscle and/or bone and/or nerve.

Complications seen in microsurgery of nerves and vessels

Failure of a nerve repair will result in local neuroma formation and failure of either sensory or motor recovery or both over the distribution of the nerves' territory. The major complication following microvascular surgery is, of course, thrombosis. These will be considered separately, together with their diagnosis and management. However, several general factors must be considered important in the prevention of complications in any form of microsurgery.

Predisposing factors

Facilities   To carry out microsurgery, magnifying loupes and a microscope are essential and the operator should be experienced in their use. There are many varieties on the market now, covering a wide price range. These can be free-standing or attached as a permanent fixture to the theatre ceiling. Cases involving free transfer of tissue can take a considerable time, using up valuable theatre time and personnel. Theatre time and space must therefore be available. Inadequate facilities may compromise the success of an operation such as this.

Operative team   For most free-flap surgery and nerve work (when a graft is required), team work is essential. Complications can arise resulting from sheer fatigue if a single individual has to carry our a major resection, e.g. for head and neck cancer, and then start a meticulous dissection of the flap, after which he is carrying out a delicate vascular anastomosis. This may also prolong the anaesthesia unnecessarily in a frail patient. Even in the best hands, anastomoses need to be revised; thrombosis can occur in the early postoperative hours, requiring a further prolonged period in the operating theatre. This form of reconstruction is, therefore, best carried out in centres where there are at least two trained microvascular surgeons.

Training   Manipulation of microsurgical instruments and sutures under microscope requires training and practice. Without good control, the inexperienced surgeon is likely to cause damage to the fine vessels, with resulting damage to the intima, poor suture ligation technique and almost certain thrombosis.

Before contemplating this surgery, therefore, the intending surgeon should train himself in the animal laboratory and by attendance at one of several training courses held each year. Vessels in the postpartum placenta or chicken carcass have proved a useful and readily available source for practising microsurgical techniques.

Instruments   Fine instruments, initially developed from those of watchmakers, have been a major cause for advances in this specialty over the last twenty years. It is important that they be kept in optimal condition. A slightly blunted end on a pair of micro-forceps results in poor apposition of the blades, which can cause vessel-wall damage when used as an aid in suturing. Inadequately cleaned needle holders will become stiff, interfering wih the precise control required in the handling of the needle and suture during anastomosis. All instruments should be cleaned after the operation, preferably by the surgeon.

Sutures Along with improvements in microinstrument manufacture, major advances in suture developments, in particular of the needles used, have increased the scope and possibilities of microsurgery of nerves and vessels. Sutures of 10-0 and 11-0 are commonly used. Any suture will inevitably cause some damage to the intimal lining of a vessel, and even the finest available can appear very traumatic in the vessel when seen under the electron microscope. Investigators continue to search for other methods of 'fusing' small vessels. The use of heavy sutures should, therefore, be avoided in this type of surgery.

Prevention of complications

Pre-operative *Patient*
factors It is evident from the preceding discussion that careful patient selection in this type of surgery is all important. Obviously in the emergency situation where a patient presents with a severed thumb or hand, for example, one must attempt replantation wherever possible. But a self-employed patient who wants to return to work as soon as possible with, for example, two severed fingers, may better be served by formalizing the amputation with minimal hospitalization and rehabilitation, provided his employment or particular interests will not be jeopardized by so doing. Several factors must be taken into account before embarking on this type of surgery.

History. Any condition that is likely to be adversely affected by a prolonged anaesthetic is likely to be a contraindication to elective microsurgery, e.g. severe ischaemic heart disease, chronic obstructive airway disease, etc. Significant past psychiatric problems must be taken into consideration. Co-operation from the patient postoperatively is vital. Regular attendance for physiotherapy over a prolonged period of time may be necessary in digit or limb replantation. It is important to record drug history. In the acute traumatic situation, the nature of the injury is important. Is it a clean-cut laceration or an avulsion injury, etc.?

Examination. Particular examination of the cardiovascular system is important. Free-flap surgery in the lower third of the lower limb is particularly prone to complication and the careful assessment of the peripheral circulation is mandatory here. Any scars in the site of the flap may have interfered with its vascularity and should be noted. Examination of the severed part in an amputation for replantation is important; for example, crush injuries do less well than sharp lacerations.

Investigations. In the acute situation, blood screening, ECG, chest X-ray, etc. should be carried out. In elective microsurgery, investigation of the vessel with a Doppler and possibly an arteriogram may be necessary. This is particularly true in the traumatized lower limb, where there may be only a single feeding artery to the distal extremity. In this situation, an end-to-side anastomosis will have to be carried out and planned. X-rays, if bone reconstruction is indicated, must be carried out to assess the length required; for example, up to 5 cm of bone deficit can be reconstructed using metatarsal incorporated into a dorsalis pedis flap, but a greater defect than this will require another flap such as a groin flap with iliac crest based on the deep circumflex iliac artery. Inadequate planning, therefore, can produce an unfavourable result.

The procedure planned The greater the complexity of the (elective) procedure planned, the greater must be the pre-operative planning to reduce the risk of complication. Other factors that are important in elective free flap surgery are:

1 size and length of the vascular pedicle;
2 size of the flap and skin quality;
3 donor-site defect that will result;
4 special qualities (e.g. innervation; muscle content, either for bulk or function).

In the acute traumatic situation, damage to other structures in the severed part must be taken into consideration. In particular, if viable soft tissue is not available to cover the bone and/or vascular anastomosis, the risk of failure, infection and thrombosis will be much higher. A measure of bone shortening will almost always be required and this may compromise the long-term success of the procedure, particularly in the lower limb.

Specific Complications Associated with Nerve Repair

In acute traumatic division of a major nerve, provided the injury is a laceration type of injury, primary repair should always be carried out when possible. Where the nerve has been damaged by an avulsion or crush type injury, the decision is more difficult, though most people would favour primary repair in children unless the avulsion or crush has caused considerable damage over a wide area of tissue.

Diagnosis

Failure of the repair, either primary, secondary, or following nerve graft, will present with one or more of the following features.

1 Painful neuroma at the site of repair or anastomosis.
2 Static Tinel's sign.
3 Tinel sign at the wound persistently stronger than the advancing Tinel's sign.
4 Absence of some evidence of recovery of function after a time elapse equivalent to normal nerve recovery (i.e. 1 mm per day approximately).

Prevention of complications

Having considered the clinical features of a failed nerve repair, the various factors giving rise to this situation are as follows.

Bed and cover   These factors are particularly important in the success of a free nerve graft, which will depend on the vascularity of both the bed and cover. If there is gross scarring or contamination, the graft fibroses and failure of axonal regeneration occurs. To provide a vascular bed and cover, flaps of tissue may be transferred (either pedicled or free flaps) in a first-stage procedure. Alternatively, vascularized nerve grafts have a role in this situation, where the viability of the graft is not dependent on the immediate environment.

Infection   Infection will inevitably leave scarring and fibrosis around the repair site. This will interfere with graft take and nerve regeneration. Adequate debridement of the wound in the acute situation, antibiotic cover if indicated and viable tissue to cover the repair are all important factors. In a wound presenting late, with infection, this must be treated first, leaving the nerve repair till later.

Alignment   Fascicular alignment is all-important in achieving a good final result from nerve repair. This is particularly true in a mixed nerve with both motor and sensory fibres. This matching can only be achieved under magnification and no nerve should be repaired without this. New staining methods are being developed which will help to distinguish sensory and motor nerve fibres.

   The technique used can be epineural, fascicular or perineural, or epiperineural as already described (see Fig. 6.1). Which method is used is relatively unimportant provided good alignment can be achieved. The author prefers an epiperineural repair, which combines the strength of the epineurium with the more accurate fascicular alignment of the perineural repair. The sutures used should be 9-0 or 10-0 and just sufficient to approximate the nerve ends. The nerve ends should be freshened with a sharp blade, the fascicular pattern should be seen clearly and the repaired nerve or graft at the end of the procedure should show no 'bunching' or buckling. There should be no overlapping of the nerve bundles (Fig. 6.2).

Tension   Too much tension at the site of nerve repair will result in fibrosis and a poor result. The nerve ends can be mobilized to a point, but excessive mobilization will inevitably interfere with nerve vascularity. The acceptable degree of tension is a matter of experience, but if considerable trimming back of the nerve ends is required to reach viable nerve, particularly when doing a secondary repair, then a nerve graft is usually a wiser option. (A gap of greater than 2.0–2.5 cm will generally need a nerve graft.)

Handling   The nerve ends should be handled with care, in particular avoiding crushing with the forceps. The epineurium should be grasped using fine jewellers' forceps. The more crushing there is, the greater the fibrosis at the site of anastomosis.

Immobilization   Splintage should be applied to prevent any sudden excessive movement in the area surrounding the nerve. This will result in

Figure 6.2
Diagram of nerve repair technique.

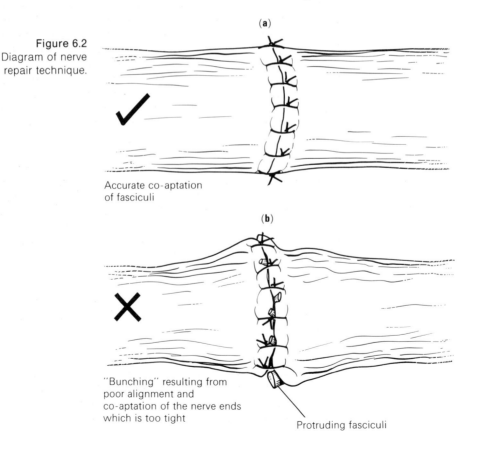

(a)

Accurate co-aptation of fasciculi

(b)

"Bunching" resulting from poor alignment and co-aptation of the nerve ends which is too tight

Protruding fasciculi

possible separation of the nerve ends at the repair site and subsequent scar formation at the interface.

Haematoma   Haemorrhage from the nerve ends should be controlled using microbipolar forceps or fine ligature. If it is not, haematoma will occur at the interface, causing scarring and an inferior result. Haemorrhage from the surrounding structures may also interfere with the repair and will certainly heighten the risk of infection. The use of magnification greatly facilitates the surgeon in identifying these small intraneural vessels.

Donor site   Where a nerve graft is required, there will be some donor site morbidity. The commonest nerve used in nerve grafting is the sural nerve. Its sacrifice will result in an area of anaesthesia over the dorsolateral aspect of the foot. A scar on the back of the leg will also result and the patient must be made aware of these. There is no functional impairment and in practice the sensory deficit is rarely noticed by the patient.

Management of a failed nerve repair
The signs and symptoms of a failed nerve repair or reconstruction have been outlined and the severity of these coupled with the patient's requirements must be carefully considered before embarking on further procedures. Secondary nerve surgery can be difficult, with significant improvement often difficult to achieve, e.g. minimal recovery of sensation on the ulnar side of the middle finger following attempted repair of a digital nerve eighteen months previously with no significant discomfort at the injury site would seldom justify re-exploration. However, the requirements for each individual patient must be carefully assessed.

Conservative   With time, the pain associated with cutaneous neuromata will
management   often decrease. Various densitization treatments are available, including transcutaneous nerve stimulation, biofeedback or simple frequent massaging of the tender area, and all can be helpful in reducing the discomfort. Return of motor function (often incomplete) usually takes longer than sensory return and time should be allowed for this.

Operative   *Neurolysis*
management   This involves exploration of the repair site and freeing the fasciculi from the surrounding scar tissue. Its clinical place is very limited and its role is not clearly defined.

Secondary repair/nerve grafting
It is rarely possible to carry out a secondary nerve repair following neuroma excision. Occasionally, however, the nerve ends can be mobilized sufficiently to facilitate this and provided the repair is free of tension, then this is a suitable method of

management. More commonly, however, after resecting the neuroma and the nerve on either side has been trimmed back to 'healthy' fascicular tissue, the resulting gap requires grafting to achieve a tension-free repair.

Relocation—painful stump neuroma
This is a relatively common problem seen in amputation stumps, particularly where the causative injury has been crushing in nature. Simple excision will result in recurrence of the neuroma and recurrence of symptoms. Many ingenious methods of dealing with the freshly excised nerve end have been devised and claim some measure of success: relocating in an adjacent bone (through a drill hole); excising back the fasciculi within an epineural collar and enclosing the fasciculi within this epineural cap with a suture; burying the nerve within a small block of embedded silicon, or capping it with an isolated piece of vein; etc.

Tendon transfer
When an important motor component fails to regenerate, then the options available are either to explore the nerve repair (as above) or to carry out a tendon transfer. Before performing a transfer, however, a careful assessment of the patient's disability and requirements must be made; for example, a common consequence of median nerve division and repair at the wrist is loss of thumb opposition (owing to lack of reinnervation of opponens pollicis). However, the reason the patient does not use his thumb may be loss of sensation over the thumb and/or index finger or hypersensitivity of this area also, supplied by the median nerve, rather than as a result of motor weakness. In this instance, carrying out an opponensplasty using, for example, the sublimis from the ring finger, could prove to be counterproductive.

Specific Complications Associated with Small-vessel Anastomosis

Early   The major complication of microvascular surgery is thrombosis of either the arterial input or venous outlet, or both, in the replanted part or transferred free flap (Fig. 6.3). Salvage of the part or flap is dependent on early diagnosis of the problem and rapid re-exploration of the anastomosis once other factors have been eliminated, e.g. dressings too tight, underlying respiratory disease leading to central cyanosis, etc. Several different methods for monitoring flap circulation have been developed, including temperature and colour monitoring, Doppler flow meters and electromagnetic flow meters. It has proved correct on many occasions that 'Most vascular complications are postoperative confirmations of intra-operative suspicions—they should be

Figure 6.3
Failed replant.

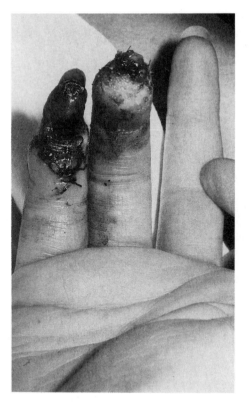

recognized and corrected at the initial operation, not 6–12 hours later.' Hence derives the need for constant monitoring of the patency of the vessel, intra-operatively as well as postoperatively, in order to avoid failure of the procedure.

Late Particularly following replantation, functional recovery of digits and limbs may be incomplete. Owing to scarring and adhesions, tendons may become adherent, or poor nerve regeneration may result in muscle weakness or imbalance (Fig. 6.4). Pain may be a problem; this is particularly seen in proximal upper-limb replantations in adults, occasionally necessitating re-amputation. Treatment with tenolysis, tendon transfers, etc. may be carried out. Poor sensory recovery may result in secondary injury (Fig. 6.5).

Predisposing factors

Poor selection Extensive damage, particularly resulting from a crush injury will considerably reduce the chances of a successful replantation (Fig. 6.6). Particularly when carrying out a delayed reconstruction, scarring around damaged vessels must be

Figure 6.4
Swan-neck deformity
in replanted index
finger.

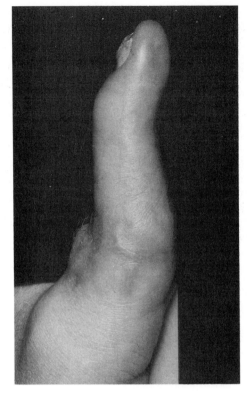

Figure 6.5
Successful
revascularization;
patient developed
frostbite (as a result of
reduced sensory
recovery) with
resulting necrosis and
subsequent
reamputation.

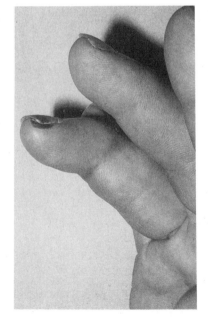 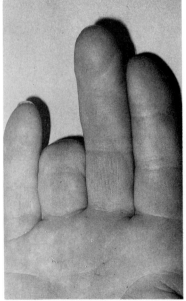

Figure 6.6
Multiple level injury
(unsuitable for
replantation).

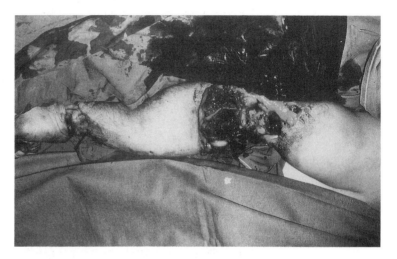

carefully assessed before selecting the best site for anastomosis. The flow characteristics of an end-to-side anastomosis are more favourable in this situation and should be used in preference to an end-to-end anastomosis.

Poor technique   Poor handling of the tissues will damage these small vessels. Intimal tears, holes in vessel walls, poor alignment of sutures and knots will all greatly increase the risk of anastomotic failure.

Poor postoperative care   Inadequate postoperative monitoring of flap or digit circulation may result in early detection of anastomotic problems being missed. Dressings may be too tight. Injudicious administration of opiates may cause sudden drops in blood pressure and failure to maintain a warm environment may cause the patient's temperature to fall, with resulting reduced peripheral circulation and subsequent thrombosis.

Prevention of failure in microvascular anastomosis
There are three factors concerned in the causation of thrombosis. Derangements of these constitute Virchow's triad of factors that determine the occurrence of thrombosis (Fig. 6.7).

The vessel wall   *Damaged intima*
Clean cut injuries, i.e. a sharp laceration from glass or a knife or carefully conducted division of a vessel during flap dissection will cause minimal damage to the vessel wall. Crush and avulsion injuries, on the other hand, result in considerable damage, sometimes with intimal separation and this damage can extend well beyond the immediate site of division. The attempt to anastomose this type of damaged vessel wall in vessels of 1 mm diameter and smaller is doomed to failure. The damaged vessel

Figure 6.7
Virchow's triad
diagram to show
clotting factors.

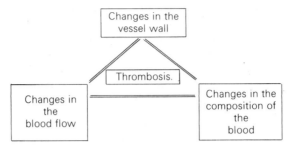

must be trimmed back until healthy tissue is seen and a good flow from the proximal artery is demonstrated on release of the clamp. The amount of vessel to be resected must not be compromised—it is frequently necessary to use a vein graft in this situation. The vessel wall can also be damaged by rough handling during the repair. When preparing the vessels for anastomosis, only the adventitia should be grasped, using fine jeweller's forceps.

Poor apposition
The aim of suturing together the vessel ends should be to achieve as perfect an apposition as possible of all layers of the vessel wall, in particular the intima. Damage to this, or large defects in it, will inevitably lead to thrombosis and failure of the anastomosis. For an end-to-end anastomosis, generally speaking, two stay sutures are placed with 120° between them (approximately one-third of the vessel circumference). The vessel wall can then be sutured between these sutures till a satisfactory closure is obtained. It is particularly important to check constantly that the posterior wall has not inadvertently been picked up with the needle. This is particularly a risk with small, thin-walled veins. The vessel is then turned over and its posterior wall is closed in a similar manner.

Removal of adventitia
It is important to remove any adventitial debris from the vessel ends. Where this becomes trapped in the lumen, the collagen fibres, tissue thromboplastin and Hageman's factor in the adventitia produce very rapid and profuse platelet aggregation and fibrin deposition. A careful balance must be obtained here, as 'excessive cleaning' of the vessels traumatizes the vessel wall.

The flow of blood
According to Poiseuille's law, flow in a hollow tube is proportional to the fourth power of the tube's radius, under standard conditions. Reduction in the flow can be caused by central (systemic) factors and local factors.

Systemic factors

Blood volume. A shocked patient compensates the central

circulation by increasing the peripheral resistance in an attempt to increase cardiac output. This results in a significant reduction in peripheral blood flow that may be critical at the site of anastomosis. It is important, therefore, that the patient is well perfused, particularly following completion of the anastomosis. Blood pressure should not be allowed to fall at this stage and in the postoperative period, small frequent dosages of analgesia, as required, must be given to avoid sudden unexpected drops in pressure such as would result from large doses of potent opiates.

Temperature. As the body cools, the cutaneous circulation is reduced in an attempt to conserve heat. This will lower the rate of flow through the anastomosis and jeopardize the result. The patient's temperature must be carefully monitored throughout the procedure and maintained around 37°C.

Nicotine. It has been shown that even smoking a single cigarette can decrease the digital blood flow by 42% with no significant change in the heart rate. Replanted digits have been lost after several days when the patient started smoking, following which the digit went blue and the anastomosis thrombosed.

Local factors

Poor anastomosis. A poorly performed anastomosis can result in constriction at the site of repair resulting in reduced flow.

Spasm. This may be caused by cold, a reduction in blood pressure, etc., or from local factors such as rough handling of the tissues. It can often be relieved by the application of a solution of plain lignocaine applied topically. Other agents have been investigated, including prostacyclin and naftidrofuryl oxalate (Praxilene)—which may have a more prolonged effect—and verapamil hydrochloride.

Turbulence. Any bends or kinks around the anastomosis will tend to cause eddy currents and other types of turbulent flow that can predispose to thrombus formation. Proper alignment of the vessels at surgery is very important and avoidance of kinking where the vessels are too long, particularly a problem in free-flap surgery, should be avoided. The flow characteristics tend to be more favourable when an end-to-side anastomosis is carried out. This is particularly important in unfavourable situations following trauma in the lower limb, where the rate of flow is somewhat less in any event, e.g. free-flap surgery to the lower third of the leg.

Dressings. Following either replantation or free-flap surgery, dressings should be applied in such a way as to give stability but not compression to the affected area. This means, in practice, a bulky dressing applied fairly loosely. There will inevitably be some swelling and oozing into the dressings, which can become progressively tighter leading to congestion of the affected tissue.

Coagulation factors in the blood

Following any trauma there is a thrombocytosis together with an increase in platelet adhesiveness. The clotting time is also shortened after haemorrhage and it is also found in relation to certain drugs, in particular, glucocorticosteroids and oestrogen. These are, therefore, important factors to consider in these patients. Around the anastomosis and damaged tissues, thrombogenic factors are released from the devascularized flap or severed part. The use of antithrombotic agents may prove beneficial though there is wide variation in different units as to which agents and which regimes are used. Inhibitors of platelet aggregation such as aspirin and dipyridamole are commonly used clinically, particularly in replant surgery. Low-molecular-weight dextran has been shown to increase flow and is useful. Throughout the operation, while carrying out the anastomosis, the tissue should be irrigated with heparinized saline solution. Administration of heparin to the patient should be reserved very much as a last resort because there are obviously considerable problems associated with anticoagulation, particularly following trauma. Other agents are under investigation.

Management of complications following microvascular anastomosis

The importance of early detection of problems at the site of anastomosis has already been stressed.

Arterial complications

This can be detected with a flowmeter or reduction in temperature of the flap or replanted tissue, which clinically will develop a pale avascular appearance.

Spasm

Excessive manipulation of the vessel or leaving it exposed in a cold environment can cause this.

Prevention. The operating theatre should be as warm as is comfortable. Endeavour to keep the vessel covered as much as possible and avoid desiccation in the wound. Irrigating solutions should all be warmed, as should intravenous fluids administered during the operation. The patient should not be allowed to cool down—a 'space blanket' is helpful.

Treatment. Topical application of an antispasmodic agent such as lignocaine is useful and should be applied if the vessel is in spasm. It should be applied at the completion of an anastomosis as there is usually a degree of spasm resulting from the unavoidable manipulation of the vessel during preparation and insertion of the sutures.

Kinking
This is liable to occur particularly where there is a long pedicle. Torsion may also occur if the alignment of the vessels, prior to application of the approximating clamps, has not been checked.

Prevention. Proper alignment of the vessels before anastomosis and careful choice of the exact site to carry out the anastomosis are important. The pedicle may need to be anchored with a fine suture through the adventitia in a position to hold the pedicle and prevent kinking. Careful positioning of drains (particularly suction drains) at the conclusion of the operation is also important.

Treatment. Sudden alteration in the vascularity of the flap or replant when closing the skin would suggest that kinking may have occurred. Early exploration is mandatory and positioning of the pedicle more securely is indicated.

Poor flow
This may be due to spasm and/or kinking, or it may be due to the patient being hypovolaemic.

Prevention. Following release of the clamps after vessel anastomosis, the patient should be maintained with an adequate fluid load to prevent hypovolaemia. Hourly urine output should be recorded and IV fluids increased if this fails.

Treatment. Poor flow, after the factors already mentioned have been checked and corrected where necessary, can be improved by administering dextran over several hours. The author's preference is dextran 40 in saline over 4 hours, repeated every 24 hours. (More rapid infusion can be given if the clinical condition necessitates.)

Venous complications A reduction in venous flow coupled with a flap that progressively becomes more engorged and purple in colour are signs of a poor venous flow.

Constricting dressings
A dressing that is too tight can cause venous engorgement. Although seemingly satisfactory at the conclusion of the operation, oozing into the dressing can progressively cause the dressing to become tight around the operation site.

Prevention. Dressings, if used, should always be applied loosely and frequently inspected postoperatively. Oozing of blood into dressings will cause the dressings to become tighter. They should never be tightly applied *around* the operation site but simply *laid on* it to absorb any drainage and changed as required.

Treatment. Removal of dressings and simple elevation of the flap/replant and covering with a green towel or light dressing should be carried out.

Inadequate vein
The vein chosen for anastomosis may be of insufficient size to adequately drain the vascularized tissue.

Prevention. Inspection of the replant/flap after completion of arterial and venous anastomoses (and after releasing the clamps) will give a good idea as to the adequacy of the venous drainage. If inadequate, the tissues will become progressively more engorged.

Treatment. A further venous anastomosis must be undertaken. Selection of the vein is all-important; one that is 'full' and whose end flows freely on trimming, resulting in decongestion of the replant/flap, is the ideal vein to use if possible. Particularly in a distal replant, e.g. distal amputation of a finger, it can sometimes be difficult to find another suitable vein. Alternatives are to anastomose the other digital artery to a (proximal) vein or simply to allow oozing into the dressings until venous connections have developed. Leeches have also been used successfully in this situation.

Surgery of Facial Palsy

Some of the best results from surgery for this condition have come from the use of cross-facial nerve grafts, with or without a free vascularized muscle graft, and hence its consideration in this chapter under microsurgery. Many different techniques have been used to reconstruct an established facial paralysis and it is one of the most demanding and challenging tasks facing the reconstructive surgeon.

The facial nerve supplies sixteen muscles of facial expression on each side of the face and these have three main functions.

Facial muscle tone This provides balance or symmetry to the face and support around the eye, nose and mouth. Loss of this tone results in watering of the eye, drooling from the corner of the mouth, and collection of food in the buccal sulcus in the mouth.

Voluntary facial movements All the voluntary movements of the face, e.g. smiling, blinking, whistling, etc., are controlled by these muscles and their motor nerve.

The face is, of course, an important communicator of inner emotions. The spontaneous smile is probably the most important example of this, and certainly the one most missed by patients with a facial palsy.

There are many different causes of facial palsy, the commonest cause being idiopathic or Bell's palsy. The mechanism of this is not fully understood but many cases go on to full recovery with no surgery being required. Others show only partial recovery and minimal procedures are often all that is required. Other cases include trauma, tumour (and tumour surgery), inflammation and vascular causes. The choice of reconstructive procedure that is used depends on several factors, but there are important questions that must be asked:

1 Is the paralysis complete or incomplete?
2 Can the facial nerve be reconstructed or not?
3 Is the paralysis recent or longstanding?
4 Is spontaneous recovery likely? (If so, perform a tarsorrhaphy and wait.)

In this discussion, the problems associated with the paralysis of long-standing duration (greater than 6 months) will be considered. In the 'acute' stage the best results will obviously be obtained from direct suture of the nerve or from nerve grafting where this is feasible. In incomplete paralysis, which is often the final outcome of an idiopathic palsy, it is important to define exactly what the major complaint of the patient is, e.g. discomfort around the eye, drooping of the eyebrow or laxity and drooping around the corner of the mouth, etc. Many patients will require a tarsorrhaphy, at least in the short term.

The types of surgical procedures that can be used in reconstruction in these long-term patients with facial paralysis include the following.

1 *Reconstruction of facial tone.* Operations here include various forms of static slings to the eye and mouth, resection of skin to increase the tone, e.g. brow lifts, elliptical excision of skin in the nasolabial region etc.
2 *Reconstruction of voluntary facial movements.* This includes muscle transfers, e.g. using masseter and temporalis muscles and also nerve transfers, e.g. hypoglossal to facial nerve anastomosis.
3 *Reconstruction of reflex facial expression.* Procedures here include two processes, i.e. neurotization and muscle transplantation. Where the facial nerve on the paralysed side is not available for reconstruction, a cross-facial nerve graft is brought across from the normal side. Viable functioning muscle is brought into the paralysed side by free microvascular transfer and this is animated by the viable facial nerve or nerve graft, e.g. using gracilis, pectoralis minor, etc.

General complications None of these procedures is entirely satisfactory in correcting the deformity. Apart from the usual complications of any procedure (haematoma, infection, etc.) the specific complications of each of these procedures will be described.

Complications of procedures for reconstruction of facial tone

Skin excision procedures These are particularly useful if the resulting weakness is minimal. The main complications are as follows.

1 *Inadequate excision.* A generous ellipse of skin should be excised, marking and then incising first along one side of the proposed ellipse, undermining of the tissue to be excised and then making a judgement on how much to remove.
2 *Scarring of the face.* Good suture technique is obviously important to minimize the scarring. This procedure works well in the nasolabial area to correct drooping of the corner of the mouth, above the eyebrow (to elevate this), and as a face-lift procedure where the incision is in the preauricular area with extensive undermining of the cheek. Suction drains should be used to minimize the risk of haematoma formation.
3 *Recurrence of laxity.* A modification of this is to de-epithelialize the flap of skin and then bury it under the other side of the incision in an attempt to give better support and prevent recurrence of the laxity. Plication of the underlying paralysed muscles can also be carried out to augment the effect of the excision.

Static slings Various materials have been used to act as a sling to elevate the drooping tissues of the paralysed cheek, particularly around the corner of the mouth and outer canthal area around the eye. These may be inserted externally or through small intra-oral incisions. The most widely used material for this is autogenous fascia lata (other materials include freeze-dried homologous fascia, autogenous tendons, Dacron, etc.).

The fascia is inserted as a loop around the upper and lower lip and involved commissure. At the same or later stage, a further strip of fascia is sutured to this and tunnelled up to a zygomatic arch, temporalis fascia or orbital rim. This procedure may be combined with a skin resection or muscle plication, etc.

Complications
1 *Infection.* Infection is one of the main problems of this procedure. It is probably better not to introduce these materials intraorally. Infection that does develop can extend the entire length of the sling and result in discharging sinuses along the cheek, frequently necessitating removal of the sling.
2 *Loosening of sling.* Loosening of the sling may be due to incorrect adjustment of the tension in the sling or loosening of

the sutures. It is generally better to introduce the loop around
the side of the mouth as a first stage and then it is easier to get
the correct tension in the sling as a second-stage procedure.

3 *Excessive tightness.* Where the sling is made too tight, difficulties may arise, e.g. at the corner of the mouth; patients may be
unable to get their dentures in. They also have a tendency to
bite their lips repeatedly. Treatment is to divide the sling
partially, a procedure that can be carried out under local
anaesthetic.

Springs and weights   Various devices can be introduced, particularly around the
eyelids, to give mechanical support to the eyelids and eyebrows.
These may be in the form of a spring or magnet. The insertion of
a small weight (e.g. of gold) into the upper lid is often helpful in
milder cases of lagophthalmos.

Complications
1 *Infection.* Infection usually requires the removal of the
material.
2 *Invariable strength.* The strength of action of the spring, etc.,
is a predetermined quantity and can only be altered by
removing the material and replacing it with another.
3 *Cosmesis.* The implant may be visible and unacceptable.
4 The spring may fail to function properly by loss of position i.e.
it may slip out of position or even ulcerate through the skin.
Treatment is to remove it and replace it in a more favourable
position when the tissues have healed.

Complications of procedures for reconstruction of voluntary facial movements

This can be carried out by either muscle transfer (usually
temporalis or masseter) or nerve transfer, e.g. hypoglossal.
Where temporalis is used, a tendon or facial extension is usually
required for attachment to the corner of the mouth, eye, etc.
Where the masseter is used, the anterior half of the muscle can
be transferred to the corner of the mouth.

Complications   Although these are dynamic procedures, unlike the static slings
previously described, patients have to learn to smile by the
voluntary acts of clenching the teeth or moving the jaws.
Further, when eating, there will be associated unwanted facial
movements. This also occurs where the hypoglossal-to-facial
nerve transfer procedure is used, with unwanted associated
movements when eating or speaking.

Complications of procedures for reconstruction of reflex facial expression

Harii in 1976 reported a case in which he transferred a gracilis
muscle on its neurovascular pedicle, anastomosing this to facial
vessels, and innervating it with the nerve to temporalis. He was

able to demonstrate contraction of this muscle. More recently, a cross-facial nerve graft (from the normal side) has been performed as a first stage. This has the great advantage of controlling the functioning of this muscle, not only by voluntary means (through the 7th nerve) but also as a reflex action the spontaneous facial expression that is so important.

Where the palsy has been of a shorter duration (and this duration is still not fully defined) it may be possible to carry out a cross-facial nerve graft and neurotize the fascicles of this into the facial muscles themselves or into the distal end of the damaged or divided facial nerve on the paralysed side. Results from this procedure, however, have generally been disappointing.

Complications

1 *Involuntary movements.* Where a nerve graft is used alone, unwanted spasmodic type movements of the muscles are often seen. Occasionally this takes the form of mass movements on the side of the face. The best results, however, are achieved with cases where this cross-facial nerve grafting is carried out in a palsy of less than 6 months' duration.

2 *Anastomotic complications.* All the complications associated with carrying out a microvascular anastomosis must be considered when a free muscle transfer is carried out on its pedicle. However, many of these patients are relatively young and healthy, and have no irradiation or previous trauma to the operation field that increase the risk of thrombosis.

3 *Muscle contracture.* One of the problems here has been to achieve the desired strength of muscle contracture (where a muscle transfer has been carried out), e.g. taking the whole of the gracilis results in a contracture which is too powerful. On the other hand, using extensor digitorum brevis, with microvascular anastomosis and cross-facial nerve grafting, has not produced a strong enough contracture in most cases. Other free muscles have been used, including pectoralis minor and serratus anterior, and Manktelow and Zuker have modified the gracilis transfer by transferring only a single fascicle muscle unit on its vascular pedicle.

Other procedures that may be used include selective myomectomies on the normal side in an attempt to make the facial expression more symmetrical. This is often satisfactory initially but denervated muscles show a remarkable ability to reinnervate in this situation and in the longer term.

Persisting controversies

- Timing of nerve repair (primary or secondary).
- Role of vascularized nerve grafts.
- Type of nerve repair.
- The role of neurolysis.

Further reading

O'Brien, B. McC. (1987) *Microvascular Reconstructive Surgery.* Edinburgh: Churchill Livingstone.

Terzis, J.K. (1984) Peripheral Nerve Microsurgery, *Clinics in Plastic Surgery 11: 1* Philadelphia, London: Saunders.

Webster, M.H.C. & Soutar, D.S. (1986) *Practical Guide to Free Tissue Transfer.* Boston, Durban, London: Butterworths.

7 Complications of Hand Repair

General Considerations

Over the last 30 years, hand surgery as a specialty interest has grown enormously and a much greater understanding and knowledge of the fine anatomy and the way the organ behaves when subjected to trauma, surgery, etc., has resulted in greatly improved methods of management, with earlier mobilization and reduced periods of time off work. The place of the hand therapist, supervising the early mobilization, splintage, etc., means that the clinically swollen, stiff hand is fortunately much less commonly seen now. It is very important to realize that what may appear as a trivial injury, such as a crush injury to a finger tip resulting in soft tissue loss, may result in many months off work with long-standing pain and discomfort. A minor cut of the skin may have divided a digital nerve leading to formation of a painful neuroma and resulting in a sensitive and uncomfortable digit with many ensuing months off work. Although rarely life-threatening, incorrect management may lead to prolonged morbidity. Large numbers of hand injuries are seen in casualty units and plastic and orthopaedic departments each year; for those dealing with these injuries, a sound working knowledge of the basic anatomy of the hand is essential. In considering complications of trauma and elective surgery of the hand, some general complications will first be considered, together with their treatment, and then a more specific outline of complications associated with each of the structures within the hand.

Prevention of Complications

General complications

Infection Infection in a wound in the hand will often lead to chronic stiffness and loss of function. Fortunately, severe infections of the hand involving the tendon sheaths extending up to the wrist are rarely seen nowadays, owing to better initial management and use of antibiotics. Infection may develop from even a very minor injury, such as a puncture wound caused by a thorn. Wounds caused by human or animal bites or lacerations caused in a heavily contaminated environment (e.g. the soil) are particularly prone to infection. Crush injuries with devitalization of tissues, are again prone to infection. As in all trauma situations involving soft tissues, correct management involves meticulous debridement and antibiotic cover where necessary. The aim in all hand injuries is to achieve primary skin healing as early as possible so that the period of immobilization is limited. Skin closure by direct suture, grafting or skin flap, either local or distant, may be required. Inadequate debridement, particularly where the wound is to be covered by a flap, may result in very severe infection with a prolonged period of dressings to the hand; fibrosis and stiffness being the long-term results. The wound should be carefully observed postoperatively with early mobilization as the goal.

Haematoma A haematoma in the hand may be a forerunner to infection. More commonly, it presents with pain in the hand. This is an early sign, since the compartments within the hand are small and even a small amount of stretching of the tissues by bleeding will result in distension of the tissues and pain. Virtually all elective surgery of the hand and most of the post-traumatic emergency surgery should be carried out under tourniquet. At the end of the operation, the tourniquet should be released before the skin is sutured and careful haemostasis with bipolar cautery should be obtained. Postoperatively, the hand should be elevated and increasing pain, particularly when this is localized, should be managed, not by stronger and more potent analgesics, but by taking down the dressings and checking for haematoma formation. Unrecognized haematoma will lead to fibrosis and scar tissue and will lead once again to stiffness and loss of function. In some procedures, such as an extensive synovectomy in rheumatoid disease, a suction drain should be left in the wound for 24–48 hours.

Stiffness The hand is, by design, an organ specifically adapted for movement, which requires not only the ability to feel and discern the shape and texture of different objects through the sensory nervous system but also the ability to carry out fine movements through the intricate mechanism of its joints and tendon systems. These are all finely balanced and controlled; stiffness can result from injury to the tendons or joints, and this in turn may result from poor splintage that causes the collateral ligaments of the joints to tighten up. Oedema may lead to fibrosis, as already discussed, and, particularly where this occurs in the flexor tendon canals ('no man's land') marked reduction in tendon excursion may result in stiffness of the digit.

Pain Pain following elective hand surgery should be minimal; when it is severe in the early postoperative period, it suggests haemorrhage within the wound. Following trauma, apart from the immediate pain, it may be non-specific, especially seen following crush injuries, or specific, for example related to neuroma formation around the injured nerve. Pain in the form of 'cold sensitivity' is extremely common in fingers following even very minor injuries. It can be extremely troublesome, often persisting for several years (over 50% extending beyond one year in a recent study) and difficult to treat.

Loss of function This may be due to a tendon which has been divided and, for example, has either been missed at the initial examination or, following repair, has become adherent (or ruptured). Loss of function may, however, result from other factors: the patient may not use a digit that has a sensitive tip following finger tip surgery. It is particularly important to decide the exact cause of this loss of function; for example, following a median nerve injury and repair, before considering a tendon transfer to reconstruct pinch to the thumb, it is important to decide whether or not the loss of function is in fact due to motor weakness (when the transfer will be appropriate) or to insensitivity or abnormal sensation in the thumb, index and middle finger tips (when a transfer would almost certainly be contra-indicated). Also, what may be a directly measurable loss of function, such as diminished range of tendon excursion, may in fact cause the patient little or no disability when it comes to everyday activities. This is particularly important when planning secondary surgery for the severely damaged hand, when the surgery should be directed towards the particular occupational needs of the patient.

Cosmesis Patients are often far more conscious of the appearance of their hands than we sometimes realize. Patients with damaged hands will often deliberately hide them from view and shaking hands often causes considerable embarrassment. As techniques for reconstruction of hand defects improve for both congenital and post-traumatic situations, so the appearance of the hand, as well as functional improvement, should always be considered when planning a reconstructive procedure.

Trauma in the hand will be considered first. Complications may arise in each of the structures making up the hand and these will be considered separately.

Skin

The skin may be simply lacerated or there may be skin loss. In degloving injuries, e.g. a ring avulsion injury, no loss may be apparent, but careful assessment may reveal devascularized tissue. A bursting wound often gapes widely, but there may be no actual skin loss.

The patient may present initially with skin loss due to the trauma, or the loss may result from debridement of necrotic tissue at operation. It is important always to bear in mind that one of the objectives in the management of hand injuries is to achieve skin healing/closure as soon as possible. Leaving wounds open to granulate is, therefore, rarely if ever the treatment of choice in these situations.

Management   *Suture*
Direct suture of the wound may be possible. However, the skin of the hand tends to be firmly bound down to the subcutaneous tissues on the palmar aspect and direct closure of even small defects may be difficult and too much tension may result in dehiscence. On the dorsum of the hand, the skin is somewhat more mobile, allowing easier closure of small defects by direct suture.

Grafts
Larger defects may require skin grafts. These will take well provided the base of the wound is a graftable surface; for example tendon stripped of its paratenon will not support a graft. Thin grafts on the flexor surface of the fingers over joint creases should be avoided where possible, as contracture is likely to occur. Split skin grafts are frequently used to repair defects in finger-tip injuries.

Flaps
Large defects, or defects where a graft is unlikely to take, are treated with skin flaps. These may be local flaps, e.g. cross-finger flaps, small VY advancement flaps or distant flaps for larger defects, of which the best known and most widely used is the groin flap (though more recently, radial forearm flaps and free flaps have been used). Cross-finger flaps are particularly useful for covering defects over flexor tendons in the digits. Using the 'reverse dermis' flap principle, when the epidermis of the flap is shaved off, the flap may be placed over the defect with the dermis side next to the defect, and the under surface and donor areas are grafted. This is particularly useful for coverage of defects on the extensor surface of the fingers and has the added advantage that it picks up a blood supply more quickly than a standard cross-finger flap (where the subcutaneous fat is next to defect base) so that division of the pedicle at 7–10 days rather than 2–3 weeks can safely be carried out and earlier mobilization can be started. The groin flap gives a good area of skin coverage to the hand. It can be raised rapidly and safely and has a reliable blood supply. The hand rests comfortably in this position and the donor site can be closed directly. Its main disadvantage is that

the hand cannot be elevated when attached in this position but with tubing of the pedicle, the fingers can be mobilized. Other distant flaps have been used, including the tensor fascia lata flap, delto-pectoral flaps and various random pattern abdominal wall flaps.

Complications and their management

Skin contracture   Any longitudinal scar crossing a flexion joint crease on the palmar aspect of the hand or web spaces can result in a contracture of the skin (Fig. 7.1). When planning incisions for elective surgery, such as in Dupytrens disease or for tendon surgery, these scars can be avoided by the initial correct planning of the incision (e.g. by Bruner's incision or using the midlateral line of the digit) or insertion of Z-plasties in a longitudinal incision (Fig. 7.2). In the trauma patient, lacerations may not oblige in this way. If the wound is clean-cut, then Z-plasty at the time of primary repair can be carried out. In most other situations it is best to close the skin and then treat with splintage, carrying out secondary Z-plasty release of the contracture if seen to develop. Thick grafts should be used where possible on the flexor side of the fingers. The risk of contractures forming is much greater in children than in adults. However, children will often respond very much better to splintage than adults and this should be attempted before embarking on any surgery.

Figure 7.1
(a) Finger with contracted scar. (b) Release of a contracted finger with multiple Y to V-plasty.

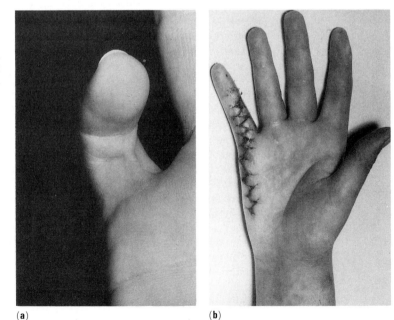

(a)   (b)

Figure 7.2
Incisions for opening
digit to prevent
contracture.

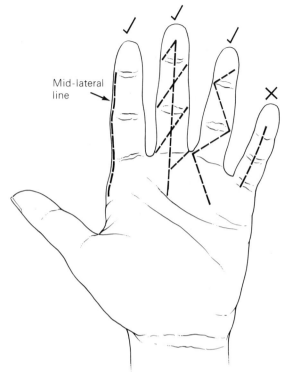

Mid-lateral
line

Instability A thin graft adherent to underlying bone and subject to repeated trauma will almost certainly eventually break down. The area involved may, therefore, need to be resurfaced with more durable tissue, e.g. a local skin flap.

Bulk Tissue loss in a particular area should, where possible, be replaced with similar tissue. This is often not easy to achieve, e.g. in a deep wound on the palm of the hand where flap cover is indicated, the flap may be too bulky. In this situation, the palmar skin is normally stabilized by septal processes from the palmar fascia that prevent excessive mobility of the skin, important in firm grip. This particular complication is difficult to correct, though subsequent thinning of the flap is helpful.

Cosmesis A large flap used for skin cover may be disfiguring, particularly in a female patient. Groin flaps in particular can be bulky and also have a different colour from the normal skin of the hand. Management consists of reducing the size of the flap where possible.

Fingertip Injuries

Fingertip injuries are amongst the commonest injuries seen in casualty departments. Often regarded as trivial injuries, they are often complicated by delayed healing and in the longer term, with discomfort or unstable scars. Deformity of the nail is commonly seen, which is cosmetically embarrassing and may present difficulty in keeping the nail trimmed. An understanding of the anatomy of the fingertip will help to show why these injuries, incorrectly treated, can result in complicated healing. The important points are indicated in Fig. 7.3. The skin of the fingertip (volar aspect) is thicker than normal skin and is abundantly supplied with sensory nerves. There are abundant sweat glands. Beneath the skin is the pulp, which is composed of fibrofatty tissue and gives stability and padding to the skin; it is connected to the terminal phalanx. Through the pulp run various cutaneous nerves and vessels to the tip. This tightly packed design acts as a very efficient sense organ but when there is swelling, even of a very minor nature within the fingertip, then it is often extremely painful. The nail lies on the nail bed which is seen to overlie the terminal phalanx. At the proximal end of the nail bed is the germinal zone from where the nail grows. The nail is supported by the nail bed as it grows distally.

Injuries of the fingertip

Laceration   Simple lacerations, in which there is no tissue loss, are best treated conservatively in children, with dressings only until healed. This may take longer than suturing but will avoid an

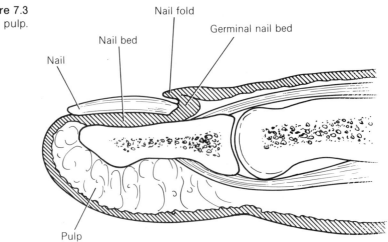

Figure 7.3
Fingertip pulp.

Nail fold

Germinal nail bed

Nail bed

Nail

Pulp

operation (usually a GA), and, more importantly in the longer term, will result in a more comfortable and cosmetically acceptable result. In adults this is not always the case and in most cases suturing under local anaesthetic is the treatment of choice. The exception in children, however, is when the nail bed is disrupted, and this should be re-aligned carefully with sutures.

Soft-tissue loss   Some fingertip injuries may present with loss of soft tissue, either skin or skin and pulp. In children, once again, these are best treated with dressings only, so good is the power of healing. In adults, when there is significant skin loss (of greater than 1 cm^2), a split-skin graft is the treatment of choice if no bone is exposed. If bone is exposed, this should be covered with surrounding soft tissue and the graft then applied or else can be trimmed back so that the soft tissue readily covers it.

Soft-tissue and bone loss   A skin graft may again be possible, but other things must be considered. For example, if the bone or nail bed or both have been shattered, then an amputation may be a better way of management. Local flaps play a useful role here, including lateral and volar VY advancement flaps; if the tissue loss is oblique in direction, a thenar flap may be useful. These have fallen into some disrepute owing to the prolonged period of immobilization of the finger in an unfavourable position (PIP joint flexion), which results in finger stiffness. However, if the reverse dermis principle is used, it need only be in this position for a week and full mobilization can usually be achieved quickly. In these more severe injuries, though, the condition of the nail bed should be considered. Often an uncomfortable nail that grows down into the soft tissues owing to lack of nail bed support will, in the long term, give the greatest discomfort to the patient. If more than half the length of the nail bed is missing then terminalization of the finger may be more appropriate, with resection of the germinal part of the nail.

Complications and their management

Poor healing   A wound that has been sutured under tension, particularly when there has been tissue loss, may necrose at the margins and dehisce when the sutures are removed. If a graft has been used, then the fingertip must be adequately immobilized with a firm, but not tight, dressing and left for 4–5 days until the graft has taken: tie-over bolus dressings are useful here. The graft should be sutured into position. Failure may be due to mobility, infection, or haematoma under the graft; or the skin graft itself may be too thick, making 'take' more difficult. The circulation to the tip may be poor due either to other disease such as peripheral vascular disease or diabetes or to local causes, the most common of which is a dressing that is too tight.

Pain and tenderness These injuries are frequently complicated by prolonged pain and tenderness. The suture line may contract, giving a tight scar on the bony end of the digit. Likewise, a graft may do the same. The wound should be tension-free, as already mentioned, to avoid this. If this is not possible, then further shortening of the bone should be carried out as necessary or some other form of reconstruction should be used. Physiotherapy can sometimes be helpful with various techniques to desensitize the tip.

Cold sensitivity This again is a common complication lasting for several months to several years. The mechanism is poorly understood, though it is thought to be linked to the sympathetic nerve supply in the damaged tip.

Unstable scar A tight scar, particularly where this is adherent to the underlying bone will tend to be unstable and liable to breakdown with even minimal trauma. Secondary flap reconstruction may be indicated if this proves a recurrent problem.

Nail deformity Without adequate support for the nail through its bed, the nail will tend to grow abnormally (Fig. 7.4). Most commonly, there is a deficiency in the distal part of the nail bed so that the nail grows curving over the end of the nail bed into the soft tissues. This can be very uncomfortable for the patient and can cause breakdown of the soft tissues. The nail is often thickened and difficult to trim and if it is not possible to keep short, then it should be removed together with the germinal nail tissue. Various procedures to reconstruct the nail bed are also possible and may be attempted in some cases, but in most cases the germinal nail bed should be ablated.

Figure 7.4
Fingertip injury, sutured. Inadequate nail support.

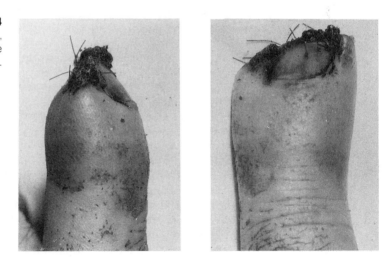

Mobility   When the tip has been reconstructed with a flap, e.g. thenar flap, excessive mobility of the reconstructed pulp area can sometimes be found, giving problems with pinch movements. One possibility here is to bring a small piece of dermis taken from, for example the groin area, as a free graft and place this beneath the flap. This has been shown to be a useful technique and is simple to carry out.

Stiffness   Delayed healing, particularly whcn the injury has been a crush type injury, can result in stiffness of the finger. Treatment should be directed at mobilizing as much as possible, though this is difficult if the tip is painful and tender.

In summary, these fingertip injuries are very common. The management, where a large number of different techniques are available, should be tailored to the particular injury, the digit involved and the patient's requirements. Age is important. Correct planning and careful surgical technique, where this is indicated, will help to reduce the significant morbidity associated with these injuries.

Nerves

Nerve injuries in the hand are particularly seen in wounds caused by sharp instruments such as glass or knives. Often the skin wound may appear minor and a careful examination of the hand as a whole is omitted, but wounds of this sort are often deep. Any injury caused by glass or other sharp objects should be carefully examined for nerve injury and in all cases explored. The most accurate test for loss of nerve function is to feel for loss of sweating in the affected area. This is particularly helpful in difficult or unco-operative patients—screaming children, or drunk adults. Proper examination of the wound should be carried out under local or general anaesthetic if indicated.

Complications and their management
1 Failure of recovery of function.
2 Neuroma formation.

In general, these are linked and are related to the degree of regeneration of the nerve occurring at the site of division. Thus, where a nerve has not been repaired or a poor approximation of the nerve ends has resulted, then the likelihood of neuroma formation is high and recovery of nerve function is reduced. These neuromata may be very sensitive and painful and the more closely related to the overlying skin or scar, then generally the greater are the symptoms. For this reason, even if the nerve lies distally on the ulnar (non-opposing) side of the finger near its distal end, repair of the nerve should be carried out wherever possible to restore continuity and prevent the formation of a tender neuroma (even if sensory restoration is relatively unimportant).

Primary repair should be carried out wherever possible. The tissues are not scarred, the nerve ends are easily dissected out and a better result, particularly in a sharp division, is always obtained. Where there has been destruction of the nerve or viability is uncertain, many would argue that a secondary repair should be done at a later stage when the proximal (viable) end of the nerve can be clearly defined. The dissection, however, is much more difficult and a nerve graft is almost always required; in a sharp injury this may have been avoided if a primary repair had been carried out. If a secondary repair is contemplated, the nerve ends should at least be approximated, making the dissection easier at the later stage. Nerve regeneration in children is very much better than adults and even avulsed nerve injuries, if treated with primary repair, have shown excellent results (Fig. 7.5). The repair should always be carried out under magnification, using either loupes or a microscope. The individual fasciculi can be visualized clearly and matching groups of fasciculi can be approximated accurately with fine sutures. This is particularly important in a mixed nerve such as the ulnar nerve at the wrist (biochemical methods of differentiating sensory and motor fasciculi are at present under investigation).

When neuromata do occur, the repair should be explored if, after a reasonable interval, regeneration of the nerve has not progressed. The fasciculi need to be carefully dissected out to preserve those fibres that are in continuity and nerve grafts used to bridge the gaps in any that are divided or connected by scar tissue. The management of the painful neuromata in an amputation stump is more difficult. These will often improve with time, but when pain and discomfort persist for many months or years, an attempt to transfer the neuroma to sites where it will not be in contact with the overlying skin, e.g. in deeper soft tissues, bone, etc., can be carried out.

Vessels

Arterial input may be interrupted either by division of the vessels or because of spasm in the vessel wall. The latter is seen particularly in crush and avulsion injuries. In the hand, a finger may survive quite normally on a single digital artery and draining vein. In most hands, the radial or ulnar artery alone is adequate to maintain good blood supply to the hand, provided the palmar arch is intact.

Complications and their management

Arterial spasm   Arterial spasm is seen in crush injuries; there may be no skin

Figure 7.5
Avulsed radial nerve in severed arm in child. Result after neurotization and replantation.

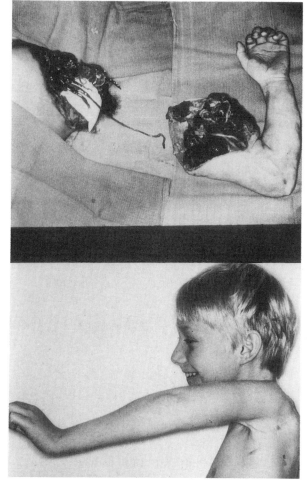

laceration but the digit may appear dusky (if the injury has been to a finger or thumb) or pallor may be the main feature. These patients should be admitted; intravenous dextran will sometimes help. Alternatively, the finger may be opened and lignocaine or other antispasmodic agents applied topically to the vessels involved.

Degloving injuries in the arm may also present with signs of vascular insufficiency in the skin. The history of the injuring force is important, and these wounds should generally be explored following injury because necrosis and infection may occur. Excision of necrotic tissue and grafting may be necessary (Fig. 7.6).

Arterial division As mentioned, a digit can readily survive on one artery provided it is uninjured. Where the digit's circulation is obviously

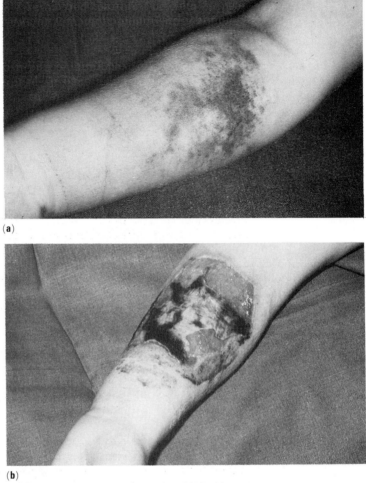

(**a**)

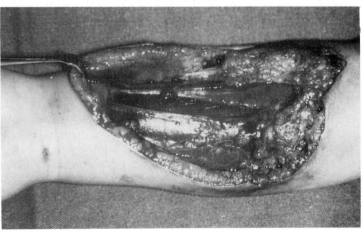

(**b**)

(**c**)

inadequate and administration of agents such as dextran, mannitol, etc., have failed to make any difference, then microvascular repair is indicated, provided other factors such as other injuries to structures in the digit have been considered: for example, it may not be worth trying to preserve a digit with multiple joint and tendon injuries. Displacement of tissues may also interfere with perfusion and replacing a displaced, but not severed, fingertip often restores the circulation to a fingertip that would otherwise appear non-viable.

Tendons

As in nerve injuries, tendon injuries are common in wounds caused by sharp objects such as glass and knives. Where the wound is clean cut and the tendon is repaired within hours of injury, then a good functional result can be obtained. A thorough understanding of the anatomy and functioning of the tendons within the wrist and hand is essential for the surgeon involved in the repair of these injuries. Much recent work has been done helping to elucidate the nutrition of digital tendons and the factors which can influence adhesion formation.

Prevention of complications

Skin cover It is useless to spend considerable time on careful tendon repair where adequate viable skin cover cannot be assured. A skin flap (e.g. cross-finger flap) may be required to cover the damaged and repaired tendon (Fig. 7.7).

Debridement An inadequately debrided wound will increase the risk of infection and scar adhesion. In a grossly contaminated wound, particularly when there is extensive skin damage/loss, then secondary tendon reconstruction is often the method of choice.

Suture technique This is very important, not only in holding the divided tendon ends in apposition, but also the way in which the tendon ends are handled. This has a bearing on the amount of scarring and adhesion formation around the repair. Several points are important here, particularly in zone II flexor tendon injuries.

Retrieval of tendon ends
Forcibly grabbing the tendon ends with heavy forceps will cause crushing. Suturing this will result in crushed tissue at the junction site with the result of inferior healing. If the tendon end has been crushed, then before suturing this end should be cleanly trimmed using a sharp razor blade. Where the proximal tendon has retracted some distance, the use of a silastic rod passed proximally from the site of injury to where the proximal tendon end has been recovered, to which this tendon end is

Figure 7.7
Cross finger flap used
for tendon graft cover
after contracture
developed in scar. (a)
Contracted finger. (b)
Cross finger flap
raised and applied to
defect. (c) Pedicle
divided.

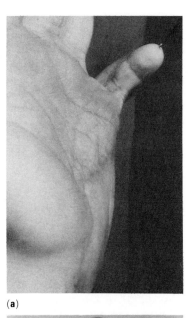

(a)

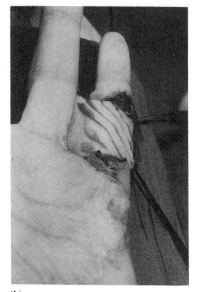

(b)

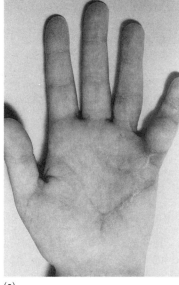

(c)

sutured and then pulled distally, is a much less traumatic method of retrieving the tendon (Fig. 7.8). 'Impaling' the retrieved tendon with a needle is a good method of preventing it slipping back during suture. Alternatively, a rubber band can be used as a 'harness' to hold the tendon, which is probably less traumatic to the tendon.

The actual repair should be carried out with the minimum of handling of the tendon ends with forceps.

Figure 7.8
Retrieval of proximal
end of divided tendon
using silastic rod.

Figure 7.8
Retrieval of proximal
end of divided tendon
using silastic rod.

Silastic rod passed
through tendon canal

Distal cut
end of tendon

Proximal cut end of
tendon sutured to
silastic rod and then
pulled distally through canal

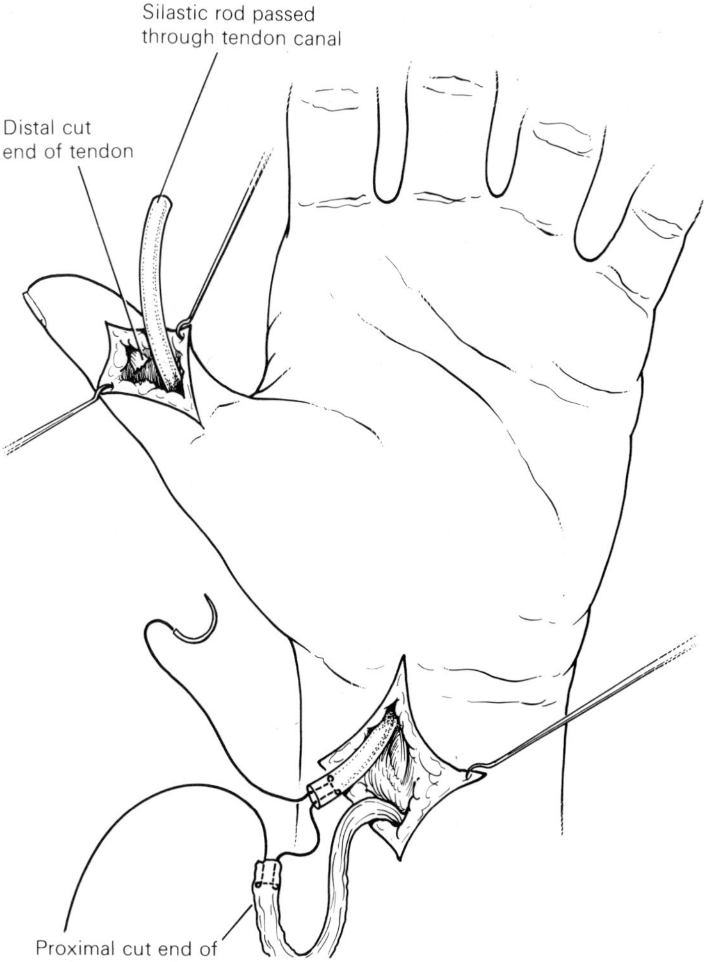

Suture material

A non-absorbable material should be used. Ejeskar has shown that 'stretching' can result at the repair site when monofilament nylon materials are used. The author's preference is 4-0 Ethibond.

Method of suture

Many different techniques have been described. To minimize the risk of adherence, the tendon ends should be in apposition with no 'bunching'. Use of the modified Kessler grasping suture technique achieves this, with the added advantage that the tension is taken up by the tendon some distance from the junction.

The synovial sheath should always be closed, as the synovial fluid is an important source of tendon nutrition. The various pulleys, so important in maintaining the normal mechanics of tendon function, should be respected. If damaged, these should be repaired and if no tissue is available locally, a free graft of, for example, retinaculum should be taken and sutured around the tendon and bone to reconstruct the pulley and prevent bowstringing of the gliding tendon.

Splintage   The tendon should be immobilized for five weeks before active movement is commenced. Alternatively, a dynamic splint (Kleinert traction) can be used and in motivated patients under close supervision, this is a very effective method of preventing adherence at the repair site. An extra week or two however, is required before active, unprotected 'exercises' are commenced, because experience has shown that, using this technique, repairs take slightly longer to achieve similar tensile strength to those incorporating non-dynamic splintage. A recent study has shown excellent results, with early controlled active mobilization (commencing after 24–48 hours) and it may be that with improved tendon suture techniques this will evolve as the method of choice for treating these difficult injuries (Zone II).

The position of the hand is important. In general, unless the specific injury dictates otherwise, the hand should be immobilized in the James position with the MP joints flexed and the IP joints straight or very slightly flexed. This prevents contraction of the collateral ligaments around these joints with the resulting stiffness after a prolonged period of immobilization.

Complications and their management

Rupture   This may result from too-early mobilization, especially against resistance. Inadequate splintage or early removal of the splint may cause this. If it is diagnosed quickly, secondary suture may be attempted. Failing this, a staged tendon graft may have to be carried out.

Adherence   Some degree of adherence is likely in Zone II flexor tendon repairs. Function often improves with time over several months. It is important to determine whether the lack of movement is secondary to joint disease or tendon adherence; for example, if there is full passive mobility of the digit but limited active motion, then carrying out a tenolysis will often help the active motion. This should not be undertaken until a sufficient trial of physiotherapy has been carried out. Tenolysis is most effective when the extent of the adherence is limited to a short length of tendon.

Failure to gain any satisfactory motion is an indication for tendon grafting, though other causes for this failure must be excluded, viz. joint disease, loss of pulley systems, etc.

Abnormal function Correct functioning of the hand and digits is dependent upon the interaction of several tendons and muscles working synchronously, e.g. the long flexors and intrinsics. Abnormal function in the presence of a repaired and functioning long flexor tendon may be abnormal or inefficient owing to injury to some other part of the mechanism. Alternatively, it may be due to a local factor, e.g. a bowstring effect from loss of an essential pulley. It is important to assess carefully the hand as a whole and define the exact nature of the deficiency, referring the patient for a specialized hand opinion.

Bones and joints

The management of fractures of the hand is a complex subject and beyond the scope of this book. Complications result not only from 'no treatment' but also from 'overtreatment' and the important point to emphasize here is the ability to diagnose and recognize those injuries liable to produce problems and treat them appropriately. For example, minor angulation deformity of metacarpal fractures rarely causes problems, but rotational deformities can result in severe disability.

Prevention of complications

Define fracture type The history of the injury is important, together with adequate X-rays. Oblique views may be required. A further useful aid is examination of the fingertips 'end on'. This is particularly useful in determining rotational deformity (this is also a key point after reduction and immobilization, and dressings covering the ends of the fingers should be avoided where possible.

Appropriate reduction Unnecessary intervention can be avoided if the surgeon is familiar with the likely outcome resulting from individual injuries; for example, the majority of phalangeal fractures have minimal displacement and 'neighbour strapping' is all that is required in treatment. However, fractures of the shaft of the proximal or middle phalanges, if displaced anteriorly, will impinge on the flexor tendons, interfering with their function. These must be accurately reduced.

Soft-tissue cover After bony reduction and stabilization, adequate soft tissue cover must be ensured. If there is doubt about this, a skin flap may be required and this is best carried out as a primary procedure after thorough debridement of the wound.

Correct immobilization Complications can arise as a result of inadequate fixation or overenthusiastic use of internal fixation. Several studies have shown that phalangeal fractures (taken as a whole) generally do worse with internal fixation. It can be extremely difficult to achieve rigid fixation by this method, whether using plates or wires. Percutaneous fixation with Kirschner wires is another possibility, but in the cases needing internal fixation, accurate reduction can often be difficult.

To avoid unnecessary trauma, careful selection of cases that do need internal fixation (estimated at about 5% of hand fractures) must be carried out (Barton, 1984, see Further Reading).

The position in which the hand is splinted is also important. James in 1970 showed that immobilizing the hand with the MP joints flexed, the IP joints extended, and the wrist slightly extended with the thumb abducted was the optimal position to avoid contracture developing (Fig. 7.9). In this position, the collateral ligaments around the MP and IP joints are under tension, thus preventing the hand from slipping into the 'position of failure'.

Early rehabilitation A stiff finger gets in the way and may well interfere with functioning of the remainder of the hand. In some cases, a stiff finger is worse than no finger at all. Early mobilization, once the fracture is stable, is very important in preventing stiffness and loss of function.

Time spent explaining to the patient what exercises are required, encouraging them to persist even though initially it may be painful, is time well spent.

Complications and their management

Stiffness This is often preventable. It is more likely following crush injuries and in which multiple tissues have been damaged. Intensive physiotherapy is worthwhile, particularly in a strongly motivated patient. Ultrasound may help. Manipulation or capsulotomy may help, but these often produce more pain and oedema. Arthroplasty in damaged joints is sometimes useful.

Figure 7.9 Position of immobilization of hand.

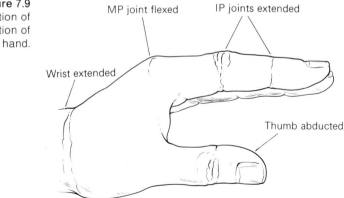

MP joint flexed IP joints extended

Wrist extended

Thumb abducted

Non-union Inadequate immobilization may result in non-union. In the case of a scaphoid fracture, bone grafting may be required, particularly if there is associated pain.

Malunion Various deformities—angulation, rotation—may result from poor reduction or immobilization. They may interfere with hand function, particularly when fingers override each other. Corrective osteotomies may be required to correct these.

Pain Long-term pain and discomfort may result from non-union. It is more commonly seen in crush injuries, particularly when there is a soft-tissue component. Cold sensitivity is particularly common. This usually improves with time, though this may take several years.

Congenital Abnormalities

A useful classification of congenital hand deformities is given in Green's text book on *Operative Hand Surgery*. It is intended only to discuss some of the complications in general terms in this chapter, in association with the surgery for these abnormalities.

Prevention of complications

Planning Where the abnormality is a relatively common defect, such as a simple syndactyly or polydactyly, the planning of the technique to be used is usually not a great problem, viz. release of the skin web or excision of the accessory digit. In more complex abnormalities, such as in various cleft-hand deformities, planning is much more critical.

Aims and objectives
As well as functional objectives, cosmetic considerations must be taken into account. The ability of children to adapt to even very gross deficiencies in abnormal anatomy is well known and when surgery is planned for the older child or adult, this must be fully taken into consideration. It may be extremely difficult for the older child or adult then to adapt to the 'new hand', no matter how adventurous or successful the surgical technique has been. In more proximal congenital abnormalities of the hand, such as the various forms of phocomelia, both proximal and distal, surgery is rarely indicated and, rather than embarking on what is often an unsatisfactory surgical procedure, use of various prosthetic devices should be considered. The more distal the 'arrest of development', the stronger is the case for surgical reconstruction, though with rapid advances being made in this field, specialist opinion should also be sought.

Functional and cosmetic

Patients are often far more conscious of the appearance of the hand than is thought. Reconstruction of absent digits by free toe transfer, for example, may be challenging surgically with a purely functional objective in mind. The appearance of toes on the hand may be difficult for the patient to accept and a prosthesis might be more appropriate. Pinch grip between thumb and index fingers and tripod grip between thumb, index and another digit are important if the patient is to be able to pick up small objects readily. To achieve this, the digits should be of a comparable length, with good sensation and adequate joint flexibility and stability. All these factors must be considered in the planning stage, together with the child's age and ability to adapt and to be trained in the rehabilitation phase postoperatively.

Timing

This has already been mentioned in general terms with regard to the patient's being able to adapt to a new anatomical hand. Patterns of hand function are usually established between 6 and 24 months; retraining is usually required after this time. However, at very young ages there may be more complications with anaesthesia, though this is very much less of a problem nowadays with modern techniques. When the deformity is left too long, secondary deformities may develop, e.g. in a syndactyly, a short digit attached to a longer digit may result in a rotational abnormality of the longer digit unless the web is released at an early stage. However, too-early surgery may result in a less satisfactory result. Flatt showed inferior results in syndactyly cases operated on under the age of 18 months and indicated that this should be the minimum age for most cases. Another factor to be borne in mind is that several procedures may have to be carried out over many months and even years. It is desirable, therefore, to commence the surgery as early as possible, though in most cases probably not before 12–18 months.

Technique To illustrate the complications that can arise in congenital hand surgery, two of the most commonly encountered congenital hand problems will be discussed. First, syndactyly and then polydactyly of the thumb.

Syndactyly

Syndactyly, or webbed fingers, is classified as complete or incomplete (depending on the extent of the interconnection) and as simple or complex. In simple syndactyly the interconnection consists of skin and fibrous tissue (or ligaments); in complex syndactyly the interconnection involves bone. Normal digital development occurs at about 6–8 weeks of intrauterine life, digits appearing as buds from the hand plate. These elongate, and it is thought that failure of separation at this stage results in syndactyly. Although it is not essential to operate on this condition, most cases of syndactyly will benefit from release of the interconnection, both functionally and cosmetically. However, the more complex the interconnection, the more careful this decision has to be. Complications include skin necrosis, infection and stiffness. These are common with all hand surgery, but several principles should be observed pertaining to syndactyly surgery to avoid specific complications associated with this condition.

Complications and their management

Web 'creep'. It is important when reconstructing the new web base, or commissure, to use a skin flap, usually taken from the dorsal aspect of the adjacent tissue as opposed to a skin graft. Using a graft may lead to some contracture or even rewebbing at the base of the release. Use of a flap brings in soft pliable tissue to the site where it is most required. Therefore, plan the skin incision so as to incorporate a skin flap at the base or commissure.

Flap necrosis. Poor design and excessive tension in the skin flaps will result in poor healing or even flap necrosis, with increase in scarring. With delayed healing, delayed mobilization is likely and there may be some functional loss.

Contracture. To minimize secondary contracture, thick grafts should always be used. These should be carefully sutured into place and a tie-over type dressing used to further stabilize the graft and enhance healing.

Several different techniques of skin flap design are used as described by Bauer, Tondra, Trusler and Colville. The aim of any of these methods, apart from commissure reconstruction as already described, is to avoid a longitudinal scar extending on the flexor surface over a joint crease, which will result in contracture. Where grafting is required on the digits, it is always preferable to cover the radial side of the digit with skin flap in preference to the ulnar side, i.e. to achieve better quality skin cover (and hopefully sensation) to the side used for opposition with the thumb.

In complex syndactyly, the decision as to which procedure is carried out is often more difficult, and depends on the skeletal anatomy. Problems particular to complex syndactyly include the following.

Malalignment. Malalignment will result in overriding of adjacent digits with reduction in function. To avoid this it may be necessary to sacrifice one of the digits. The number of digits is not so important as their disposition, functional capabilities and non-interference with each other.

Digit viability. Often in complex syndactyly a neurovascular bundle may be shared between two connected digits. If there are more than two digits connected, then the viability of the central digit may be impaired and a decision has to be made as to which digit may be sacrificed in preference to another.

Polydactyly (thumb duplication)

This again is one of the most common congenital abnormalities involving the hand. There are several different classifications used, but that most commonly used is based on the degree of skeletal union involved in the duplication (Wassel). Thumb polydactyly is not usually associated with other syndromes but may be (including the musculoskeletal system, viscera, haematopoietic and nervous systems). Indications for surgery include:

1 *Restoration of correct number of digits.*
2 *Functional benefits.* These include improvement in the position of the thumb, better stability, better length for opposition with the fingers, correction of bulk (where this is initially too great) and reconstruction of a more adequate first web space.

Techniques   It is not proposed to discuss every procedure available but rather to illustrate the principles of surgical treatment and the complications that can arise. All the techniques used can be categorized into three groups.

Excision. Simple excision of a duplicate thumb is rarely sufficient unless the remaining thumb is completely or nearly completely normal. Secondary deformity and instability is commonly seen when this simple approach only is carried out. This is particularly true when a joint is involved in the duplication.

Combination. In combination, elements from both parts of the duplication are used in the reconstruction. In the simplest form, in a duplication at distal phalangeal level, when the duplicated segments are of equal size, a triangular-shaped wedge of tissue from the centre of the defect is removed and the two lateral elements are brought together. There are any number of variations on this principle, of course, and the choice will depend on the anatomical variation of the anomaly—for example, one of the segments may have better joints whilst the other has greater soft-tissue bulk.

Revision. This includes transfer of abnormally sited tendons, osteotomies of malaligned bones, etc. Revisionary surgery may be indicated at various intervals following the initial reconstruction.

Complications and their management

Neurovascular injury This is rarely seen but will be avoided if technique is good and surgery is carried out under tourniquet. Immediate nerve repair is carried out if the nerve has been damaged or divided.

Infection This again is extremely rare but is a disaster when it does occur. Treatment with the appropriate antibiotic is indicated.

Inadequate motor tendon units If the surgery interferes with function, then tendon transfers may be indicated.

Joint instability Lateral instability is a common complication as time progresses and may require stabilization using ligament reconstruction. Arthrodesis may be required if this continues to be a problem.

Bony malalignment Rotation and angulation deformities of the bones are corrected with osteotomies, depending on the exact deformity.

Growth discrepancy Obviously, growth of the thumb must be monitored carefully. Reduction in size of a thumb that is too large can be carried out by soft-tissue or bony reduction. Lengthening procedures, e.g. Matev technique, may be used for thumbs that are too short.

Dupytren's Contracture

Dupytren's contracture that affects the palmar and plantar fascia of hands and feet, respectively. Its incidence increases with age and it is much commoner in males. It is predominantly a disease of caucasians. Its aetiology is uncertain, though it is well recognized as being associated with such diseases as epilepsy and chronic alcohol abuse. Family history is also important. It usually occurs on the ulnar side of the palm of the hand, extending as bands into the ring finger and little finger, causing progressive contracture, this usually being why the patient consults medical opinion. Treatment is directed towards correction of the digital flexion deformity. Less commonly, pain in the hand is the predominant feature for which treatment is sought; alternatively, if the skin is wrinkled in the palm with extensive involvement there, it can become macerated or infected, necessitating treatment.

Indications for operative treatment
A simple nodule in the palm rarely causes symptoms and therefore is not on its own an indication for surgery. Early contracture of the MP joint rarely causes inconvenience and can almost always be fully corrected, even when quite advanced. PIP contracture, however, is much more difficult to correct and

as soon as contracture commences here surgery should be undertaken.

Surgical technique Several techniques are used and in most cases that chosen will be according to the surgeon's preference. However, the more aggressive the disease, e.g. in a young epileptic or a patient with a strong diathesis, the more radical the operation that should be planned. In an older patient with slowly progressive disease, especially when the main problem is a single longitudinal band, a simple fasciotomy will often lead to a major improvement with minimal associated morbidity, operative time, etc. Some believe in the importance of excising the overlying skin together with the fascia to prevent recurrence. This will require a skin graft in most cases. Important consideration must also be given to the type of skin incision to be used. The wound should never be closed in such a way as to leave a longitudinal scar over a transverse skin crease, as a contracture within the skin is likely to result. The finger may be opened with a straight-line incision but Z-plasties should be inserted at the level of the joint creases for closure. Other possibilities include multiple V to Y advancement flaps, multiple zig-zag incisions, etc. The palm may be left open along the wound, allowing the wound to heal by secondary intention (McCash technique).

Complications of operative treatment
These may be operative or postoperative.

Operative *Neurovascular injury*
The surgeon operating on this condition must be conversant with the anatomy of the palmar fascia, both in the palm but more importantly with the extensions of the fascia within the digits. In the digits as the spiral bands contract, the neurovascular bundles are frequently displaced and great care must be taken to avoid injury to them. The nerve and contracting bands should be clearly visualized. In a very tight contracture it may be necessary to do a fasciotomy early in the operation to improve visualization. At the end of the operation the course of the nerves should be clearly identified. Primary repair, if the nerve has been divided, is the treatment of choice to restore sensation as well as to prevent painful neuroma formation. The dangers are much greater, of course, in recurrent disease with scar tissue from the previous surgery complicating the picture.

Missed band
Failure to be able to straighten a digit following surgery may be due to contracture of the ligaments around the joints or due to a missed contracture band. These often lie deeply in the digit and palpation in the depths of the wound whilst extending the finger will often reveal its presence. Failure to do so is likely to result

in early recurrence. If all the bands have been released, then tightened collateral ligaments or volar plate may be released; this is particularly seen in PIP joint contracture.

Postoperative   *Early*

Haematoma. The more extensive the dissection, the higher the risk of haematoma, though this is greatly reduced if all the points mentioned earlier are taken into consideration: meticulous haemostasis, elevation, etc. Even a small amount of haematoma formation in a closed wound will cause considerable pain. The treatment is to evacuate the haematoma and achieve haemostasis.

Delayed healing or necrosis. This may result from poor planning of the incisions, e.g. Z-plasties incorrectly placed leading to excessive tension in the wound or where the skin flaps are too thin owing to tight adherence of the resected, diseased fascia. It may be due to pressure from either underlying haematoma or dressings that have been applied too tightly. As in all hand surgery, the aim should be to achieve skin healing as soon as possible to enable early mobilization to commence. At the end of the operation, after the Z-plasties have been created and haemostasis has been achieved, with the tourniquet applied, the surgeon should be able to satisfy himself as to the viability of all the skin flaps before applying the final dressings. If necessary, non-viable skin should be excised and the area grafted. If there is any doubt, the dressings should be removed after 24 hours to check the wounds.

Infection. This is usually associated with haematoma or delayed healing/necrosis or both. It must be actively treated with appropriate antibiotics. Dressings should be changed frequently and antibiotic-impregnated tulle-gras is useful. If underlying flap necrosis is the cause, necrotic tissue should be debrided and when the infection has settled any residual areas of skin defect may require grafting or local skin flap repair.

Late

Recurrence. This may be due to inadequate surgery initially, when a band of tissue has been missed. Recurrent contracture may also arise from misplaced skin incisions (longitudinal scars over transverse creases). If skin grafts have been used on the fingers, these should be either full-thickness or thick split-skin grafts, as these grafts will tend not to contract as much as thin grafts. Many cases will require splintage for several weeks postoperatively (perhaps intermittently, e.g. at night) to achieve full straightening of the digits. Treatment of recurrent disease may be very difficult in previously scarred digits. Adequate exposure to enable identification of contracting bands is essential.

Sympathetic dystrophy. This complication, though not very common is particularly difficult to treat and may result in permanently reduced hand function. It is essential to try to keep the hand moving as much as possible and close supervision by the hand therapist is indicated.

Persisting controversies
- The role of the dermis (and its excision) in the prevention of recurrent Dupytren's contracture.
- The place of internal fixation in fractures of the hand.

Further reading
Barton, H.J. (1984) Fractures of the hand. *J. Bone and Joint Surg., 66.B* 159.

Green, D.P. (1988) *Operative Hand Surgery* (2nd edn). Edinburgh: Churchill Livingstone.

Lister, G. (1984) *The Hand: Diagnosis and Indications.* Edinburgh: Churchill Livingstone.

Acknowledgement
Figure 7.5 shown by kind permision of Dr R.M. Zuker, Toronto.

8 Facial Soft-tissue Repair

Any significant trauma or surgical procedure to the face will inevitably leave some scarring or contour defect that, unlike most other parts of the body, is exposed throughout the patient's life, frequently drawing comment from relations and friends and causing embarrassment throughout the life of the patient. There is, therefore, great responsibility on those dealing with these injuries or carrying out elective procedures on the face to be well versed in the anatomy of the area together with the specialized methods of repair frequently utilized to gain an optimal cosmetic result.

The face is frequently involved in injury, particularly in road-traffic accidents, though the incidence of major facial trauma has reduced considerably since the introduction of compulsory wearing of seat-belts for front-seat passengers. The blood supply to the soft tissues of the face is excellent, as is demonstrated not only by the often copious haemorrhage associated with even relatively small facial lacerations, but also by the rapid healing of facial wounds. Even small undermined flaps of skin will often survive on the face, flaps that in many other regions would not heal or take a great length of time to do so. The surgeon dealing with these wounds, therefore, can afford to be more conservative in his debridement of compromised skin than elsewhere in the body and can consequently minimize the scarring to some extent. Another feature of facial trauma is the frequency of multiple tissue injury in the area, including injury to the eyes, ears, nose, facial nerve, lacrimal and parotid ducts and associated bony injuries. Skull fractures and fractures of the cervical spine must always be borne in mind when dealing with these patients. Facial wounds often bleed profusely and patients presenting with even quite small lacerations of the face may be in shock with severe haemorrhage. Small, deep lacerations of the neck may also injure the major arteries or veins, again leading to significant blood loss. It may be necessary to apply a vascular clamp or sutures around the vessel in the wound before any other procedure is carried out. This is likely to be much more effective than piling on layer upon layer of dressings that simply become more saturated with blood.

Prevention of Complications

Accurate assessment

The importance of facial soft-tissue trauma being complicated by other multiple injuries cannot be overemphasized. The history is all-important in assessing these patients before deciding on priorities when it comes to treatment; for example, a patient with a facial laceration giving a history of having cut his face in a broken glass window is unlikely to have a skull fracture or injury of the cervical spine. On the other hand, another patient presenting with a similar facial laceration following a road-traffic accident will need careful assessment, including information on the nature of the accident.

Investigations

Fractures of the skull and cervical spine are much more likely following, for example, a road-traffic accident, and X-rays of the skull, cervical spine and facial bones are indicated. CT scans are important if the patient's level of consciousness has altered. Often, multiple specialties will be involved in the management of such patients with facial injuries: neurosurgeons, plastic surgeons, oral surgeons, etc., and unless a full and careful assessment is carried out initially and the priorities of treatment are carried out in the correct order, then important injuries may be overlooked.

Debridement

Thorough debridement of the wound will help reduce complications such as infection, delayed healing and tattooing of scars (in the longer term).

The management of the various soft-tissue structures damaged following trauma will now be discussed and the main complications associated with each of these, together with their treatment will be outlined.

Skin

Skin lacerations, as with lacerations elsewhere, should be repaired as soon as possible. Where these are small, this can be carried out in the casualty department under local anaesthetic. When they are more extensive, or when wounds present in difficult areas, e.g. the eyelids or in young children, then a general anaesthetic is administered. This may necessitate waiting if the patient has recently had a meal or if some other injury takes precedence: for example, if the patient has been unconscious, CNS observations for up to 24 hours may have to be carried out. In these circumstances the wounds should be kept slightly moist with saline or povidone iodine soaks, as this will facilitate easier debridement later. Thorough debridement of the wound is carried out. Where the laceration has been caused by shattered windscreens, multiple tiny fragments of glass are frequently found and these should be removed. Any devitalized tissue is excised. The wound should be sutured carefully in layers if multiple layers are involved and the aim should always be to complete the repair with fine 5-0 or 6-0 nylon sutures to the skin layer itself. Tension should be avoided (this should be taken up by the deeper subcutaneous sutures). The wounds may be left exposed or a light dressing may be applied; sutures should be removed at 5–7 days.

Where there is skin loss in the wound, it may be possible to approximate the margins of the remaining wound if the loss is minimal. Otherwise, a skin graft may have to be carried out. Alternatively, a small local skin flap may be used, particularly where major structures such as nerves or bones are exposed. The choice of flap will depend on the site of the injury and the tissue available.

Prevention of complications

Debridement This must be thoroughly and carefully undertaken. Foreign bodies (fragments of glass, etc.) must be removed. Non-viable tissue should be excised. This may take a considerable time, but in the typical injury caused by the shattered glass from a vehicle windscreen, multiple fragments of glass are frequently found. Caution must be exercised in deep wounds to avoid damage to branches of the facial nerve.

Haemostasis Vessels should be coagulated or ligated. It is important to ensure that this is carried out at the patient's normal mean blood pressure, otherwise postoperative haemorrhage may be a problem when the pressure rises. Where significant undermining of tissue is present, a drain should be inserted to avoid haematoma formation.

Recognize skin loss Delayed healing, wound dehiscence and unsightly scars can all result from a wound sutured under tension, often when tissue loss, necessitating reconstruction by graft or local flap, has not been recognized.

Suture technique Poor suture technique can also contribute to inferior scars. This is particularly important in the face (see Fig. 8.1). Failure to evert the skin margins can result in delayed healing and early removal of the sutures, which is desirable, can result in wound dehiscence. Incorrect approximation of certain particular features on the face can be very obvious, causing very noticeable disfigurement, e.g. the red–white (mucosal-skin) margin of the lip (see Fig. 8.2).

Complications and their management

Haematoma The skin of the face is extremely vascular. Haematomas are most

Figure 8.1
Bad scar on face.

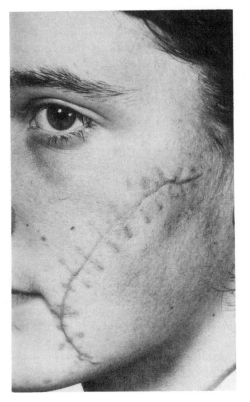

Figure 8.2
Incorrectly aligned
red–white margin.

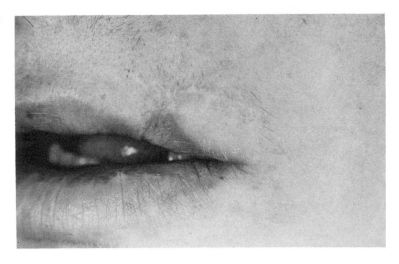

likely to occur in an injury resulting in extensive undermining of the skin. Careful haemostasis and use of drains are very important. An enlarging haematoma will eventually compromise the circulation to the overlying skin and subsequent necrosis will occur.

Early diagnosis and evacuation of the haematoma, removal of several strategic sutures and application of a firm bandage may be sufficient, though care should be exercised, since a bandage that is too tight can itself cause ischaemia to the flap.

Infection Infection usually results from inadequate wound debridement and/or haematoma. Early diagnosis and active treatment with antibiotics should be commenced.

Particular wounds are more susceptible to infection, e.g. through and through wounds into the mouth, and animal and human bites. Prophylactic antibiotics should be used in these cases, e.g. metronidazole and flucloxacillin.

The presence of pus necessitates drainage.

Delayed healing Wound dehiscence will result from poor suture technique combined with early suture removal. Suturing poorly vascularized tissue (which should have been debrided) will also result in poor healing. An infected wound will also result in delayed healing.

Dehiscence at the time of suture removal is best treated by immediate resuturing, provided the wound is not grossly infected. This will offer the best chance of a good scar. Tapes, e.g. sterstrips, can be used but it is very difficult to evert the wound margins, which is important in achieving the optimum scar. An infected wound should be treated with antibiotics and topical antibacterial dressings.

Disfigurement Scars can be disfiguring for several reasons. They may become thickened or hypertrophic. They may widen if lying across rather than parallel to natural crease lines. They may be tattooed with small particles of grit (see Fig. 8.3), and so on. The management depends on the careful assessment of the cause of the disfigurement.

Conservative

Many scars will improve with time alone. Massaging the scar regularly with a bland cream helps to soften the scar tissue. Normal maturation of a scar takes 12–18 months. During this time the scar can be expected to fade in colour and be smoother in texture. Various creams can be applied, particularly to mask the colour of an unsightly scar.

Steroid injection

A scar that becomes hypertrophic can sometimes be improved by steroid injection, e.g. triamcinolone. This must be injected into

Figure 8.3
Tattooed scar on face.

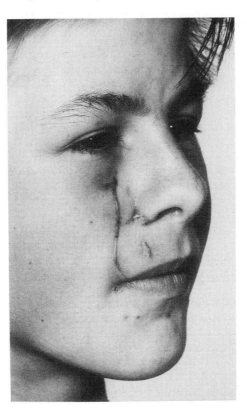

the scar itself, producing a 'blanching' effect. Treatment should be repeated every 3–4 weeks for about three treatments. Care should be taken to avoid the scar becoming too thin, when there is the risk of it breaking down.

Steroid tape
An adhesive tape impregnated with a mild steroid (flurandrenolone) is available and some patients have reported a good response to this. The pressure effect of the tape may also be beneficial.

Revisionary surgery
Where a contracture develops resulting in, e.g. ectropion or distortion of the alar base, revisionary surgery is often helpful. Z-plasties can both elongate and realign a scar, positioning it closer to the direction of the natural crease lines.

Contracture Contracture is part of the natural healing process, but inappropriate management of the initial wound can accentuate it. For example, an unrepaired skin deficit, or a split-skin graft applied to the cheek below the eye, can contract and result in an ectropion (see Fig. 8.4).

Figure 8.4
Ectropion following
tissue loss on cheek
laceration.

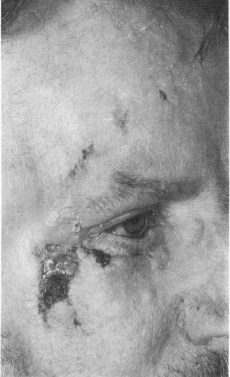

Figure 8.4
Ectropion following
tissue loss on cheek
laceration.

Tissue loss must be recognized and repaired by local flaps or grafts, full-thickness grafts being used in situations where contracture is likely to be a problem.

Nerve

Injuries to the facial nerve in the face are most frequently seen in deep lacerations associated with glass and knife wounds. The diagnosis may not be immediately apparent if there is associated swelling or there are other injuries, such as fractures, present. However, unrecognized and untreated, a facial nerve injury is one of the most disfiguring of all facial defects. The facial nerve enters the face from the stylomastoid foramen. It courses through the parotid gland, dividing into several branches. There is a certain amount of cross-over between these branches. Consequently, as a general rule, laceration of the nerve lateral to an imaginary vertical line running from the outer canthal area must be repaired if function is to be restored; but medial to this line, although the nerve should be repaired, this is probably not so critical as function usually returns. The nerve should be repaired under magnification with fine nylon sutures (10-0 or

11-0). Sensory nerves—trigeminal, supraorbital and supra-trochlear—may also be injured.

Prevention of complications

Diagnosis It can be very difficult on occasions to diagnose a facial nerve injury, particularly when the face is swollen or there are associated fractures, intracranial injuries, etc. Suspicion should be aroused, however, by a deep penetrating wound in the face. At operation, a nerve stimulator is helpful.

Magnification The divided branches of the facial nerve can be extremely difficult to locate at operation. They tend to retract into the soft tissues. Blood clot, oedema and a contaminated wound can all combine to make repair of the nerve very difficult. Use of operating loupes for magnification can aid in the location (and subsequent repair) of these branches.

Careful debridement Debridement must be meticulous. Injudicious debridement may result in nerve damage. Glass fragments should be removed with great care.

Complications of nerve injury in facial trauma and their management

No recovery Complete division of the main trunk of the facial nerve is a major deformity; when it occurs, referral for specialist treatment as soon as possible must be carried out. A 'primary' repair, provided there is no nerve loss, can generally be carried out within 10–14 days of injury. Thereafter the nerve ends are difficult to approximate without undue tension and a nerve graft is usually necessary. After approximately 12–18 months it is seldom worthwhile carrying out a nerve repair, except in the possible exception of children, as irreversible changes in the motor nerve end plates occur. Pedicled muscle transfers or free vascularized muscle grafts in conjunction with cross facial nerve grafts should then be considered. Complete absence of sensory recovery in the face is unusual and seldom requires treatment. However, patients with loss of sensation over the supraorbital distribution often complain about this and it is frequently associated with a painful neuroma at the site of injury.

Partial recovery Even in optimal conditions, complete recovery of normal facial nerve function may be difficult to achieve. A recent long-term survey of patients who underwent primary repair of facial nerve injuries showed poorer than expected recovery of brow and lower-lip function.

Abnormal recovery Synkinesis may occur and be very difficult to treat. The commonest example of this is probably linking of eye and mouth function—when the patient smiles there is a tendency for the orbicularis oculi to contract simultaneously.

Eyelids

Laceration involving the eyelids necessitates careful examination of the eye itself. This is particularly the case when the patient may be unconscious and will not immediately complain of any loss or interference with vision. Glass fragments may have entered the eye. Simple lacerations of the lids are best repaired under a general anaesthetic with careful approximation of the corresponding tissues, with particular attention being paid to alignment of the grey line. Continuous subconjunctival sutures are used for full-thickness lacerations so as to avoid irritation of the globe by the suture material. Management of eyelid injuries when there is tissue loss will be discussed in Chapter 15. A light dressing may be applied, but if there is any concern about vision in the eye, vision should be checked at frequent intervals.

Complications

A poor repair can often result in overlapping of the wound margins with discomfort in the eye. Failure to recognize tissue loss and deal with it adequately may lead to watering of the eye and ectropion. Penetrating injuries, particularly around the lateral part of the lid, may cause scarring and tethering of the external ocular muscles with diplopia resulting. This may require operative release if spontaneous improvement does not take place.

Ears

Total reconstruction of an ear is one of the most formidable of all plastic surgery reconstructive challenges and excellent results are difficult to achieve. Preservation of the parts of a lacerated or damaged ear is, therefore, very important. Where there is extensive soft-tissue loss, attempts should be made to preserve the cartilaginous framework. Several techniques are available for this: for example covering the cartilage with temporalis fascia, raised as a pedicled flap on the superficial temporal artery, a skin graft then being applied over this. A totally avulsed ear, attached to the scalp, has been reported as being successfully replanted using microvascular techniques. Where this is not possible, one method is to remove the posteromedial skin from the amputated part, followed by fenestration of the cartilage. The amputated part is then sutured back and the posteromedial part is applied against a vascular bed created by raising a retroauricular flap. After several weeks the ear is sufficiently vascularized to enable a posterior margin to be elevated and grafted to create a new postauricular fold.

Complications
The blood supply to the ear is normally very good so that lacerations of the ear generally heal well. Haematomas may form and these should be aggressively treated, as the ear may become deformed and thickened. It may also be very painful in the acute stage. Simple needle aspiration is rarely successful and recurrence is common. Release, using a small incision, is the treatment of choice with a firm, conforming bandage applied following this.

Nose

The skin on the dorsum of the nose is fairly tight, so that tissue loss here often requires reconstruction with skin grafts or flaps. Full-thickness lacerations should be repaired in layers and a small nasal pack should be inserted for 24–48 hours to avoid adhesions. Extensive lacerations of the nose are often associated with fractures of the nasal bones or more extensive fractures of the facial skeleton.

Complications
Scarring is the main complication seen following purely soft tissue injuries to the nose (i.e. excluding cartilaginous injuries). Scarring is often very obvious on the nose owing to its prominent site. More extensive reconstruction of nasal defects will be discussed later.

Specific techniques relating to reconstruction of the eyelids, ear and nose are covered in more detail in the relevant chapters.

Ducts

The lacrimal and parotid ducts may be injured in facial lacerations. Failure to repair injuries of the lacrimal ducts may lead to epiphora. These should be carefully repaired (under magnification) over a small nylon stent or fine-bore silastic tube, which is later removed. Failure to identify parotid duct injuries may lead to stenosis of this with recurrent pain and parotitis in the gland. The duct can either be ligated completely (causing the gland to atrophy) or it can be repaired again with fine sutures over a nylon stent.

Mucosal Lacerations

Small lacerations of the mucosa heal rapidly and, apart from maintaining good oral hygiene, no treatment is required. Larger lacertations should be sutured with absorbable material such as catgut or one of the synthetic absorbable sutures. Full-thickness injuries of the cheek or lips involving skin, muscle and mucosa are liable to become infected. These are often caused by penetration of the teeth, tending to contaminate the wound. Treatment consists of careful debridement and repair in layers. Oral hygiene postoperatively must be meticulous and antibiotics should be given. A combination of antibiotics can be used and should include metronidozole, as this has been shown to be highly effective in countering infections originating in the mouth.

Head and Neck Cancer

The management of skin tumours of the face is covered in Chapter 12 and this section is, therefore, confined to intraoral malignancy—of lips, buccal mucosa, floor of mouth (and alveolus), upper alveolus and hard palate and tongue. In the UK these tumours account for only 2–3% of all human cancers. They are often associated with heavy smoking, excessive alcohol consumption, poor dental hygiene, etc. Recently there has been a rise in the incidence of these tumours in a younger age group (especially females), reported in the United States in non-smokers and non-drinkers (particularly of tumours involving the tongue) with no obvious cause as yet identified.

Many potential complications are associated with the surgical management of these patients, in view not only of the complex anatomy and accessibility, but also of the spread of the disease. Recent work (Sharp, 1981, see Further Reading) has helped in predicting the likely lymphatic spread of these tumours according to the primary site, thus modifying the approach to neck dissection and reducing some of the complications associated with this procedure. A greater understanding of the spread of floor of mouth and lower alveolar tumours has led to procedures in which the lower border of the mandible can safely be preserved, thus reducing the morbidity of total mandibulectomy.

Complications of Tumour Resection

Prevention of complications

Pre-operative factors   In this difficult and complex field of surgery, pre-operative assessment of the patient is extremely important; many patients are elderly and frail, often poorly nourished, frequently showing the effects of excess alcohol and cigarette smoking affecting liver and respiratory function. Thorough pre-operative assessment and planning will help prevent many unnecessary complications.

History and examination
This must be directed at the site of involvement to ascertain the extent of the disease, e.g. an anterior floor of mouth tumour may be associated with altered sensation over the mental nerve distribution on the chin, suggesting involvement of the inferior alveolar nerve within the mandible. Rapid progression of symptoms suggests an aggressive tumour. Examination should take into account the state of the dentition, as teeth may need to be extracted at the time of surgery. An assessment of the likely extent of the resection necessary should be made, though further information from investigations will be necessary and a final decision can not be made until the time of surgery. Careful examination of the lymph glands in the neck is important, as this helps in staging the disease and preventing the complication of inadequate tumour resection. A neck dissection combined with excision of the tumour may be required. It is a great mistake to have too-fixed an idea as to the likely method of reconstruction prior to the resection being carried out and the surgeon performing the operation should be well versed in various options that may be required.

Investigations
Apart from routine blood screening, specific X-rays of the mandible, maxilla and chest may be required. Wide-angle X-rays of the mandible are particularly helpful. CT scans and NMR scans have greatly increased the scope of accurate localization of intraoral tumours. Further advances in this field, e.g. three-dimensional CT scans, will further add to the surgeon's preoperative information. All these techniques, however, have their limitations: for example, CT scans cannot discriminate between tumour and oedema. A chest X-ray must always be taken to exclude lung metastases.

Biopsy examination under anaesthetic (EUA)
A biopsy should be taken as a preliminary measure to establish a tissue diagnosis. This may reveal a lymphoma better treated with radiotherapy. The majority of intraoral tumours are squamous cell. An EUA is often helpful in determining the extent of the disease, particularly if the patient has trismus, making clinical assessment difficult.

Nutrition
Pre-operative enteral feeding in a cachectic patient will better prepare the patient for major surgery and help reduce postoperative complications resulting from poor wound healing, etc.

Combined consultation
Several studies have shown that combined use of surgery and radiotherapy significantly enhance local/regional control of these tumours (though not, as yet, long-term survival). As local

recurrence is one of the major complications, these patients are best assessed initially at a combined clinic between surgeon and radiotherapist (Fig. 8.5). Owing to the significant complications that can arise when operating in an irradiated field, the author's view is that in the majority of cases surgery should precede radiotherapy wherever possible. It is, however, important for the radiotherapist to assess the extent and site of the tumour before surgical treatment.

In different cases, especially when the cancer is advanced, and operability is in doubt, a decision to treat with radiotherapy alone may be made.

Planning treatment

Careful planning in the light of the above factors will again reduce the risk of preventable complications such as unnecessary radical surgery in an obviously inoperable tumour. The final decision on postoperative radiotherapy will rest on the operative findings, final histology report, etc. If indicated, the earlier this can be initiated, the more effective it is likely to be. Studies have shown that the effect of radiotherapy is enhanced when therapy can start within 6 weeks of surgery.

An operation complicated by delayed healing or poor flap section or design will inevitably delay postoperative radiotherapy and thereby reduce the overall effectiveness of the total treatment. Free vascularized flaps have shown superior healing qualities, enabling even earlier postoperative radiotherapy.

Figure 8.5
Diagram for combined clinics.

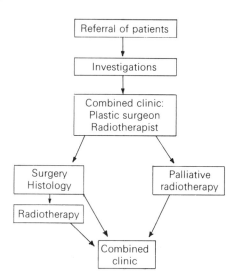

Operative factors

Planning the incision

Since adequate excision is crucial to success in controlling local recurrence, accessibility and, therefore, exposure of the tumour are all important. Respect for the natural crease lines so as to minimize the facial and neck scars is also important. Unless the tumour is small, lying anteriorly in the floor of mouth, the lip must generally be split. This is best done through a midline incision extending in a curved manner around the chin (Fig. 8.6). If a neck dissection is required, the incision is extended in a curved direction across the neck to the mastoid region at a level of approximately two finger breadths below the angle of the mandible. A vertical incision joining to an inverted V enables flaps to be raised exposing the neck. The McFee incision is often advocated in the post-irradiated neck to reduce the risk of neck flap necrosis.

Splitting the lip enables greater visualization of the intraoral tumour.

Osteotomy

For tumours lying posteriorly in the mouth, a mandibular 'swing' greatly facilitates exposure and thereby adequate resection. McGregor has shown that by siting the osteotomy away from the midline, i.e. between the first and second premolars just anteromedial to the mental foramen, the amount of muscle dissection is greatly reduced (Fig. 8.7). Healing is also likely to be enhanced because the osteotomy does not lie immediately deep to the lip scar. Failure of the osteotomy to unite is a

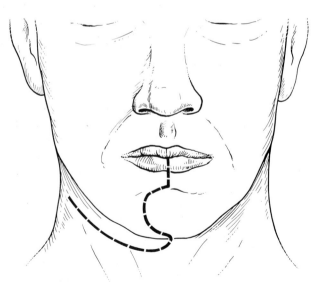

Figure 8.6
Incision to split lower lip.

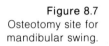

Figure 8.7
Osteotomy site for
mandibular swing.

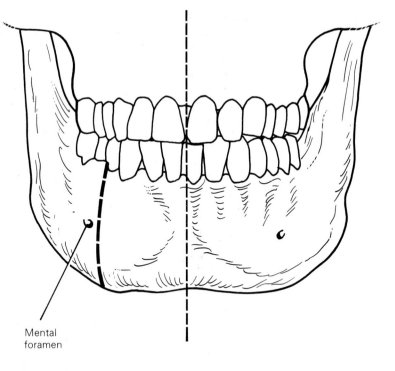

Mental
foramen

complication partially related to vascularity of the mandible at the site of division. This can be lessened by avoiding stripping back the periosteum excessively. The mucosa should be incised between the teeth (if present) and an attempt made to preserve the papilla. Decayed and infected teeth should be extracted.

Adequate stabilization of the osteotomy at the end of the procedure is important. Various techniques are available, e.g. combined lower border loop combined with a Kirshner wire, plating, etc.

Resection margin
An adequate resection margin to prevent local recurrence is vital. A margin of 1.5 cm should be aimed at all around the tumour. Several factors are helpful here.

1 *Magnification.* Use of operating loupes can be of assistance where the margin is otherwise indistinct.
2 *Site.* A knowledge of the likely pattern of spread of the tumour is important; for example, in the tongue, tumour can spread extensively posteriorly in a submucosal plane and also deeply through the extensive interlacing muscle fibres.
3 *Frozen section.* This has proved extremely helpful where there is any uncertainty about margins, and in helping confirm adequate clearance before embarking on reconstruction.

Other operative factors
Considerable morbidity can be associated with the surgery of these tumours as already mentioned, but this can be minimized partially by preserving form and function where possible without, of course, compromising the adequacy of tumour resection.

Resection of the full thickness of the mandible can produce a significant cosmetic defect and interfere with oral function. Often the lower border of the mandible can be preserved, carrying out a 'rim' resection only.

The anterior free segment of the tongue is very important in speech and control of saliva in the mouth and should be preserved where possible. In reconstruction, an attempt should always be made to reconstruct this 'free tip'.

Antibiotics
Use of intra- and postoperative antibiotics is useful in preventing infection. The author's preference is a combination of flucloxacillin and metronidazole continued over a 5-day period.

Postoperative factors

Airway maintenance
Postoperative oedema may compromise the upper airway. If this is anticipated, the patient should have a tracheotomy at the time of surgery or remain intubated until such time as the swelling subsides.

Prevention of infection
Oral hygiene is the single most important factor here. Different mouthwashes are available (e.g. Corsodyl, Betadine). Antibiotics (e.g. metronidazole) are particularly useful. Any blood clots should be removed.

Enteral feeding
This should be commenced as soon as possible, progressing to normal feeding as the mouth heals. This should be gradually increased, starting with clear fluids, progressing to a soft diet as tolerated by the patient.

General complications and their management

Early

Haemorrhage
This will usually present with oozing from the suture line or obvious haematoma formation beneath the reconstruction. Major haemorrhage may occur from a vessel in the neck and result in sudden onset of shock.

The patient should be returned to theatre for evaluation of the haematoma and ligation of the vessel involved.

Airway obstruction
Extensive surgery, particularly in the oro-pharyngeal region

may result in oedema causing airway obstruction. This may also result from haemorrhage in this region. For these reasons many would advocate routine tracheotomy at the time of operation in these patients.

Depending on the cause, the airway should be cleared, an endotracheal tube inserted, or tracheotomy carried out.

Carotid sinus syndrome

Where, in particular, a radical neck dissection has been carried out, the carotid sinus may lie superficially beneath the skin flaps. Pressure to this area, either during or after the operation, may result in a sudden drop in pressure and bradycardia.

At operation, applying lignocaine around the sinus helps to block the afferent fibres.

Soon ### Seroma

Suction drains should always be inserted at the end of the operation to prevent seroma formation. Fluid will collect beneath the flaps and may become infected, with resulting wound breakdown.

Sunction should be maintained in the drains for at least 7 days. If the drain blocks, then aspiration may need to be carried out until the fluid stops collecting.

Chylous leak

The thoracic duct is most likely to be damaged when dissecting out the lymph nodes low down in the neck on the L side. At the time of injury, a dilute milky fluid is usually seen 'welling up' in the wound. Failure to recognize this complication will result in the patient becoming progressively more cachectic over several weeks. If missed at the time of operation, excessive drainage is noted in the suction drains, especially after enteral feeding has commenced.

At operation, if the thoracic duct is divided, it must be securely ligated. If the fault is diagnosed later, the patient should be returned to theatre for ligation of the duct.

Fistula

A small fistula may occur in the early postoperative phase before the wounds are securely healed. Later fistula may be related to poor healing, e.g. following radiotherapy in a poorly nourished patient, associated with diabetes or when the skin flaps necrose.

An early, small fistula will generally close spontaneously. Oral hygiene and antibiotics should be continued and full oral feeding delayed. Later treatment should be directed to the cause, e.g. skin necrosis. The dead tissue should be debrided and if the fistula is small, the wound packed and allowed to close in itself. Larger fistulae may need more definitive flap repair. The patient's nutritional state should be carefully monitored.

Necrosis

This is a serious complication, particularly if it occurs in the neck over major vessels. 'Carotid blow-out' may occur with catastrophic haemorrhage. This potential complication underlines the need for careful pre-operative planning of skin incisions, particularly in irradiated patients.

Excision of the necrotic tissue and flap repair should be carried out when the neck vessels are in danger of being exposed. Minor flap necrosis should otherwise be treated conservatively; one advantage of using myocutaneous flaps is that, when skin necrosis occurs, often the underlying muscle remains viable and the wound subsequently heals.

Infection

This may complicate any of the above situations. Treatment with appropriate antibiotics is indicated.

Late   *Recurrence*

This may occur locally or in the neck glands or as distant metastases. Full assessment of the extent of the recurrence should be undertaken.

This should once again be undertaken at a joint clinic, with factors such as the age and general condition of the patient, symptoms and previous therapy being taken into consideration. Radical radiotherapy cannot be repeated if recurrence occurs within the previously irradiated field. Surgery in this situation can be exceedingly hazardous.

Metastatic glands appearing in the neck are best treated initially with surgery, but if recurrence of disease occurs in a neck previously treated surgically, then radiotherapy is the treatment of choice.

To date, chemotherapy has proved disappointing, having significant side-effects.

Complications of Reconstruction in Different Anatomical Sites

Lips

Malignant tumours of the lips are virtually always carcinomas. Characteristically affecting older men, the incidence is much commoner in the lower than the upper lip. Anatomically, the lip consists of skin, muscle and mucosa and in reconstructing the lip the best results are obtained by reconstructing each of these layers, preferably with functioning (innervated) muscle. The vast majority of lip cancers occur singly and involve the lower lip. They are usually situated between the midline and one commissure. In general, defects involving one-third of the lip or less can be treated satisfactorily by wedge excision and direct suture. This is often combined with a 'lip shave' procedure or vermilionectomy, as the adjacent mucosa often shows instability and the presence of leucoplakia. Defects between one-third and the whole of the lip are usually treated satisfactorily by a redistribution of the remaining circumference of the oral stoma. Such reconstructions are best performed in one stage with full-thickness flaps (skin, muscle, mucosa) of local tissue. Resections involving the whole of one lip and a portion of the other normally require additional tissue—a distant flap of some sort. The ideal reconstruction should produce a normal-looking lip, not too tight, with a vermilion border, an adequate sulcus between the lip and alveolar margin, good sensation and good muscle tone. It should ideally be able to permit chewing, prevent drooling and perform labial consonant formation. This ideal is rarely achieved.

Methods of repair

Up to one-third resection
Simple wedge excision is carried out either as a V or as a W. The labial artery is cauterized or ligated and the defect is repaired in layers. Particular attention should be paid to the mucocutaneous junction so as to achieve accurate alignment—a feature which, if not correct, is particularly noticeable postoperatively.

Greater than one-third to whole length
Many different operations have been described to reconstruct these defects. There are basically three categories of these operations:

1 those that use cross-lip pedicles from the opposite lip (almost always from the lower to reconstruct defects in the upper lip);
2 those in which tissue from the opposite lip is mobilized around the commissure to facilitate closure;
3 those that use sliding horizontal cheek flaps.

The third group is actually introducing new tissue into the lips and, therefore, reducing the size of the stoma is not an inevitable conseqence as is the case with operations in the first two groups. Most of the operations described are excellent for introducing skin muscle and mucosal reconstructions, but the muscle is at best only partially functional as a result of denervation. Karapandzic showed that by careful dissection the orbicularis oris muscle could be freed from the surrounding musculature with its nerve supply intact to produce a reconstruction with viable functioning muscle.

Whole of one lip plus adjacent opposite lip
If there is insufficient local tissue, distant flaps may have to be used in lip reconstruction. The results are usually poor because lip is best reconstructed with lip tissue or adjacent cheek. A deltopectoral flap may be used for this, or any of the myocutaneous flaps used for major head and neck reconstruction.

Complications **Microstomia**

Operations using adjacent lip tissue can lead to microstomia. Although there is no definite measurement of what constitutes a normal oral stoma and what is classified as microstomia, if the patient has difficulty getting a fork or spoon filled with food into his mouth then he will require a secondary mouth-widening procedure. Patients may also have difficulty inserting or removing dentures, as well as a feeling of tightness in the mouth. If it is not of too great severity, the mouth will often stretch sufficiently, so that no further procedure is required. If the microstomia is more marked, however, extension of the commissure will be required. A procedure for doing this is outlined (Fig. 8.8).

Figure 8.8
Mouth-widening procedure.

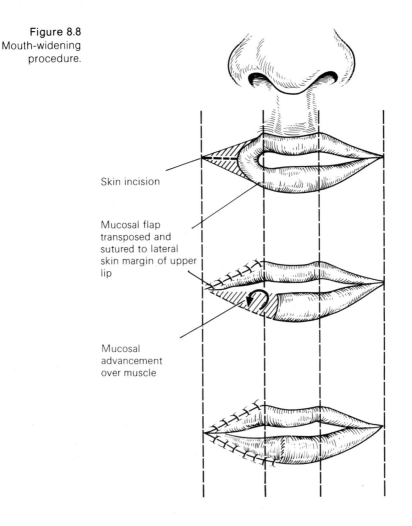

Skin incision

Mucosal flap transposed and sutured to lateral skin margin of upper lip

Mucosal advancement over muscle

Drooling

This may result from too little tone in the lower lip, either from muscle that has no function or from too much tissue without adequate support. It is frequently a sequela of reconstruction using distant flaps. It may also result from an inadequate sulcus between the alveolus and the lower lip. Tightening up of the reconstruction is most easily achieved by carrying out a wedge excision if there is too much tissue present and, within limits, if it is due to lack of muscle tone. Obviously, too great a resection will lead to microstomia, but the gain achieved (namely, lack of drooling) will usually outweigh the degree of microstomia that will ultimately result. Inadequate sulcus can be reconstructed using a skin graft after freeing the lip from the alveolus. Excessive freeing here, however, in the absence of adequate tone in the lower lip, may only partially relieve the symptoms.

Speech deficiency

The formation of labial consonants is an important function of the orbicularis muscle. Where the Karapandzic principle is utilized in the reconstruction, then obviously motor function is preserved and speech problems are less marked. Where full muscle function is not restored, speech therapy may be useful. In most patients speech deficiency is rarely a problem, except where distant flaps are used.

Sensory loss

There is inevitably some local sensory loss around the scars at the site of repair. Some patients find this irritating and uncomfortable. Most of the sensation will recover in the ensuing months.

Cosmesis

Simple wedge excisions generally heal with minimal obvious scarring. Attention to correct alignment of the mucocutaneous junction has already been referred to. A lip with functioning muscle will again be aesthetically better than one without. The commissure of the mouth is a particular site that is often aesthetically deficient following reconstruction: for example, where an Estlander-type flap is used, this will result in a rather rounded appearance to the commissure. This can be avoided (provided it will not compromise the tumour resection) if the flap is designed to avoid using the commissure tissue. A two-stage procedure is required (for division of the vascular pedicle), but the specialized tissue of the commissure is preserved and an aesthetically superior result obtained. Alternatively, using the procedure described for widening the mouth, a new commissure can be reconstructed.

Tongue

Carcinoma of the tongue is a disease of the middle-aged and

elderly. The majority of malignant tumours of the tongue are squamous carcinomas. Carcinomas of the lateral border of the tongue accounts for about 90% of all tumours of the anterior two-thirds of the tongue. Surgical treatment involves partial glossectomy. On the lateral border of the tongue this frequently involves resection of the adjacent floor of mouth or buccal mucosa or incontinuity resection of the glands in the neck to where the spreading occurs. Methods of reconstruction depend on the extent of the resection. It may be possible to approximate the side of the tongue to the cheek mucosa, particularly towards the posterior end of the tongue. At the anterior end, maintaining a mobile tip to the tongue is of great importance with regard to articulation, etc. Use of skin grafts in the mouth has proven very satisfactory. Where these lie against hard tissues such as mandible, a mould of, say, guttapercha may be taken and used to help immobilize the graft initially. On soft tissues, the graft may be quilted; perforations should be inserted in the graft to prevent it lifting off the bed in the event of oozing. For larger resections, reconstruction using forehead flaps, deltopectoral flaps, myocutaneous flaps can be used. More recently, free flaps have been used extensively. The radial forearm flap, which is now widely used, has proved a superior method of reconstructing these defects owing to its thin quality, requiring microvascular techniques for transfer.

Complications   *Haemorrhage*
The tongue is very vascular and this is a particular problem following surgery to it. Meticulous haemostasis is important. If hypotensive anaesthesia has been used during the resection, the pressure must be brought up before closure of the defect to ensure that all bleeding points are coagulated or ligated.

Speech difficulties
The tongue has a major function in speech production. It is particularly important to maintain the mobility of the tip of the tongue and this must be borne in mind when planning the reconstruction. Tissue around the tip should not be used for reconstruction itself.

Swallowing
When extensive resection involving the posterior parts of the tongue are involved, there may be problems with swallowing. Tube feeding may be required postoperatively.

Buccal mucosa
This is an ideal site to reconstruct with split skin grafts where the defect is partial thickness. Full-thickness defects will require flap coverage for outer and lining layers: for example, radial forearm or forehead flap for lining, local cheek rotation,

pectoralis major musculocutaneous or deltopectoral for outer surface.

Complications   The main complication is collection of food in the vestibule of the mouth with full-thickness defects when no buccinator function is present. Flap necrosis is always a risk when the patient has had previous radiotherapy. Healing may be delayed and fistula formation may be a problem. Fistulae will usually close spontaneously, though this may take several weeks. Tube feeding may occasionally be indicated, together with further surgery.

Anterior floor of mouth
This is a common site for tumour. Split-skin grafts can again be used for reconstructing small defects. If larger defects are grafted, however, this will extend up onto the tongue and tethering of the tip occurs as the graft contracts. Nasolabial flaps are particularly useful in this situation for small anterior defects, though it is important to avoid using hair-bearing skin. Free flaps can be used with great advantage here owing to the thin nature of the skin (e.g. radial forearm, dorsalis pedis) and the relative ease of designing them to fit the defect's size and shape.

Complications   If extensive, skin grafts used in reconstruction here can contract, reducing tongue mobility. Bulky flaps, particularly when myocutaneous flaps are used, can be very uncomfortable for the patient and require later thinning. Nasolabial flaps are best avoided in the male because hair growth can occur in the mouth. If postoperative radiotherapy is being carried out, however, it will usually correct this complication.

Tonsillar fossa (retromolar area, posterior one-third of tongue, lateral pharyngeal wall)
In virtually all cases the mandible will have to be divided to allow access to this area. Owing to the convolution and folds in this area, reconstruction with grafts is difficult and flaps are the method of choice. Free flaps are particularly useful here owing to their flexibility in adapting to the shape of the defect. Musculocutaneous flaps, such as pectoralis major and latissimus dorsi have proved reliable and useful; deltopectoral flaps can also be used.

Complications   Complications include difficulty in swallowing. Prolonged tube feeding may be required, particularly when the tumour resection and subsequent reconstruction has been extensive.

Lower alveolus
Tumours involving the floor of the mouth frequently necessitate rim resection of the mandible with subsequent loss of the

alveolar ridge. Preservation of the lower border of the mandible, where possible, greatly reduces the cosmetic disfigurement normally associated with total mandibulectomy.

Complications The main complications are loss of a ridge on which to place a denture. This can be very disfiguring for the patient. Bulky flaps, such as pectoralis major musculocutaneous flaps make it very difficult to fit a denture subsequently. It is sometimes possible, with a thinner flap such as a radial forearm flap, to create a ridge by using a fold in the flap. However, great care must be taken because, with no sensation in these flaps, a poorly fitting denture will cause breakdown of the tissue.

Palate
This is one of the commonest sites for malignant tumours arising from the minor salivary glands. Extensive resection involves excision of the hard palate and a dental plate is used to reconstruct the defect and obturate the roof of the mouth to facilitate eating and speech.

Complications These mainly relate to feeding and speech, but a well-fitting obturator is usually effective in reconstructing the defect following excision.

Persisting controversies
- Choice of flap for intraoral reconstruction.
- Timing of surgery and radiotherapy for intraoral tumours.
- Excision margin required.

Further reading
McGregor, I.A. & McGregor, F.M. (1986) *Cancer of the Face and Mouth.* Edinburgh: Churchill Livingstone.
Sharpe, D.T. (1981) The pattern of lymph node metastases in intraoral squamous cell carcinoma. *Br. J. Plastic Surgery 34,* 97.

9 Complications of Burns

Introduction

A burn is an injury caused, except in special circumstances, by heat. Heat destroys tissue and damages tissue beyond the zone of complete destruction. Similar injury can be caused by electricity or corrosive chemicals.

The two most important factors that influence the outcome of a burn are its depth and its size.

The overwhelming majority of burns are small and most never reach hospital. In dealing with burns of less than 10% in children and 15% in adults, the problems are restricted to the burn wound itself. Larger burns lead to serious systemic upset. The aim in treating a patient with a burn is to ensure the patient's well-being and to enable the burn to heal as quickly as possible with minimum loss of function and disfigurement; complications of healing interfere with these goals.

Normal Healing

Healing depends on the depth of the burn (Fig. 9.1), which is related to the temperature of the burning agent and the length of time it has been in contact with the skin. In partial-thickness

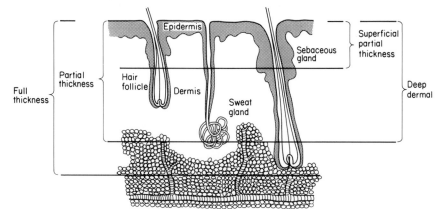

Figure 9.1
Cross-section of the skin indicating the classification of burn depth.

burns, the deeper layers of the dermis survive and healing will take place from outgrowth of epithelial cells in the hair follicles and sweat glands. The superficial partial-thickness burn should heal in less than three weeks and leave few or no long-term traces. The deep partial-thickness or deep dermal burn takes longer than three weeks to heal because there are fewer surviving epithelial appendages, and the quality of the healed skin is poor, with hypertrophic scarring (see below).

Full-thickness burns can only heal from the edges unless they are skin-grafted. If unexcised, the dead skin ('eschar') softens and separates, exposing granulation tissue that has been forming beneath it. The resulting ulcer—for that is what it is—heals by secondary intention, that is by a combination of epithelial cells growing across the surface from the edges and *contraction* of the base. This process may take many weeks or even months and results in poor-quality skin cover and shortage of skin, which can lead to *contracture* of joints.

Assessment
Successful treatment of a burned patient depends on an accurate assessment of depth and size of the burn and an appreciation of other factors that may affect the patient's recovery. Mistakes in any of these areas can lead to problems.

Mistakes in assessment of depth and extent

The clinician should disregard erythema when assessing the extent of a burn as there is no associated tissue destruction or fluid loss. A superficial burn is blistered and if the blisters are broken the base is pink, weeping and very painful. Such a burn is usually easy to identify but if the patient has been well sedated or the burn is very oedematous it may not be particularly painful or tender. Blisters may not develop for some hours, so that if the burn is seen early its extent may be underestimated. A careful search should be made of the scalp after a scald as it is easy to miss blisters hidden by hair.

Full-thickness burns are usually easily identified by being dry, completely insensitive and often depressed. They may be white, a fixed red or charred, and coagulated subdermal veins may be visible. Occasionally pale full-thickness burns may be confused with unburned skin.

Deep dermal burns are often difficult to diagnose but may appear as pale or dull red areas in the centre of a superficial burn. They may be easier to recognize after two or three days under a dressing but may not be identified until they are found to be unhealed three weeks after the injury. At this stage they can be distinguished from full-thickness burns, which should be covered in an even layer of granulation tissue as the slough separates, by their network of deep dermal collagen with beads of granulation tissue appearing throughthe interstices and scattered epithelial islands.

The extent of the burn is often misjudged. Burn units and

casualty departments should be equipped with Lund and Browder charts on which an accurate map of the burn can be drawn and the percentage body surface area calculated. In the absence of such charts, the Rule of Nines can be applied to burned adults, but it is inappropriate for children, whose heads are relatively much larger than those of adults and whose lower limbs are much smaller. In practice, the most useful guide is the patient's hand, which, with the fingers together, is about 1% of the body surface area. This is accurate enough to allow the clinician to decide whether intravenous resuscitation is necessary (see below). Remember that erythema should be disregarded when making this assessment.

Complications of Healing

Factors that can delay healing usually increase the depth of the burn and therefore also lead to poorer quality of the healed skin, with possible disfigurement and loss of function.

Prolonged exposure to causative agent
The effect of this is most commonly seen in scalds, when clothing soaked in hot liquids retains the heat so that the typical toddler scald, caused by pulling a container of hot liquid down from a cooker or table, is deeper on the chest than on the face.

Prevention The proper First Aid treatment is to separate the patient from the source of the heat as quickly as possible and to remove all clothing from the burned area. If it is stuck it must be trimmed. The immediate application of cool water, either by immersing the burned part or with wet dressings, can cool the area and may diminish the depth of the burn. It is also a very effective analgesic. However, if the burn is large or the patient is a small child the risk of causing hypothermia must be recognized and avoided.

Chemical burns
Chemical burns should be washed with copious quantities of running water. This may be under a tap, in a shower or with a hose, depending on the severity and situation of the accident. Thereafter an antidote, if available, may be of help; sodium bicarbonate for acid burns and vinegar or ammonium chloride for alkali burns. Certain agents penetrate deeply and the burn must be excised; for example, burns from phenol, hydrofluoric acid (which should be treated initially with a calcium gluconate gel or soaks) and phosphorus (where 10% copper sulphate will identify the phosphorus particles by turning them black).

Infection
Infection is the commonest and most serious complication of the

burn wound. Although bacteria in the burned skin are destroyed, the surrounding skin remains colonized and the dead tissue and blister fluid are ideal culture media for contaminating organisms. Infection delays the healing of partial-thickness burns and can increase the depth of tissue destruction.

Infection of a full-thickness burn is almost inevitable unless it is excised within the first few days. Early infection readily becomes invasive. Granulation tissue, once it has formed, is an effective barrier to the passage of bacteria but can be penetrated if the numbers are large, if they are particularly virulent or if the body's immune response is depressed. In other circumstances, surface infection is not necessarily a clinical problem. Indeed, it may speed the separation of slough and does not necessarily interfere with the 'take' of skin grafts.

Infecting organisms   *Staphylococcus aureus* is the commonest pathogen found on a burn wound in hospital. In small numbers, on a granulating surface, it does not usually cause problems but if it becomes invasive it can be dangerous. In some burn units, antibiotic-resistant strains have appeared.

β-Haemolytic streptococcus infection, particularly Lancefield Group A, can cause more local tissue destruction than any other, increasing the depth of a burn and destroying granulations and skin grafts.

Gram-negative bacteria appear on burns of the lower half of the body and after treatment of Gram-positive organisms with antibiotics. The most dangerous to patients with large burns is *Pseudomonas aeruginosa*, which can cause a frequently fatal septicaemia. *Proteus* and *E. coli* are also commonly found.

Fungal infection is seen in large burns after prolonged courses of antibiotics. It is difficult to treat and if it becomes invasive it is usually fatal.

Invasive infection
If treatment of the burn wound is delayed, cellulitis is common, usually caused by a staphylococcus. Invasive infection is uncommon in small burns that have been promptly and properly treated but is frequent in patients with large full-thickness burns whose immune response has been depressed. In these patients it may lead to septicaemia and metastatic infection— pneumonia, carditis, meningitis, arthritis (Fig. 9.2) and abscesses in many different sites.

Prevention of infection   This is one of the most important aims of treatment of the burn wound.

1 *First Aid*. Contamination can be minimized by covering the burn with a clean cloth or 'cling' film.

Figure 9.2
A child with an
infected burn and a
septic arthritis of the
right hip following a
staphylococcal
septicaemia.

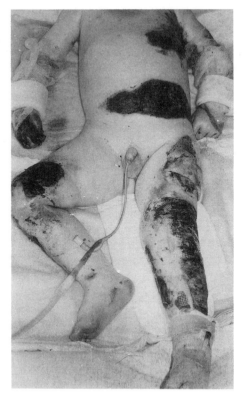

2 *Cleaning and debridement of the burn wound.* At the earliest opportunity the burn should be gently cleaned with normal saline or a mild antiseptic such as cetrimide, chlorhexidine or povidone iodine. Loose epithelium should be removed and blisters deroofed, because the epithelium and trapped blister fluid nourish bacteria. It is permissible to leave the epithelium over intact blisters if there are no broken ones near it, since, under these circumstances, the wound is closed and unconta- minated.

3 *Prevention of further contamination.* Bacteria must be kept from the wound until it has healed. This is difficult because of the copious outpouring of fluid, since bacteria can pass through a wet dressing. A number of techniques are available.

Evaporative dressing. The standard method of care is an inner single layer of tulle gras, gauze swabs and a bulky layer of cotton wool or gamgee extending well beyond the limits of the burn and held in place with a crepe bandage. It must contain no impervious layer and should not be covered with anything (such as adhesive tape) that will interfere with evaporation through it (Fig. 9.3). If it becomes soaked through, it must be changed down

Figure 9.3
An evaporative
dressing that has
soaked through. Note
the soakage under the
adhesive tape, which
should not have been
applied over the burn.

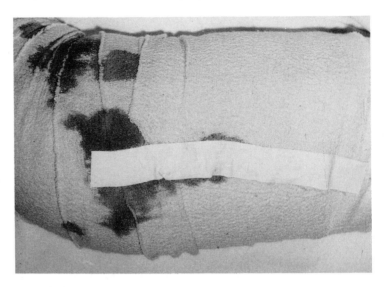

to the inner layer. Synthetic cellulose swabs are inappropriate as they do not allow evaporation and hold a sodden layer next to the burn that readily becomes infected. An evaporative dressing should be left in place for a week to ten days.

Antibacterial applications. Local antibacterial agents are often used as an inner layer of the dressing. They are very valuable in the treatment of large burns where the risks of overwhelming infection are serious, but are probably unnecssary in small burns. These, if partial thickness, should not become infected if promptly and properly treated as described above. Antibacterials retain their activity for only a limited period and need to be renewed daily or more frequently if they are to be effective. Except in certain specific situations such as the hand (see below), such frequent dressing changes are not justifiable for small burns. They take up a great deal of nursing time, are expensive and are distressing and inconvenient for the patient.

Local application of most antibiotics is contra-indicated because of the risks of producing bacterial resistance, patient sensitivity or toxicity. They are readily absorbed through the burn wound and a number of disasters have occurred, such as the production of permanent nerve deafness following the use of local neomycin/bacitracin sprays.

Silver nitrate and sulfamylon have been popular in the past; both have their disadvantages. Silver sulfadiazine cream (Flamazine) is now most commonly used and is effective against both Gram-positive and Gram-negative bacteria. In spite of its use, most large full-thickness burns eventually become colonized with bacteria unless they are excised early; the agent helps by keeping the numbers of bacteria low.

Exposure

The exposure of a burn wound after thorough debridement allows a crust to form from the solids left by the evaporating exudate. If this crust forms, covers the whole wound, is adherent and has no cracks, then it forms an excellent barrier to bacteria.

The technique is an old one but was popularized by A. B. Wallace after the Second World War. It fell into disfavour after Winter showed that drying a burn can increase its depth and delay its healing. However, it is still a very useful method of treating burns of the face, buttocks and perineum, which are difficult to dress effectively.

Exposure is a difficult technique and if not carried out properly will lead to potentially disastrous infection (Fig. 9.4). It must be instituted within the first few hours; all blisters must be completely deroofed and shreds of epithelium removed; nothing must touch the surface and any related joints must be immobilized. The crust should be fully formed by 48 hours and should begin to separate during the second week. If any raw areas are exposed, bacteria can get under the crust and the method must be abandoned.

Apart from very superficial facial burns, the use of exposure should be restricted to burn units where nursing staff are familiar with it and can cope with its difficulties.

Prophylaxis with systemic antibiotics

The indiscriminate prophylactic use of systemic antibiotics in the treatment of burns causes more problems than it solves and

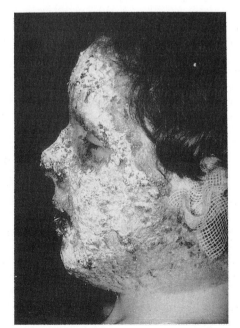

Figure 9.4
A badly exposed facial burn. The infected crust had been sprayed daily with Polybactrin (risking deafness) while it floated on a sea of pus. Note the piece of tulle gras serving no useful purpose.

must be avoided. Superinfection with resistant organisms is common and can be disastrous. Probably the only situations in which it is justified are (i) when infection with *β-Haemolytic streptococci* is a particular risk because of its prevalence in the community or in the hospital environment; (ii) when a deep burn is contaminated with soil; and (iii) following very deep burns such as high-tension electrical injuries, in which muscle necrosis is likely. In the last two instances, there is a risk of clostridial infection. In all three, penicillin is the antibiotic of choice, or erythromycin if the patient is allergic to penicillin.

Early excision of the burn wound
Early excision of the dead tissue and closure of the wound with split skin grafts is the surest way to avoid infection and, where the condition of the patient allows it, should be the treatment of first choice. This applies to deep dermal burns, which can be excised tangentially with a skin-grafting knife, and to full-thickness burns, which can be excised tangentially or with a scalpel. Early excision is practical within the first four or five days; thereafter, softening of the slough makes it difficult.

Treatment of established infection
The growth of most organisms on the surface of a full-thickness, unexcised burn wound usually does not require any specific treatment. *β-Haemolytic streptococcus* can be so destructive that it should be treated with antibiotics immediately if it is known to be present. Penicillin G is the antibiotic of choice but should be given with flucloxacillin if there is also a staphylococcus present.

Cellulitis around a burn wound is an indication for systemic antibiotic treatment, the choice of drug depending on the organisms grown from the surface. If the patient presents with an obviously infected burn, it is likely to be due to a staphylococcus, and flucloxacillin should be given until the organism has been cultured and sensitivities are known.

Septicaemia must be treated vigorously with the appropriate antibiotics intravenously, but systemic antibiotic treatment should not be prolonged because of the risk of superinfection with resistant bacteria or fungi, which can be impossible to treat effectively.

Local antibacterials will not eradicate established infection from a granulating surface but can keep the number of bacteria down and so reduce the risk of invasive infection.

Chondritis

A full-thickness burn of the ear is liable to lead to chronic infection of the cartilage. It is very painful and leads to destruction of the cartilaginous framework (Fig. 9.5).

Prevention
If infection can be prevented by early excision and grafting or by using local antibacterial agents, then chondritis will not occur

Figure 9.5
Chronic chondritis of
the right ear following
a burn. Note the
destruction of
cartilage.

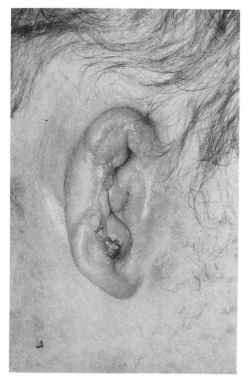

and loss of cartilage will be limited to those areas where it is exposed and devitalized.

Treatment Established chondritis must be treated by wide exposure through an incision round the periphery of the ear, curetting and excision of all affected cartilage, and drainage. Antibiotics should be given.

Cross-infection
An infected burn presents a risk of cross-infection to other, non-infected patients and in an environment such as a burn unit, which may contain a number of patients with infected burns, the risk to a new patient is high.

Prevention Patients with large burns should be segregated from other patients, particularly from those admitted for elective, clean operations, and from those with infection. Burn dressings should be carried out in a dressing room separate from the ward area and in a strict order of priority, with the uninfected ones first. Patients carrying *β-Haemolytic streptococcus* and others with severe infections should be isolated and barrier-nursed.

Burns units are designed to reduce the risk of cross-infection, some by elaborate air-conditioning and others by less sophisticated means. Air-conditioning in these circumstances is not without its problems, as bacteria tend to colonize the system and can be difficult to eradicate. The most important preventive measure is for personnel to be aware of the risks and to take the appropriate precautions.

Trauma to the burn wound

A healing burn is easily damaged. The new epithelium growing to cover a partial thickness burn can be torn or lifted off by a knock or a dressing change and a new skin graft can be sheared off by a poorly applied dressing.

Prevention   The inner layer of a dressing should be as little adherent as is consistent with its ability to allow exudate to pass through it. The most generally accepted compromise is some form of lightly impregnated petroleum jelly gauze. This does adhere to some extent so it should not be removed from a partial-thickness burn for about ten days, by which time a superficial burn should be well on the way to healing. Even at this stage it must be removed very carefully and, if still adherent, should be left longer.

An inner layer of antibacterial cream will remain non-adherent for about 48 hours but tends to dry out if left longer. Plastic film will not stick, but exudate collects under it and tends to leak from the edges. In practice, a film such as Opsite^R that adheres to the dry surrounding skin is useful in treating small superficial burns and has the benefit of making them pain-free. When used for larger burns it tends to leak and cause problems. Plastic bags on the hands do not adhere and allow active exercises and the use of the hands; they need to be changed daily and the hands are usually washed and smeared with silver sulfadiazine cream.

Dressings must be held firmly in place to prevent shearing forces damaging the healing skin. Grafts may be sutured and tie-over dressings can be used. Alternatively, grafts can be exposed in suitable situations. This prevents their being damaged by dressings, but the technique requires careful nursing supervision.

Ischaemia

Circumferential full-thickness burns around a limb or digit cause a rigid, constricting eschar which cannot stretch to accommodate the oedema developing beneath it. The resulting rise in tissue pressure can cut off the circulation to the distal part of the limb after some hours and loss of fingers and toes is common.

A similar phenomenon in the trunk can restrict respiratory excursion and lead to respiratory failure.

Prevention and treatment   Escharotomy or release incisions down the whole length of the circumferential deep burn can be carried out without anaesthesia, although it can be a very bloody procedure. The incisions gape widely and pressure is released (Fig. 9.6).

Systemic Complications

These can arise in patients with severe burns. Some are an immediate result of the injury; others occur later in the burn illness.

Fluid and electrolyte disturbance

Thermal injury causes damage to the capillary walls and leakage of fluid from the circulation into the tissues. This is of normal electrolyte content and is rich in protein. The loss of this fluid causes burn shock.

Figure 9.6
(a) Constricting, full thickness electrical and flame burns of the trunk and arms. (b) After escharotomies. Note the gaping of the incisions.

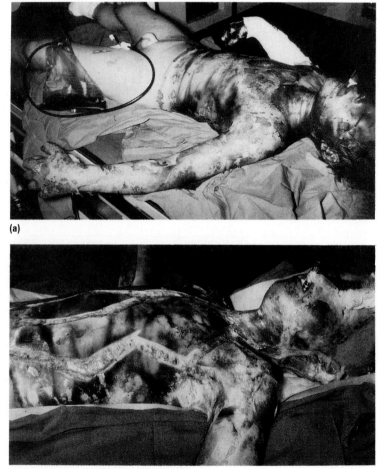

(a)

(b)

Prevention Burns of more than 15% body surface area in adults and 10% in children (excluding any erythema) require intravenous resuscitation. Many different salt-containing fluids have been advocated, but in the UK nearly all burn units use a purified protein solution (PPS). The quantity required is judged by the patient's response to resuscitation but the Muir and Barclay formula, originally described for resuscitation with freeze-dried plasma, remains a valuable practical guide to the volumes that are likely to be needed (Fig. 9.7).

Muir and Barclay The time after the burn is divided into six successive periods of 4,
(Mount Vernon) 4, 4, 6, 6 and 12 hours. During each period, the patient is likely to
formula require.

$$\frac{\text{Total percentage of burn} \times \text{weight in kg}}{2}$$

In addition to this, the normal daily intake of fluid must be given.

Formulae are only a guide to the amount of fluid replacement and must not be rigidly adhered to if the patient's condition suggests that either more or less is required. Pulse, blood pressure (when possible), peripheral circulation and urinary output must be carefully monitored as guides to the patient's response to resuscitation.

Sick-cell syndrome
Severely burned patients may develop this condition, characterized by a breakdown of the function of the cell membrane that allows potassium to leak out of the cells and sodium to enter them. The patient becomes very ill; serum sodium may be normal

Figure 9.7
Resuscitation requirements for 6 ft 4 in, 16-stone man with 46% burns; 58 units of plasma were needed in the first 48 hours.

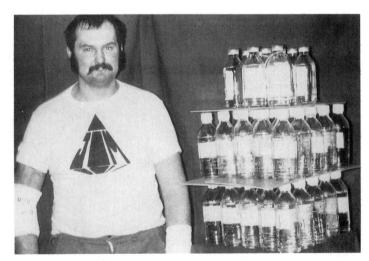

or low and potassium normal or high; urinary sodium is low and potassium is high.

Prevention Prevention of tissue hypoxia by maintaining a good circulating fluid volume and transfusing blood as required should help to prevent this condition.

Treatment Infusion of insulin 150–200 units and 5% glucose 1–2 litres should be given daily.

Anaemia

Anaemia has two causes.

1 *Red cell destruction.* This occurs following a full-thickness burn. Many cells are disrupted by the heat and free haemoglobin is released. Excessive destruction continues after the acute injury.
2 *Marrow depression.* The body fails to replace destroyed red cells due to toxic depression of the bone marrow. This results in a progressive anaemia that persists until healing is almost complete.

Prevention Large full-thickness burns require repeated transfusions, preferably of whole fresh blood. The first of these should be on the second day of resuscitation. Regular checks on haemoglobin and haematocrit are required.

Renal impairment

Renal impairment may be due to acute tubular necrosis. Inadequate or delayed resuscitation allows the development of burn shock which in turn leads to poor renal perfusion. Unless quickly corrected, this can result in acute tubular necrosis. Blood pigments from red cell breakdown and myoglobin can block the tubules and cause renal failure.

Severe renal failure is characterized by a very low urinary output (less than 10 ml/h) in spite of adequate resuscitation, rising blood urea and a fixed urine osmolality of about 350 milliosmol/litre. If it is caused by haemoglobinuria, the urine becomes dark red or dark brown as the volume falls. Less severe renal failure may be of a 'high-output' type associated with an inability to concentrate the urine.

Prevention Prompt and efficient resuscitation will maintain renal perfusion. Falling urinary output associated with haemoglobinuria can be corrected by giving mannitol 20% 1 g/kg body weight over 30 minutes.

Treatment Established renal failure must be treated by dialysis. Peritoneal dialysis may be used for a short time, but haemodialysis is required if the failure is more than transient. In the presence of a major burn, this poses severe problems of management and close co-operation is required between burn clinician and renal physician. The mortality is high.

Urinary infection

Infection of the renal tract is very common in the presence of an indwelling catheter, which may have been used to monitor resuscitation, or if the burn involves the genitalia or surrounding area. It may be present as a high pyrexia or be unnoticed if the patient is very sick with an infected burn wound.

Prevention   Urinary catheters should be removed as soon as possible. The male child can often be fitted with Paul's tubing and the adult male can use a urinal. Female patients with perineal burns present a more difficult problem but can often manage to use a bedpan.

Catheter specimens of urine must be sent daily for culture.

Treatment   A urinary infection cannot be successfully treated in the presence of an indwelling catheter and, if possible, it should be removed and appropriate antibiotics should be given. If it has to remain in place, an attempt must be made to keep the infection under control with antibiotics until the catheter can be removed.

Peptic ulceration

Haematemesis is nearly always due to superficial gastric erosions. Curling's ulcer (acute duodenal ulceration associated with burns), is extremely rare in the UK but seems to be commoner in the United States.

Prevention   The early institution of oral feeding, at about 48 hours, and the use of plasma or PPS for resuscitation may be reasons for the lower incidence of this problem in the UK.

Cimetidine should be given prophylactically to all major burns.

Treatment   General supportive measures and transfusion are adequate in managing most episodes of bleeding peptic ulcer in burns, but if bleeding persists and laparotomy is required, the prognosis is poor.

Respiratory failure

Lung damage due to the inhalation of hot or toxic gases is commonly associated with burns occurring in house fires and is often fatal. If less severe, it may not become apparent for up to eight hours after exposure. A relevant history coupled with facial or intraoral burns (Fig. 9.8a, b) and black sputum should make one suspicious. Serial blood gas estimations show a falling pO_2 and usually a normal pCO_2. COHb level is high at first and

Figure 9.8
A patient with smoke
inhalation and
respiratory tract injury.
(a) Face showing soot,
especially around
nostrils and lips. (b)
Soot and blisters of
palate. (c) Inhaling
humidified oxygen.

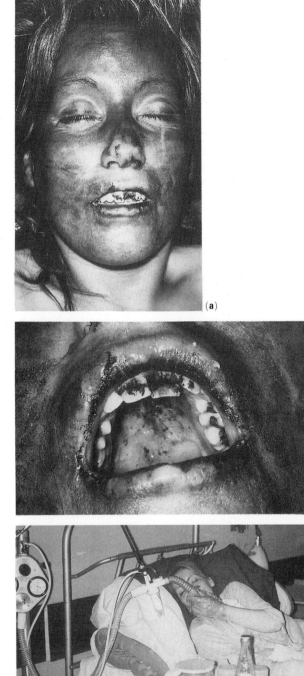

(a)

(b)

(c)

falls. A level over 15% three hours after exposure is diagnostic of smoke inhalation.

Respiratory failure may occur in the absence of smoke inhalation. The increased capillary permeability coupled with a large obligatory fluid load during resuscitation can lead to pulmonary oedema, particularly if salt-free water is given and if there is renal or cardiac failure. Pneumonia is a common complication later in the burn illness, often secondary to infection of the burn wound, and is a frequent cause of death.

Prevention Awareness of the likelihood of inhalation injury, and frequent blood gas estimations, will allow treatment. Early and well-controlled resuscitation reduces the risk of pulmonary complications during this early period. Measures to prevent and control infection of the burn wound and regular chest physiotherapy during the subsequent weeks are important in avoiding later respiratory problems.

Treatment Recognition of acute respiratory failure due to inhalation injury or other causes should lead to prompt intubation and assisted ventilation. If it is prolonged, tracheostomy may be necessary, but if it has to be done through burned tissue it increases the risk of infection. Sometimes less severe smoke damage can be treated by oxygen and humidification alone (Fig. 9.8c) but it is better to intubate early than to be in doubt.

Pneumonia should be treated with appropriate antibiotics and ventilatory support as needed.

Burn encephalopathy

This occurs most commonly in small children during resuscitation, often for relatively small burns. It is characterized by drowsiness and twitching, or, when it is severe, by full-blown epileptic fits, coma and hyperpyrexia, and can be fatal. It is due to cerebral oedema and may sometimes be the result of excess sodium-free water being given in the hours before its onset.

Prevention Sodium-free water should not be given orally to burned children. Their normal water requirements should be given as an electrolyte-containing oral preparation such a Dioralyte, which contains 1 g NaCl, 1.5 g $NaHCO_3$, 1.5 g KCl and 4 g glucose, each per litre. These solutions can be flavoured, for example, with fruit squash. If given intravenously as 5% dextrose, the metabolic water requirement should be spread evenly over the 24 hours and not given in large boluses.

Treatment Convulsions in the burned child should be treated with the following regime:

Mannitol 20%	4 ml/kg IV
Diazepam	1 mg/year of age + 1 mg IV (slowly)
Phenytoin	4 mg/kg at once IV, then 4 mg/kg in next 24 hours
	Dexamethasone 2 mg IM.

Weight loss

After a major burn, the body is in a catabolic state and negative nitrogen balance. An increase in metabolic rate is thought to be due to a combination of excessive evaporative fluid loss, increased catechol amine secretion and a change in central temperature regulation, so that body temperature is elevated even in the absence of infection. Caloric requirements to replace this energy loss may be as high as 7000 kilocal.

At the same time as he has this increased requirement, the patient is ill, with a poor appetite, and will be receiving repeated sedation or anaesthesia. As a result, his intake is likely to be low and weight loss can be very great (Fig. 9.9). If this happens, resistance to infection is poor, healing is retarded, and the patient may easily succumb.

Prevention   It is impossible to prevent all weight loss in a patient with a large burn. However, with care it should be possible to keep this below 10%. The requirements can be calculated as follows (Sutherland, 1985).

Figure 9.9
Same patient as in Fig. 9.6. (a) Healed at 10 weeks, showing cachexia. (b) 5 years later.

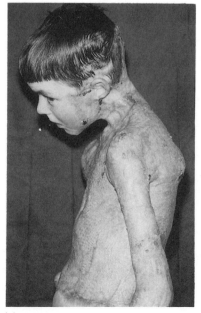
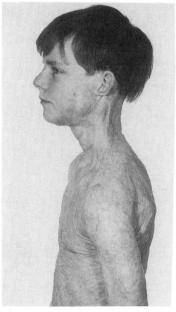

(a)   (b)

Adults	Calories	20 cal/kg body weight + 50 cal per % burn
	Protein	1 g/kg body weight + 2 g per % burn
Children	Calories	40 cal/kg body weight
	Protein	2 g/kg body weight

The most effective way of ensuring that this intake is achieved is to pass a fine-bore nasogastric tube within 48 hours of the burn and commence dietary supplements, but patients with burns of less than 30% may be able to achieve the required amount orally.

A number of different proprietary preparations are available for the supplementary feeds; alternatively, they can be made up by the dietician. They should be introduced well diluted and only gradually be built up to full strength, or they may cause intractable diarrhoea. Over-nutrition should be avoided as it may precipitate diabetes, fatty degeneration of the liver or uraemia.

Pressure sores
A patient with a large burn, lying supine, in a catabolic state and with poor peripheral circulation, is at particular risk of developing pressure sores. If such sores occur, they can cause further debilitation and set up a vicious circle.

Prevention Good nursing care with frequent turning of the patient, attention to his general condition and nutrition should prevent pressure sores developing. Low-air-loss or Clinitron beds can be invaluable for such patients.

Treatment The sore must be laid open, debrided and grafted along with the burn. Consideration of bone excision and flap cover must be left until the patient is fit enough to undergo these more major procedures.

Long-term Complications of Burns

Scars and contractures
There are always scars after all but superficial burns. Proper treatment of the injury will ensure that the scars are minimized, but they may still be disfiguring or disabling.

Hypertrophic scars occur particularly after deep dermal burns (Figs. 9.10 and 9.11a) but junctional scars between skin grafts can become hypertrophic (Fig. 9.12a). They are raised, red, thickened and itchy. They usually soften and flatten over a period of several years but if there is significant skin tension they may persist.

Figure 9.10
Scald of chest. (a) On
admission. Central
area, deep dermal. (b)
Healed. Hypertrophic
scarring of deep
dermal area.

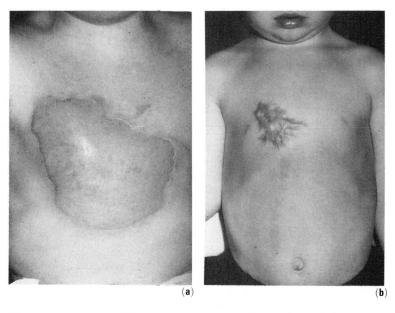

(a)   (b)

Figure 9.10
Scald of chest. (a) On
admission. Central
area, deep dermal. (b)
Healed. Hypertrophic
scarring of deep
dermal area.

Scar contractures. All scars shorten, grafts tend to shrink and a burn that heals by secondary intention results in a great shortage of skin in all directions. Skin shortage in the region of a joint will cause a limitation of movement and a contracture of the joint. These are usually found on the flexor sides of joints because flexor muscle pull is stronger than extensor and many joints tend to be held in flexion.

Prevention   Both hypertrophic scars and contractures can be minimized by constant pressure over the scars, which allows them to soften and relax more quickly than they would naturally (Fig. 9.11). Special elastic pressure garments are available and can be made to measure. They must be worn continually for many months for best effect. Joints need to be splinted and necks supported in a rigid collar to prevent contraction (Fig. 9.12b); physiotherapy can prevent joint stiffness.

Treatment   Established hypertrophic scars can be treated by pressure and, if small, by injections of triamcinolone, not more than 1 ml of the 10 mg/ml suspension being injected into the scar at one time. Silicone gel has recently been found to be effective in resolving hypertrophic scars; its action seems to be independent of pressure.

Mild contractures will respond to physiotherapy and splinting but, if severe, they need to be released and thick split-skin or full-thickness grafts inserted (Fig. 9.12c). Frequently, hypertrophic scars adjacent to the graft resolve once the tension has been released. Incisions should be designed so that junctional scars do not themselves cause contractures when they shorten.

Figure 9.11
Hypertrophic scar
around left knee
treated with a tubigrip
pressure bandage. (a)
Three months after
healing. (b) The
tubigrip in place. (c) A
year later.

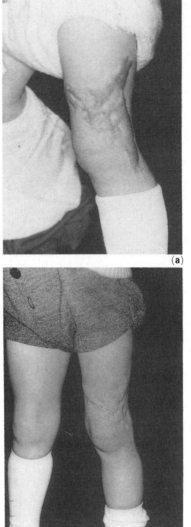

Figure 9.11
Hypertrophic scar
around left knee
treated with a tubigrip
pressure bandage. (a)
Three months after
healing. (b) The
tubigrip in place. (c) A
year later.

(a)

(b)

(c)

A patient who has recovered from severe burns is likely to need a series of reconstructive procedures over many years for the release of contractures and improvement of appearance.

Malignant change in burn scars

Long-standing and unstable burn scars, like other scars, can eventually undergo malignant change and develop squamous carcinoma (Marjolin's ulcer). Distant spread is unusual while the tumour is confined to the scarred area; thereafter, it behaves like any other squamous carcinoma of the skin.

Figure 9.12
Neck contracture and
hypertrophic junctional
scars after excision
and grafting of full-
thickness burns. (a)
Three months after
.healing. (b) Rigid
collar worn for 6
months after release
and grafting of neck
contracture. (c) A year
later. Good correction
of neck. Hypertrophic
scars have resolved.

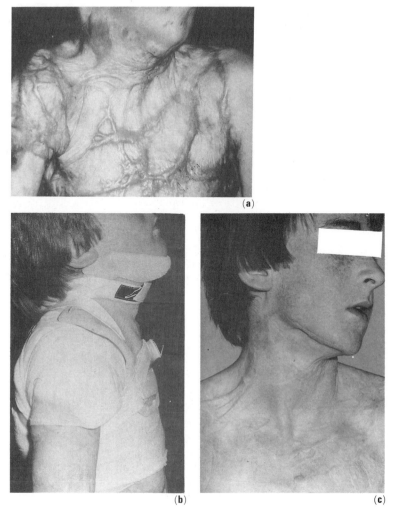

Prevention   Unstable scars should be excised and replaced by skin grafts long before there is a risk of malignant change.

Treatment   The tumour, once recognized, should be excised with a margin of at least 1 cm and the defect skin grafted.

Further reading

Muir, F.K., Barclay, T.L. & Settle, J.A.D. (1987) *Burns and Their Treatment* (3rd edn). London: Butterworths.

Sutherland, A.B. (1985) Nutrition and General Factors Influencing Infection in Burns. *Journal of Hospital Infection 6 (Supplement B) 31*: 42.

10 Complications of Cleft Lip and Palate Repair

Clefts of the lip and palate are a continuum of deformities and an individual may present with complete clefts of both or a partial cleft of one or other. Although the primary management of the lip and of the palate is nearly always carried out in two stages, there are certain problems shared by both and a number of early complications that can be considered together.

Wound Dehiscence

Predisposing factors

Infection   It is impossible to sterilize the mucous membrane of the mouth and nose by pre-operative preparation. Fortunately, the tissues usually heal well in spite of their exposure to bacteria, but wound breakdown may occur in the presence of pathogens. As in other sites, the most dangerous organism is the *Group A haemolytic streptococcus* and this frequently colonizes the throat, particularly in children and in the winter.

Prevention   It is important to establish pre-operatively what organisms are in the patient's nose and throat. Swabs should be taken and sent for culture two days beforehand; if the patient lives close to hospital this can be done at an out-patient visit, or the family doctor or a nurse may do it at the patient's home. Alternatively, the patient may be admitted two days pre-operatively, but this is expensive and carries the hazard of cross-infection with hospital organisms. The swabs should be repeated on the day before operation and again on the morning of surgery, since sometimes organisms are grown from the later swabs that failed to appear on the first. Although the results appear postoperatively, institution of appropriate antibiotic treatment is still usually followed by primary healing.

    If a report is received pre-operatively that a Group A haemolytic streptococcus is present, it is wise to delay the operation until swabs are clear after antibiotic treatment. Other pathogens such as other streptococci, *Staphylococcus aureus, Pneumococcus, Haemophilus influenzae* or coliforms should be treated with a course of the appropriate antibiotic, but the operation can proceed. If only non-pathogenic bacteria are grown, then no antibiotic need be given.

Tension on suture lines

The minimizing of tension is a fundamental principle of wound closure, but there are particular problems associated with the closure of a congenital cleft, associated as it is with both a deficiency and a displacement of tissue. The muscles of the cleft lip and soft palate, denied their normal attachment across the midline, pull the two soft-tissue elements apart. When the cleft is complete, splitting the alveolus and hard palate, the pull of the muscles, together with unopposed pressure from the tongue, force the two halves of the maxilla apart as well, creating a wide gap that is difficult to bridge.

Prevention   In order to bridge the gap without tension, the muscles must be widely mobilized and freed from their abnormal attachments, and flaps designed to allow skin and mucous membrane or mucoperiosteum to move across the cleft. If, in spite of these manoeuvres, closure can only be achieved under tension, then wound dehiscence is likely. Much of the improvement in the results of operations on cleft lip and palate has been due to the development of techniques that allow more effective, tension-free closure while restoring normal muscle function.

Haematoma

The development of a haematoma in any wound can lead to breakdown by increasing tension and by providing a medium in which pathogenic bacteria can grow. The vascular nature of the tissues and the wide undermining often required to close a cleft contribute to the risk in these procedures.

Prevention   Meticulous haemostasis and a careful, layered repair of lip and soft palate are essential. Although closure of the hard palate leaves a potential dead space between bone and mucoperiosteal flaps, almost all operative techniques leave unsutured gaps laterally that will allow haematoma to escape.

Ischaemia

Ischaemia of the wound edges will prevent healing. Infection, closure under tension and haematoma can all contribute to ischaemia, but poor operative planning, crude technique and the tying of sutures too tightly are other factors. Successful closure of the hard-palate cleft was not achieved for many years after repair of the soft palate because of the poor vascularity of mucosal flaps of the hard palate. It was only when von Langenbeck began to raise thick, vascular flaps of mucoperiosteum from the hard palate that success was assured.

Trauma

The constant movement of the lips against the teeth and of the tongue against the palate cannot be prevented and, unless alternative means of nutrition are provided, the patient must eat and drink in the postoperative period. Fortunately, repairs of cleft lip and palate can almost always withstand this sort of trauma provided sensible precautions are taken, and neither nasogastric tube feeding nor parenteral nutrition are required. However, if fingers or other hard objects get into the mouth or if the lip is knocked, breakdown of the repair can easily occur. This is especially likely in areas where there may be only a single layer closure, as in some techniques of repair of the alveolus and hard palate.

Prevention On return from the operating theatre, the patient's arms must be restrained to prevent the hands getting to the mouth. Once the child is awake, elbow splints achieve this while allowing normal play activities (Fig. 10.1). These splints should be worn for three weeks. While oral intake can begin within hours of the opera-

Figure 10.1
Elbow splints, made from fine cotton with wooden spatulae inserted into the pockets.

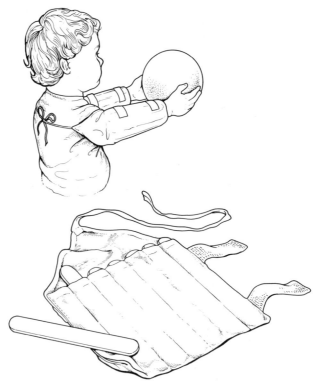

tion, it should be restricted to liquids for the first few days and then, if the child is old enough, he can move on to a soft diet. Nothing hard should be given for three weeks and every meal should conclude with a drink of water to remove debris. It is wise to avoid the use of a bottle and teat and of cups with spouts, particularly after repair of the hard palate; while a spoon is the safest way of feeding, breast feeding can continue after lip repair without danger to the suture line. In some centres, the repaired palate and alveolus are protected with an acrylic splint.

Treatment of wound dehiscence   If a cleft lip repair breaks down in the early postoperative period—usually due to trauma—the wound should, if possible, be resutured immediately. If there is only a minor gaping of part of the wound or if there is significant delay, it may be left to heal by secondary intention. Later revision can be carried out, for example at the time of palate repair.

It is unusual to attempt immediate closure of dehiscence of a palate repair. This is most often due to infection; diagnosis is delayed and the tissues are vascular and friable. They are left to heal by secondary intention and the timing of secondary correction depends very much on the extent of the breakdown and the symptoms it is causing. A fistula, if small, may close spontaneously. If it does not, it should be left as long as possible unless it is interfering with speech or there is troublesome nasal regurgitation of food and drink. Early closure causes more scarring of the palate, which interferes with its growth and repair is best delayed until the later part of childhood, when it may sometimes be combined with bone grafting the alveolar cleft.

Airway obstruction
After any intraoral operation and particularly palate repair, where raw areas are left and there is an inevitable ooze of blood, there is a risk of inhalation of blood or of upper airway obstruction due to clot. Obstruction can also occur after a pharyngoplasty if haematoma collects in the retropharyngeal space. A small baby can only breathe through its nose and if both nasal airways are blocked it may develop respiratory distress.

Occasionally repair of the palate of a child with Pierre Robin syndrome can lead to recurrence of respiratory obstruction.

Prevention   Careful haemostasis is essential. A throat pack should always be inserted at the beginning of the operation to prevent the inhalation of blood. If the operation is on the lip and nose the pack may be left to the anaesthetist but when the palate or pharynx is involved, only the surgeon can insert a pack which will not obstruct his procedure and then only after the insertion of the gag. Proper steps must be taken to ensure that the pack is removed at the end of the operation and the surgeon has the primary responsibility for sucking blood and clots from the oro- and nasopharynx. Flexion of the patient's neck and a shake of the head at this stage will dislodge any clots from the nasopharynx into view. When surgery involves the palate or pharynx, a tongue stitch should be inserted using, for example, 3-0 silk in the middle third of the dorsum of the tongue. A knot should be tied so that it lies outside the lips and the ends should be left long. If inserted at the beginning of the operation, this stitch is useful when centralizing the tongue under the blade of the gag and at the end of the procedure the long ends are taped to the chin where they can be used to pull forward the tongue in the event of upper airway obstruction. To prevent damage to the lower lip, a bolus of two or three dental rolls can be taped to it, over which the ends of the suture are drawn (Fig. 10.2). This tongue stitch is left in place until the patient is fully awake.

Retropharyngeal haematoma following pharyngoplasty can be prevented by never completely closing incisions in the pharyngeal walls. Often, defects are left open and allowed to heal by secondary intention, but even when they are sutured—which, when appropriate, can reduce postoperative discomfort—the lower ends should be left open to allow haematoma to escape.

In the small baby, care should be taken to ensure that at least one nasal airway is clear. Packs should never be inserted into both nostrils and after bilateral lip repair it is better to use lengths of polyethylene or silastic tube to maintain the contour of the nostrils and to provide an airway.

In the immediate postoperative period the patient should be nursed three-quarters prone with a head-down tilt, but, as soon as he is awake and able to swallow, the head should be raised to reduce venous pressure. Any bleeding usually stops quickly once this has been done.

Treatment   If the patient's respiration should become acutely obstructed,

Figure 10.2
Tongue stitch left long and taped over a bolus of dental rolls.

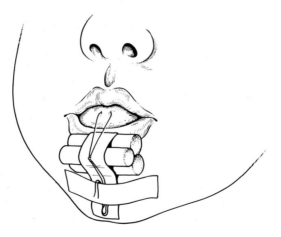

traction on the tongue stitch will open up the oropharyngeal airway. Suction, which must be available at the bedside, should be used to clear blood and secretions and this is usually sufficient to relieve the emergency. If obstruction persists, manifested by snoring even though the patient may be awake, the anaesthetist should carefully, and under direct vision, insert a nasopharyngeal airway that can be left in place for as long as may be necessary; this may be for a week, until oedema has subsided. On two occasions the author has had to carry out tracheostomies after pharyngeal flap procedures on patients who had had the Pierre Robin syndrome. They were needed for several months but both were eventually closed.

Haemorrhage

The inevitable ooze after palate repair or pharyngoplasty has been referred to. While it is almost always slight and stops within an hour or two, occasionally it can persist or a reactionary haemorrhage occur several hours later. In the presence of pathogenic bacteria, the tissues can be congested and tend to bleed excessively. Secondary haemorrhage is also the result of infection; fortunately it is rare, but the writer can recall one particularly frightening case. The bleeding may not be immediately apparent as the blood may be swallowed, sometimes to reappear as a massive haematemesis, and the only signs may be an increasing pulse rate and indication of impending circulatory collapse.

A minor bleed occurring about a week postoperatively may indicate an area of wound breakdown and the possibility of a fistula.

Prevention Pre-operative bacteriological reports on nose and throat swabs should prevent the surgeon from operating on a patient harbouring a β-haemolytic streptococcus and ensure that antibiotics are given if pathogens are present, reducing the risk of bleeding due to infection.

The importance of haemostasis should not need to be stressed. While most surgeons inject a haemostatic agent into the tissues pre-operatively, a minority do not do so because of the reactive vasodilatation that occurs when its effect wears off that gives a possibility of an increased risk of haemorrhage. Postoperatively, sedation, a head-up tilt once the patient can swallow, and the avoidance of intraoral trauma are important.

Blood should always be available for transfusion for a child, who is having a palate operation.

Treatment Blood must be replaced quickly in the presence of persistent or severe reactive or secondary haemorrhage. This should not be difficult if the patient has already been cross-matched and an intravenous drip is running—as it should be for 24 hours after the operation. The patient must be returned to theatre, anaesthetized, an endotracheal tube passed, a gag inserted and the mouth and pharynx sucked out. If major bleeding points can be identified, they may be undersewn or diathermied but, as is common elsewhere, there is often a generalized ooze that can only be dealt with by firm packing. If necessary, the pack can be left in place with an endotracheal tube for 24 hours, after which both can be safely removed with little risk of recurrence of the haemorrhage. It is a wise precaution to pass a nasogastric tube to empty the stomach of swallowed blood, but this should be done under direct vision in the operating theatre to avoid damage to the cleft repair and the tube should be removed at the end of the operation.

Complications Specific to Site

Lip

A cleft of the lip is a hideous deformity (Fig. 10.3) and its repair has been a challenge to surgeons for many centuries. The aim of the surgeon is to reproduce as closely as possible all the features of the normal upper lip and nasal tip; the operation falls short of complete success to the extent that he fails to do this. The lip is repaired by most surgeons when the baby is between 3 and 6 months old; old enough to allow a careful and comprehensive operation and not leaving the ugly deformity for too long.

The history of cleft-lip surgery is of an increasing understanding of its anatomy, which has led to better surgery and better results. However, not all the problems have been solved and the challenge to surgical ingenuity is still there.

Complications of lip repair
Early attempts to close the cleft involved simply paring the edges and dragging them together with heavy tension sutures. Breakdown was frequent and even a successful result produced a tight upper lip with an ugly scar, none of the normal landmarks, and maximal tightness at the free border. Difficulty in closing the cleft was made worse if it was very wide.

Prevention
The surgeon can achieve more with the tissue available to him if he does not have to drag it across a wide gap. The cleft can be narrowed before definitive surgery in one of two ways.

1 *Presurgical orthopaedics.* The orthodontist can fit a series of plates during the first few months of life that mould the soft bones of the maxilla to form a satisfactory dental arch and bring the halves of the maxilla together (Fig. 10.4).
2 *Lip adhesion* (Fig. 10.5). This is a preliminary operation carried out within the first two or three weeks of life, in which the edges of the cleft lip are pared and joined to convert a complete into an incomplete cleft. The resulting pull of the

Figure 10.3
Unilateral cleft of lip
and palate.

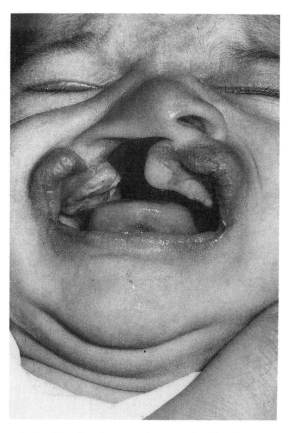

joined soft tissues draws the halves of the cleft maxilla together so that by the time of the definitive operation it is narrow. Care is taken at the time of the adhesion not to disturb tissue that will be used later.

Flap repair   The results of cleft-lip repair improved with the development of a variety of techniques that introduced flaps into the lower part of the lip to reduce tension in this area. The most sophisticated was that of Le Mesurier, who constructed a cupid's bow, until Tennison realized that two-thirds of the cupid's bow and one philtral column were already present, and made use of this in his triangular flap procedure.

Rotation advancement technique   Millard developed the rotation advancement technique, which also uses these structures and has the added advantages of better positioning of scars, rolling in the ala of the nose on the cleft side and, in particular, that it can be carried out without discarding any tissue (Figs. 10.6 and 10.7). This is important when one is dealing with a condition in which tissue is missing and the tight upper lips of days gone by are now rarely seen. Millard describes his technique as a 'cut as you go' method, by

Figure 10.4
Presurgical oral
orthopaedics. (a) The
appliance. (b) The
appliance in place
(same patient as Fig.
10.3). (c) Same patient
after three months.
Note narrowing of
cleft (compare with
Fig. 10.3).

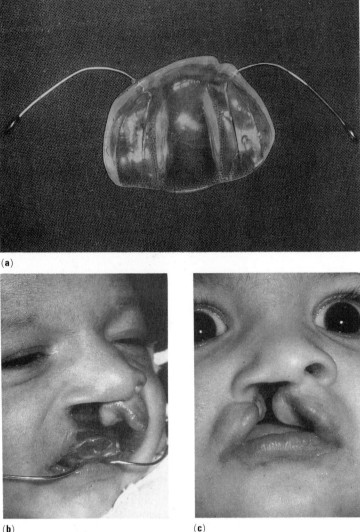

Figure 10.4
Presurgical oral orthopaedics. (a) The appliance. (b) The appliance in place (same patient as Fig. 10.3). (c) Same patient after three months. Note narrowing of cleft (compare with Fig. 10.3).

(a)

(b)   (c)

which he means that the surgeon can make adjustments up to the last moment of the operation, in contrast to most other procedures, in which the result is determined at the time the flaps are first cut. This allows for 'fine tuning' in the Millard method, which is another advantage, and it has steadily gained in popularity. The main criticism of it is that, when the lateral element is deficient, it can produce a lip in which the distance from midline to angle can be short on the cleft side.

Some problems remain unsolved; a scar is inevitable and although it is usually inconspicuous it may sometimes remain red and thickened. In spite of numerous attempts, no-one has been able to reproduce consistently the philtral column on the

Figure 10.5
Lip adhesion (after
Millard). (a) Incisions.
(b) The medial element
of the lip elevated from
the maxilla. Mucosal
flap raised from lateral
element. (c) Lateral
flap sutured to
posterior edge of raw
area on medial lip. (d)
Muscles have been
sutured and mucosa
stitched to skin.

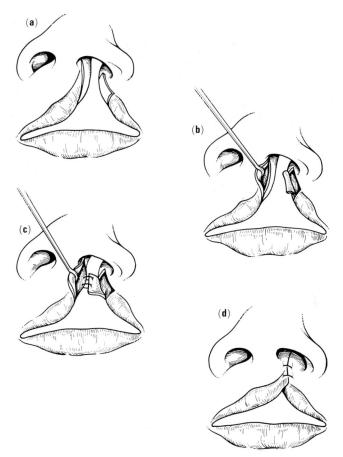

cleft side. Perhaps the biggest problem with the lip is to produce symmetrical movement.

Muscle repair   Dissections by Fara and others have shown that the orbicularis oris muscle is attached abnormally, especially in the complete cleft, to the margins of the piriform fossa (Fig. 10.8). The muscle has to be freed from these bony attachments and mobilized enough to allow its fibres to be transposed horizontally and sutured to those on the other side of the cleft, so restoring the continuity of the circumoral sphincter. If this is not done, the orbicularis is noticeable as a bulge on each side of the cleft when the muscle contracts. By proper mobilization it is possible to produce a lip that can be pursed in a natural manner but, unfortunately, the deformity is often revealed when the patient smiles, as the cleft side of the lip does not lift symmetrically. This is due to failure of the action of the levator labii superioris, either through its hypoplasia or its division during muscle dissection.

Figure 10.6
Rotation-advancement
repair of unilateral
cleft lip. (a) Incisions
marked. (b) A, flap
rotated downwards;
B, advancement flap;
C, flap used for
lengthening columella.
(c) Flaps sutured.

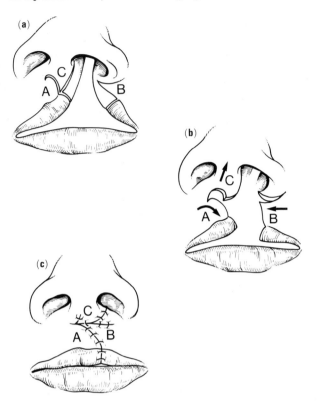

Figure 10.6
Rotation-advancement
repair of unilateral
cleft lip. (a) Incisions
marked. (b) A, flap
rotated downwards;
B, advancement flap;
C, flap used for
lengthening columella.
(c) Flaps sutured.

Bilateral cleft lip

The bilateral cleft lip is a much more severe deformity and the results of even the most skilful repair fall far short of normal.

Predisposing factors   In the complete cleft, there is a great shortage of tissue. The prolabium lacks muscle; it is suspended from the nasal tip so that there is no columella, and is attached to the front of the premaxilla so that it has no mucosal lining (Fig. 10.8).

Prevention   There are several techniques of repair, all of whch are staged. One side of the lip may be repaired at a time, using a unilateral method of repair such as rotation advancement. This is very appealing in theory, particularly when the prolabium is so far in front of the lateral lip elements that bilateral closure would be difficult. It is usual, if the premaxilla is deviated, to close the wider side of the cleft first, as the muscle repair will narrow the cleft and improve symmetry, so making the second procedure easier. Although excellent results can be obtained, the technique is not as straightforward as it may seem and symmetry can be difficult to achieve.

The alternative approach is to close both sides of the cleft at the same time and lengthen the columella at a separate proced-

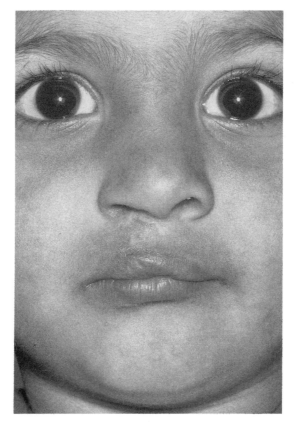

ure, either before or, more usually, afterwards. In a symmetrical cleft, the bilateral procedure helps to maintain symmetry. The surgeon has a choice of methods but, whichever he uses, once the primary operations are complete the repaired lip should have a complete orbicularis muscle sphincter and mucosal lining, its contour should be reasonably normal, and the nasal tip should project naturally. An attempt is often made to narrow the prolabium so as to place the scars in the line of the missing philtral columns, where they are somewhat disguised (Fig. 10.9 and 10.10).

The deficiencies in the aesthetic results of cleft lip repair have led to many variations of technique, none of which has overcome all the problems. However, these failures to reach perfection cannot really be termed complications and it is not the purpose of this chapter to review the advantages and disadvantages of the different operations. Complications are due to errors in planning, management or technique and can occur irrespective of the method of repair used.

Figure 10.8
Orbicularis oris. (a)
Normal. (b) Unilateral
cleft. (c) Bilateral cleft.

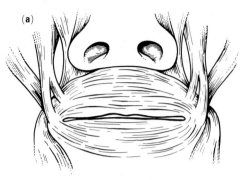

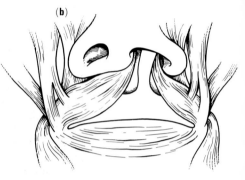

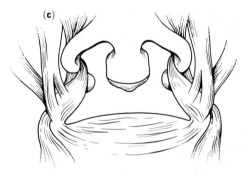

Errors of planning   Many poor results of lip repair are determined before the knife touches the skin. There is no branch of plastic surgery for which meticulous pre-operative measurement and planning is so vital or where an artist's eye can so convert an adequate result to an excellent one. It is here that the rotation advancement technique has an advantage over most others as adjustments can be made up to the end of the operation to refine the result. However, the inexperienced surgeon can get into trouble with this somewhat freehand method and may be happier with the comforting support of measurements and angles that are a feature of some other procedures. Whichever operation is cho-

Figure 10.9
Bilateral cleft lip and
palate.

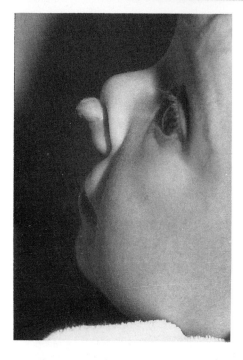

sen, careful marking with a fine pen, with checking and rechecking before the first incision is made, will prevent many disasters, and pricking ink dots to identify landmarks—particularly the mucocutaneous junction—will avoid misalignment of wound edges at the end of the operation.

Errors of technique   The operative field in a cleft lip repair is small and there is little margin for error in making incisions; a millimetre can make all the difference. Magnifying loupes are of great help in improving

Figure 10.10
Same patient after lip
repair and columellar
lengthening. (a)
Anterior. (b) Lateral.

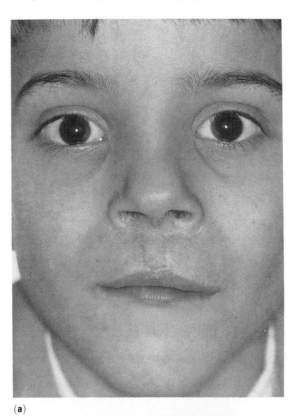

(**a**)

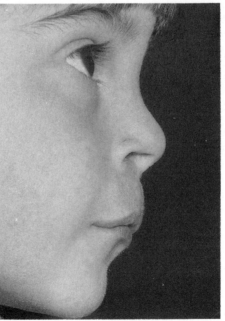

(**b**)

the accuracy of cutting and suturing. Fine, sharp instruments, proper mobilization of the tissues, careful haemostasis and closure with 5-0 or 6-0 sutures all contribute to success.

If, during the repair, it becomes apparent that all is not going well, the surgeon must be prepared to remove as many sutures as necessary to allow him to put matters right.

The nose

It is much more difficult to correct the deformities of the cleft lip *nose* than those of the lip itself and it is the abnormal nose rather than the lip that usually gives rise to comments at school. There is still no agreement on whether it is better to do a radical nasal correction at the time of the primary operation or to wait until the child is four or five years old. The deformity is very complex, involving deviation of the septum to the non-cleft side, slumping of the alar cartilage on the cleft side and splaying of the alar base, with lack of bony support to the nostril floor (Fig. 10.3). Many people feel that the radical surgery required to correct these abnormalities is likely to cause scarring that will inhibit normal growth and that it is better left until the child is older. Nevertheless, good results are being reported from early radical surgery.

Failure to correct the deformity — There is almost always a degree of failure to correct the deformity in all but the mild, incomplete cleft. In particular, some widening of the nostril floor and shortness of the cleft side of the columella may persist (Fig. 10.7).

Treatment — Treatment may have to wait until the child is older, when a more extensive procedure, perhaps including septoplasty and onlay bone grafting around the piriform margin or cartilage graft to the ala can give greatly improved results without compromising growth.

Stenosis of the nostril — Stenosis of the nostril can result from the contraction of a circumferential scar within the nostril, from overcorrection of the splaying of the ala, or from the loss of a lining flap. It may obstruct the airway, but there can be other reasons for such an obstruction, particularly septal deviation.

Correction — Nostril stenosis is notoriously difficult to correct. Surgery, by introducing more skin, either with local flaps or a full-thickness skin graft, must be followed by continuous dilatation for many months, using some form of plastic stent, and requires a degree of co-operation from the patient that is not always forthcoming. However, dilatation without surgery may be all that is required if the deformity is mild and the patient is well-motivated.

It is better to prevent the risk of this complication by avoiding circumferential scars and by undercorrecting rather than over-correcting the wide nostril.

The alveolus

Closure of the alveolar cleft is usually carried out at the time of primary lip repair. Some surgeons prefer to wait until growth is complete to avoid scarring in this area that will restrict growth. A single-layer closure that leaves a raw area on the under-surface inevitably leads to scar contraction and narrowing of the alveolar gap; Burian and Muir devised buccal mucosal flaps, which have proved very popular, to line the oral side of the alveolar cleft and prevent this collapse. However, bone grafting of the cleft between the ages of 8 and 11 years has been shown, particularly by the Oslo group, to allow the orthodontist to move teeth into the line of the cleft and produce an almost normal dental arch, and teeth will not erupt through a buccal mucosal flap. It may be that these flaps have had their day.

Damage to tooth buds   The chief complication of operating in the line of the alveolar cleft is damage to unerupted teeth and great care must be taken to avoid breaking through the thin alveolar bone while elevating mucoperiosteum.

Fistula

The repair may break down, leaving a fistula: this will be considered with those of the palate.

Palate

The aim of palate repair is to produce an intact palate with a soft palate of sufficient length and mobility to allow normal speech and swallowing. Unfortunately, in order to achieve this, tissue normally has to be mobilized from the palatal shelves and nasal septum; this produces raw areas that are usually left to heal by secondary intention, thus causing scars that can restrict maxillary growth. In general terms, radical surgery carried out early seems to produce better speech at the expense of less satisfactory dental arch form, while more conservative operations performed later lead to children who may look better but cannot speak so clearly. This dilemma has for many years fuelled arguments about the management of cleft palate and will continue to do so for a long time to come. While refinements of technique will undoubtedly occur, the surgeon's choice will ultimately depend on whether he believes speech or appearance to be more important.

Fistula   The repair of palate or alveolus may sometimes break down, leaving a fistula between nose and mouth (Fig. 10.11). Fistulae may be left deliberately for some years, but those that occur after attempted closure are associated with scarring that makes later repair more uncertain. Fistulae may allow nasal escape of air during speech and allow food and drink to get into the nose, which can be both uncomfortable and embarrassing. If they

Figure 10.11
Palatal fistula.

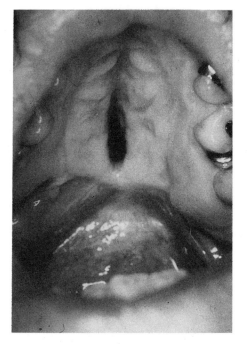

persist until teeth are lost, they make retention of dentures very difficult.

Fistulae can be caused by closure under tension, poorly vascularized wound edges, haematoma or infection. They are commonly found at or behind the alveolus, where closure can be technically difficult and is often only of a single layer, or at the junction of hard and soft palate, where there may be tension. Usually these fistulae are small and may close spontaneously but occasionally, perhaps as the result of infection, a large part of the repair may break down.

Prevention Careful technique, adequate mobilization and tension-free closure of well-vascularized flaps, using two layers wherever possible, should make fistulae unlikely. Use of a figure-of-eight suture to approximate nasal and oral mucosa at the junction of hard and soft palate obliterates dead space and reduces the risk at this site.

Treatment If a fistula occurs after primary palate repair, no attempt should be made to re-operate until the child is considerably older, because of the extra scarring and growth inhibition that would result. There is urgency only if it is causing significant symptoms during eating, drinking or speech; otherwise closure can be delayed and may be combined with bone grafting.

Velopharyngeal incompetence

A normal palate allows complete separation of the mouth from the nose by closure of the soft palate against the pharyngeal walls. This is particularly important during speech and swallowing and if a repaired cleft palate cannot do this efficiently, then the operation has failed. This failure shows itself by audible nasal escape of air through the nose during speech and often leads to complex secondary faults of articulation that can be very difficult for the speech therapist to correct. There can also be leakage of food or drink down the nose, and middle ear disease may be caused by contamination of the Eustachean tube orifices. Velopharyngeal incompetence is the usual presenting feature of an unoperated submucous cleft palate and can occur in the absence of a cleft if there is neuromuscular dysfunction or palatopharyngeal disproportion. It is commonest after cleft palate repair in those patients with the most severe shortage of tissue; that is, bilateral clefts and some wide, isolated cleft palates. Its incidence increases the older the patient is at the time of repair.

Prevention Early repair of the cleft palate using a technique incorporating an *intravelar veloplasty* will give it the best chance of functioning normally. In this procedure, the muscles of the soft palate are freed from their abnormal bony attachments to the posterior edge of the hard palate and the cleft margins, and are mobilized to allow them to be sutured together across the midline. In this way they form the muscle slings that pull the soft palate backwards and upwards to close against the posterior pharyngeal wall.

Treatment Speech therapy alone cannot correct any but the mildest velopharyngeal incompetence and surgery is needed to eliminate or reduce the incompetent gap. This may be limited to re-operating on the palate but, more often, the surgeon manipulates the pharyngeal walls. Many different operations have been devised, generically known as 'pharyngoplasties' and it is likely that the best results from these procedures can be obtained if they are tailored to the individual patient's anatomical defect after careful assessment, using nasopharyngoscopy and multiview videofluoroscopy. Surgery can influence only the function of the palate and nasopharynx but can thereby create an anatomical environment that will allow the speech therapist to correct the other, more complex, secondary articulatory faults.

Choice of operation *Reoperation on the palate.* This has been advocated by Sommerlad for patients who are believed to have had inadequate muscle mobilization at their original operation. A very extensive dissection is carried out, completely mobilizing the levator palati from all its attachments in the palate before reconstituting the muscle sling. He reports excellent results, but other surgeons, who are perhaps not so radical, have been less successful.

Midline pharyngeal flaps. These may be superiorly or inferiorly based. A superiorly based flap may be let into a defect in the nasal mucosa created by a palatal lengthening procedure (Honig) (Fig. 10.12). There are many other variations but all create a midline sagittal bar between posterior pharyngeal wall and soft palate. The nasal airway is maintained on each side but

Figure 10.12 Honig pharyngoplasty. (a) Flaps raised. (b) Pharyngeal flap sutured, muscle mobilized.

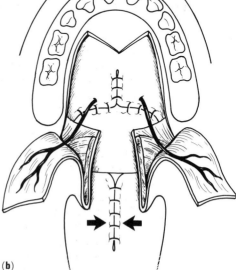

(a)

(b)

can be closed off by inward movement of the lateral pharyngeal walls during speech. Complete velopharyngeal competence can therefore be expected with such procedures only if there is active lateral wall movement, and this can be demonstrated endoscopically or by videofluoroscopy.

Posterior wall implants. If the soft palate moves moderately well and there is little or no lateral pharyngeal wall movement, so that a transverse incompetent gap is left in the nasopharynx, the posterior pharyngeal wall can be brought forward to meet the raised soft palate. This can be done by implanting a block of cartilage or a prosthetic material such as silastic behind the posterior pharyngeal wall. Such implants can be effective but have fallen out of favour as they tend to be extruded.

Sphincter operations. Both Hynes and Orticochea devised operations in which superiorly based musculomucosal flaps of lateral pharyngeal walls are transposed into the posterior wall. Hynes inserted his as high as possible and overlapped the flaps to produce a transverse ridge to meet the raised soft palate, while Orticochea emphasized the active role of the palatopharyngeus muscles in the flaps to produce sphincteric closure. He inserted his flaps at a low level into a defect produced by raising a small midline flap. Most surgeons now using this type of procedure try to put the palatopharyngeus flaps as high as possible. Active sphincteric closure cannot be relied upon but the operations do cause a permanent narrowing of the pharynx from side to side as well as bringing the posterior wall forward (Fig. 10.13).

Figure 10.13
Sphincter
pharyngoplasty.

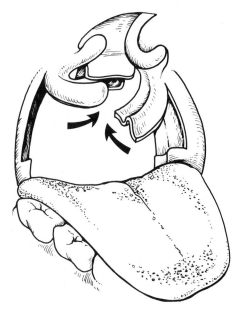

Complications The narrowing of the nasopharynx produced by all pharyngo-plasties can lead to postoperative hyponasality. If mild, this is of little significance; but if severe, it can cause snoring, chronic catarrh, difficulty of breathing while eating and drinking and, at worst, obstructive sleep apnoea which is potentially fatal.

Prevention Wide, obstructive flaps are effective in curing nasal escape but should be avoided because of the hyponasality they cause. An attempt should be made to tailor the flap to the defect and not overcorrect it, although one has to recognize that surgery in this area is not sophisticated enough to allow pre-operative measurements to give an accurate prediction of the final dimensions of a flap. Re-operation on the palate without pharyngo-plasty avoids the risk of hyponasality while making correction of the hypernasality less certain.

Treatment of hyponasality Mild hyponasality does not need treatment and often gradually resolves spontaneously. An excessively wide pharyngeal flap can be narrowed by using Z-plasties on each side, or it can be completely divided. Lateral wall flaps can be returned to their original position and implants can be removed. However, if any raw areas are left, there is a high incidence of reattachment of the flaps or recurrence of the stenosis. Raw areas should be avoided.

Often, if the pharyngoplasty is followed by an improvement in speech, this does not relapse to its pre-operative state after the pharyngoplasty has been taken down.

Maxillary hypoplasia

A small, underdeveloped, retrusive maxilla with severely collapsed upper dental arch used to be the hallmark of the adult with a repaired cleft palate (Fig. 10.14). Adults with unrepaired cleft palates were known to have well developed maxillae and the blame for this deformity therefore fell on the surgeon who closed the cleft at an early age and produced scars that tethered the growing bone. Nowadays, such severe deformities are rarely seen but some degree of maxillary hypoplasia and cross-bite are still common.

Prevention Schweckendiek of Marburg has, for many decades, avoided operating on the hard palate until his patients are in their early teens. He has produced very impressive results in terms of maxillary growth but, it has recently become clear that his results with speech are much less satisfactory. Are the aims of achieving normal growth and normal speech mutually exclusive? This dilemma has already been alluded to and has not been resolved. Fashion appears to be moving towards early, complete closure of the hard and soft palates using techniques that leave less scarring than earlier methods, in the hope that these will

Figure 10.14
Collapsed maxillary
arch.

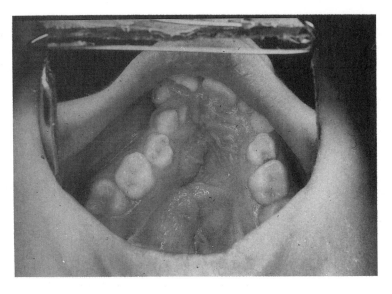

cause less impairment of growth and still allow the development of normal speech.

Treatment   Minor degrees of malocclusion can be corrected by the orthodontist, usually between the ages of 8 and 15 years. Bone grafting of the alveolar cleft during this period may allow him to move teeth into the line of the cleft and achieve a virtually normal dental arch.

It is not possible to correct more severe degrees of maxillary hypoplasia orthodontically, particularly in an anteroposterior direction, but these patients can be helped by means of maxillary osteotomies. These are usually at the le Fort 1 or, less commonly, le Fort 2 level.

Deafness

This is a potential complication of the cleft palate deformity rather than its treatment.

The tensor palati muscle, which opens the Eustachean tube orifice, is hypoplastic in cleft palates and fails to function properly so that secretions cannot drain, leading to middle ear effusion or 'glue ear'. In the unrepaired cleft, there is nothing to stop food going into the nasopharynx and the irritation and inflammation this produces around the Eustachean orifices can add to the problem. In addition, infection can more easily travel up the Eustachean tube from the nasopharynx and there is a greater chance than normal of suppurative otitis media which may lead to perforation of the tympanic membrane and permanent deafness.

Prevention   Early closure of the cleft palate may reduce the incidence of middle-ear disease but certainly does not prevent it altogether. An awareness of the risk, regular ENT monitoring and hearing tests will lead to early diagnosis of glue ear and treatment by myringotomy and grommets. Any sign of earache in the young child must lead to immediate treatment with antibiotics.

Fortunately, middle-ear problems tend to be confined to early childhood and are uncommon after the age of six or seven years.

Conclusion

The management of the cleft lip and palate deformity is complex, involving many different specialties, and is spread over many years. One of the most important ways in which it has been improved is by the setting up of combined clinics at which plastic surgeon, ENT surgeon, orthodontist, speech therapist and other specialists can see the patients together and share their experience and expertise. There is no longer any place for the isolated surgeon to operate on clefts; if he cannot gather together a team of appropriate and interested colleagues, he should send the patient to a centre where such a team exists. In this way, patients will get the best possible management and complications of this complex condition will be kept to a minimum.

Persisting controversies

- Early radical correction of the cleft lip nose.
- Early closure of hard palate and alveolus versus delayed closure.
- Extent of palatal surgery.
- Choice of repair of bilateral cleft lip.

Further reading

Edwards, M. & Watson, A.C.H. (Eds) (1980) *Advances in the Management of Cleft Palate.* Edinburgh: Churchill Livingstone.

Hotz, M., Gnoinski, H., Perko, M. *et al.* (Eds) (1986) *Early Treatment of Cleft Lip and Palate.* Toronto: Hans Huber.

Millard, D.R. Jr. (1976) *Cleft Craft.* Boston: Little, Brown.

11 Complications of Plastic Surgery of the Ear

Congenital Ear Deformities

These range in severity across a continuous spectrum from the prominent ear through cup ear to microtia and anotia (Fig. 11.1).

Prominent ears
Though common, in some societies prominent ears are not considered undesirable. In our own, they can be the cause of much teasing and distress.

Predisposing factors Three factors contribute to the deformity: abnormal depth of the conchal cavity, poor development of the antihelix, and prominence of the lobule. The relative contribution of each varies from ear to ear, and failure to achieve a pleasing aesthetic result from surgical correction is often due to a wrong choice of operation for the particular deformity.

Prevention of complications

Pre-operative assessment Time should be taken to discuss the problem with the patient and, if appropriate, the parents. Surgical correction should, as a rule, only be offered if the patient wishes to have it; a child does not respond well to an operation, forced on him by anxious parents, when he does not feel that he has anything wrong. On the other hand, the parents' anxiety may transmit itself to the child. Under the stress of a formal consultation, a child may deny any worries while his parents report that he is seriously upset by teasing. The degree of deformity is not important; if a child is being made miserable, he should be offered help.

The surgeon should be cautious when faced with an adult requesting otoplasty, particularly for a male, as most boys, if they survive their schooldays psychologically unscathed, accept the shape of their ears. Sometimes, presentation may be delayed simply because a patient had not known before that treatment was possible, but a significant proportion of these patients have

Figure 11.1
(a) Prominent ears; no antihelical folds.
(b) Cup ear.

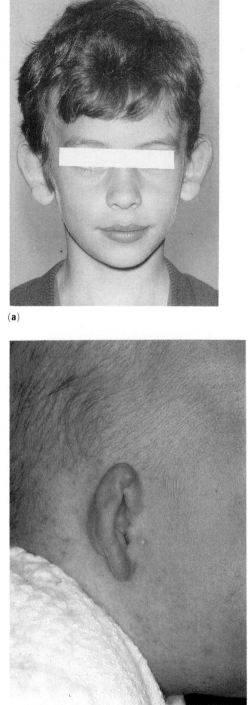

(a)

(b)

Figure 11.1 continued
(c) Microtia; no
external auditory
canal.
(d) Anotia; no pinna,
abnormal cleft.

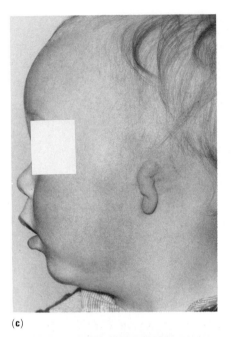

(**c**)

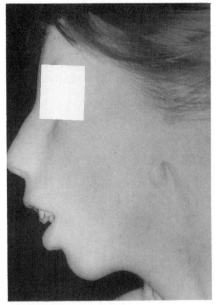

(**d**)

unrealistic expectations of surgery and should not be touched. When the surgeon is in doubt, it is sometimes helpful to offer to operate only if a psychiatrist agrees that it would be appropriate; many patients refuse such a referral but some can benefit from a combined approach.

Once the patient has been accepted for surgery, the ears must be examined carefully so that the nature of the deformity can be assessed and the operation planned. Ears with deep conchae and prominent lobules require more experience to correct than those in which the problem is confined to a poor antihelix.

If the patient complains of only one ear, the surgeon must decide whether he can achieve better symmetry by operating on both.

Timing of operation   For the reasons discussed above, surgery is usually carried out in the early years at school, or after the child has moved to secondary school. Parents presenting with babies should be reassured and asked to bring the child back if problems develop. Only if the deformity is gross, or parental anxiety so great that it is obviously communicating itself to the child, should correction be offered before the child starts primary school.

Choice of anaesthesia   In the child, the operation is performed under general anaesthesia but in adolescents and adults it can equally well be done using a local anaesthetic.

Operative techniques (otoplasty)

Most surgeons mark key points such as the crest of the desired antihelix ridge by pricking ink dots into the cartilage with a needle. A solution of adrenaline 1/100 000 is injected between skin and cartilage to decrease bleeding during surgery and to ease dissection. Incisions are almost always confined to the posterior surface of the ear and various patterns of skin excision have been advocated.

Choice of operation   Techniques of reshaping or creating an antihelix include incisions through the cartilage, scoring, thinning or abrading the anterior surface, and the insertion of non-absorbable sutures. Often a combination of these is used. A deep concha can be made shallower by the excision of a fusiform strip of its posterior wall—either cartilage alone or including skin—and it can be pinned back with sutures between cartilage and mastoid periosteum.

Once the desired shape has been achieved, haemostasis is ensured and skin is usually closed with subcuticular absorbable or pull-out sutures.

It is important that in the operation note the surgeon details the method of correction and particularly the number of any non-absorbable sutures used.

Postoperative dressing   A padded dressing is essential to maintain the position of the ear during the phase of postoperative oedema. A closely fitting dressing of flavine-impregnated or damp cotton wool is carefully applied to fill every concavity and maintain the desired shape, and held in place with a crèpe or cotton conforming bandage.

Recently a silicone foam dressing has been advocated. The dressing is kept in place for about 10 days; thereafter a head bandage is worn at night for about a month.

Complications

Early pain This is not usually severe after otoplasty. Immediate severe postoperative pain may be due to a slipped or tight dressing or to a developing haematoma.

Prevention. Pain can usually be prevented altogether by the use of bupivacaine hydrochloride either infiltrated into the ear with the adrenaline preoperatively or as a nerve block.

Treatment. Significant pain occurring in spite of this or persisting after moderate postoperative analgesia should be a signal for the dressings to be removed. If they are too tight or have slipped, they need to be adjusted. If there is a haematoma, it must be treated.

Haemorrhage This presents as blood soaking through the bandage. If the area is not extending and there is no pain, no action need be taken, since a bleeding point is rarely found.

Haematoma This presents as pain and possibly blood soaking through the dressing. It can occasionally result in infection or skin necrosis and can compromise the aesthetic result of the operation, predisposing to a cauliflower-ear deformity.

Prevention. Careful haemostasis and a well padded dressing are usually enough to prevent this complication.

Treatment. The haematoma must be evacuated under general anaesthesia, any bleeding points cauterized or ligated, and the dressing carefully reapplied.

Infection This is very rare but is suggested by pain starting 3–4 days postoperatively, possibly accompanied by a systemic upset. If it is not properly treated, it can give rise to *chondritis*—infection of the ear cartilage—which is potentially extremely damaging.

Prevention. The excellent blood supply to the ear contributes to the rarity of this complication. Routine sterile precautions during operation and measures to prevent haematoma are all that are needed to prevent it.

Treatment. Evacuation of infected haematoma and drainage of pus, as soon as they are identified, are essential. A drain should be left in the wound and a course of antibiotics commenced. Infection will usually be due to *Staphylococcus aureus* and flucloxacillin is the best first choice. Prompt treatment will prevent the development of chondritis.

If non-absorbable sutures have been used it is likely that infection will not settle until the suture or sutures concerned have been removed.

Skin necrosis The blood supply of the ear is very good and this complication is rare, but small areas of skin necrosis may occur over sharp ridges of cartilage if local pressure has been too great. Necrosis can also occur in relation to infection.

Prevention. Care to avoid sharp prominences of cartilage at the time of operation and careful application of the dressing should prevent skin necrosis.

Treatment. Small areas will heal spontaneously but, rarely, cartilage may need to be trimmed and defects sutured or closed with a local flap.

Late complications

Hypertrophic or keloid scar These are rare but the risk of them is the reason why incisions are nearly always confined to the hidden posterior surface of the ear and should not be extended to the upper or lower poles where such scars would be visible.

Treatment. Injection of triamcinolone, either alone or after scar excision. (See discussion on treatment of scars in Chapter 5.)

Exposure of sutures When buried non-absorbable sutures are used to create the antihelix fold, they tend to bridge across the concavity of the fold, deep to the post-auricular scar. They are often palpable, sometimes visible, and they occasionally become exposed through the scar or adjacent skin. They may also erode through the anterior skin.

Prevention. This risk is always present when buried sutures are used close to the skin and is one of the reasons why many surgeons prefer techniques that avoid them.

Treatment. The sutures have been passed through the cartilage and will not become completely extruded unless they are cut and withdrawn. Once one stitch has become exposed, low-grade infection is introduced and remaining sutures may have to be removed before it can be controlled.

Relapse An initial good aesthetic result may gradually relapse over several years—particularly after buried sutures have been used alone to achieve correction, because the uncorrected spring of the cartilage slowly causes the sutures to cut through. If they become exposed and have to be removed, then relapse is very likely.

Poor aesthetic results These may be due to incorrect choice of operation for the particular deformity, or to poor execution of the procedure.

An attractive result depends on the operator's aesthetic judgement. He should try to produce an ear that, seen from in front, has the whole length of the helical rim visible, passing in a smooth curve, just behind and lateral to the antihelix fold, into the lobule. The upper pole should be slightly farther from the side of the head than the lower (Fig. 11.2(a)). The lateral view should show a smoothly rounded antihelix with no sharp edges and no visible scars.

Failure of set-back

It is unusual to see a complete failure of correction as the central third of the antihelix fold seems very easy to create. However, it is common for either the upper pole or the lobule to remain prominent in the presence of a good correction (or even overcorrection) of the middle third of the ear (both together produce the so-called 'telephone ear', Fig. 11.2(b)).

Upper pole

If an anterior scoring technique has been used, failure is usually due to the scoring not being taken close enough to the helix both anterosuperiorly and posterosuperiorly. If the cartilage is incised, as in the Chongchet technique (see Further reading), this should be done close to the helix in the upper third of the ear, the incision gradually approaching the antihelix as it passes inferiorly. This allows the scoring to be taken well laterally, though it should not be too intense or the cartilage will roll too far back. During skin closure, care must be taken to ensure that the cartilage has not rolled on itself; one or two fine absorbable sutures to bring the cut edges of the cartilage together make this easier.

Figure 11.2
Anterior views of ears.
(a) Normal contour.
(b) Undercorrection of upper and lower poles. ('telephone ear')
(c) Overcorrection of helix with undercorrection of deep concha.

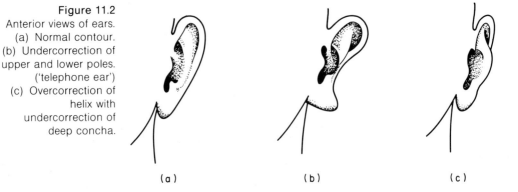

(a)   (b)   (c)

Lobule

Various ways have been recommended to overcome the problem of the protruding lobule. Posterior skin excision or a Z-plasty can be effective, but may cause distortion if overdone. Excision of the tail of the helix can also distort the rim of the ear, but the tail can be sutured behind the conchal cartilage or buried sutures can be inserted to approximate skin and conchal cartilage. Judicious use of any of these methods, or a combination of them, will allow correction of the deformity.

Over-correction

Excision of too much post-auricular skin can result in an ear lying flat against the head. It is easy to over-correct the middle third of the ear in this way. Even without excessive skin excision, if the deformity is predominantly due to a very deep concha in the presence of a well formed antihelix, any attempt to fold back the antihelix further will produce an ear that, when viewed from the front, has a helix that disappears behind the prominent posterior conchal wall. This is not a normal appearance (Fig. 11.2(c)).

Prevention

No more than a 5 mm wide strip of skin need be excised from behind the middle third of the ear, although slightly more can be taken above and below if desired. An ear with a deep concha and well formed antihelix should be corrected by an excision of the posterior conchal wall, or conchal–mastoid sutures. The antihelix should be left undisturbed unless, after conchal set-back, the upper pole still remains prominent, when the superior crus of the antihelix should be set back appropriately.

Sharp antihelix

In older techniques, such as that described by Luckett, the antihelix was created by cutting through the cartilage along the line of its crest. The resulting sharply angulated fold looked unnatural and was the reason for the great variety of operations designed to produce a smoothly rounded curve. Luckily (because it is very difficult to correct) it was nearly always accepted by patients. Attempts to disguise it by anterior scoring of the cartilage on each side of the incision are not very successful. Dermal grafts have been used to camouflage the sharpness.

Microtia

Microtia is a rare condition in Western countries and the results of construction of the microtic ear have, in general, been so disappointing that many plastic surgeons will not undertake such surgery. However, the few surgeons who have committed themselves to this work have produced remarkably good results.

The requirements for success are careful choice of patient, counselling before starting reconstruction and between stages, and meticulous planning and operative technique.

Predisposing factors

Unrealistic expectations It is impossible to reproduce the fine contours of the normal ear. The aim is to produce a structure in the right place, with an overall contour matching the normal ear, a projecting, naturally curved helix, a conchal hollow and a tragus. It should be covered with normally coloured, hairless skin and there should be the minimum of visible scars (Fig. 11.3). A lobule is usually present and should be incorporated smoothly into the reconstructed ear.

However the reconstruction is done, the presence of a framework close under the skin in an exposed position makes it vulnerable. Contact sports such as rugby football, boxing or judo are absolutely contra-indicated and this must be made clear to parents and patient before the decision for reconstruction is made. It may well make them decide against it.

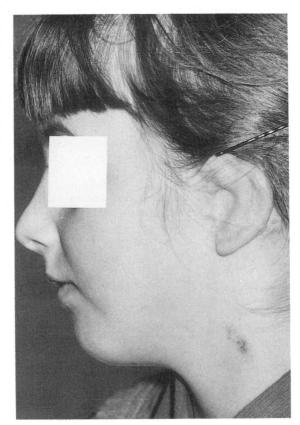

Figure 11.3
Reconstruction of microtia by Tanzer technique. Ear in good position and good inset of lobule but upper pole tilted slightly too far forward, and no tragus which mar the quality of the result.

Prevention of complications

Selection of patients Time must be spent on discussions with the parents and child before a final decision is made. The limitations of reconstruction must be made clear, preferably with photographs of an *average* result, with consideration being given to the factors mentioned above. It is in the best interests of some patients not to have a reconstruction.

Choice of technique The choice for the supporting framework lies between carved autogenous costal cartilage and preformed silastic or other implant. Each technique has its own particular complications.

Costal cartilage

The standards for this method were established by Tanzer and advanced by Brent. A block of the 6th and 7th costal cartilages from the opposite side is carved according to a pattern taken from the normal opposite ear. It is augmented by wiring on a helical rim carved from the 8th costal cartilage. This is slipped into a subcutaneous pocket over the mastoid, placed to be symmetrical with the other ear. The skin is snugged into the contours of the framework either by mattress sutures tied over boluses or by suction drainage. At subsequent procedures the framework may be elevated from the side of the head and the sulcus skin grafted and a tragus created. The lobule may be transposed into position either before or afterwards, or simultaneously.

Complications *Perforation of the pleura.* Such perforations are usually small and do not cause significant problems. As they are being closed, the anaesthetist blows up the lungs to empty the pleural cavity of air. Chest drains are unnecessary but postoperative chest X-ray is advisable.

Scarring of the chest wall. This is inevitable but can be resented by the patient when older and is a significant disadvantage of the technique.

Exposure of cartilaginous framework. As the cartilage is a living autogenous graft, this is a nuisance but not a disaster. The cartilage should be covered with a local flap.

Exposure of sutures. Sometimes sutures holding the helical rim to the main framework become exposed. The sutures can be removed under local anaesthesia and there should be no long-term problems.

Silastic implants

Absence of donor site and ready availability of silastic implants make them attractive alternatives, but there are considerable problems.

Exposure of implant Silastic implants have failed to become popular because of the very high risk of exposure. Early reports quoted 50% and, in the longer term, the great majority probably had to be removed. Ohmori protected the silastic by covering it with a flap of temporalis fascia and produced impressive results with few exposures.

Complications common to all methods of reconstruction

Positioning However good a reconstructed ear, if it is in the wrong place it looks worse than no ear. Careful planning is therefore essential but a number of factors may make positioning very difficult.

Low hair line
This must not induce the surgeon to place the ear low in order to cover it with hairless skin. Tanzer described a preliminary scalp-roll by which he tucked up the hairy scalp, closing the defect with a full-thickness skin graft. Tissue expansion can now help to overcome this problem.

Facial asymmetry
Microtia is often part of the syndrome of craniofacial micro-somia, which may make it impossible to produce a symmetrical ear reconstruction. If the asymmetry is mild then a satisfactory position for the ear can be obtained, judging by eye and not by measurements. If surgical correction of the asymmetry is planned, ear reconstruction is better postponed until that has been completed. In severe hemifacial hypoplasia there is simply no room to put an ear without it looking grotesque and it should not be attempted.

Rotation
The long axis of the ear should be parallel to the bridge of the nose. If the upper pole is too far forward relative to the lobule it will look unnatural.

Projection
A reconstructed ear should always lie close to the head. Attempts to make it project by freeing deep to the framework, inserting cartilage wedges and skin grafting are liable to make it floppy and more prone to injury. The surgeon and patient should be content with a limited freeing to define a postauricular sulcus and should set back the normal opposite ear to match the reconstructed one.

Shortage of skin cover The skin over the mastoid is inadequate to cover and follow the contours of a three-dimensional framework. Some extra skin can be provided from the microtic remnant, after the crumpled cartilage it contains has been removed. If an anterior vertical incision is used to create the pocket, tucking the skin into the contours will cause the incision to gape and the defect can be closed with a full thickness skin graft in the conchal hollow. Alternatively, preliminary tissue expansion can be used and this should avoid the need for later grafting in the retro-auricular sulcus.

Late loss of definition
After a successful reconstruction, the contours of the framework are well defined by the adherent overlying skin. On review some years later, the definition is often less obvious. Two factors may contribute to this.

1 *Absorption of cartilage.* In the absence of infection, significant absorption does not seem to occur, but a chronic low-grade infection, perhaps originating from mattress sutures or exposure of cartilage, can lead to collapse and crumpling of the graft.

2 *Tension from contracting split-skin graft in the sulcus.* This can pull the skin out of the hollows in the framework and cause collapse of the projecting helical rim. It can be avoided either by accepting the absence of a postauricular sulcus or by creating a shallow one and using a full thickness graft to line it.

Bilateral microtia
These children require middle-ear surgery to reduce their deafness. This is not easy and often results in many admissions to ENT wards. Before committing child and parents to bilateral construction of the external ears, one must balance very carefully the likely psychological benefits against the extra hospitalization and loss of schooling.

Anotia
Complete absence of the ear may be treated in the same way as microtia but the presence of a cleft, lying at a low level and passing upwards and medially, has, in this author's experience, made it impossible to produce a satisfactory reconstruction.

Further reading

Chonghet, V. (1963) A method of antihelix reconstruction. *Brit. J. Pl. Surg.*, *16*: 268.

Tanzer, R.C. (1959) Total reconstruction of the external ear. *PRS 23*: 1.

Tanzer, R.C. (1978) Microtia: a long term follow up of forty four reconstructed auricles. *PRS 61*: 161.

Brent, B. (1981) A personal approach to total auricular construction. *Clinics in Plastic Surgery 8*: 211.

12 Skin Tumours

Treatment of skin lesions is one of the major elements of plastic surgery. Skin cancer is the most common malignancy in man and its incidence is increasing. The number of complications arising must therefore be considerable, yet there is a unfortunate tendency to regard the treatment of skin lesions as minor surgery—and to delegate it to junior members of the surgical team. Careful selection must be made if patients are to receive efficient and accurate treatment, particularly in the case of malignant disease, where the penalties of inappropriate treatment can be recurrence and more major treatment for the patient. The key to successful tumour management is accurate pre-operative diagnosis, assessment and careful selection of patients for treatment, to give optimal results with a minimum of complications.

General complications

The basic complications of wound healing, such as infection, haematoma, scar formation and complication of graft and flap reconstruction, have already been discussed in Chapter 2 and in the companion volume 'Complications of Minor Surgery'.

Predisposing factors

Patient selection The patient may be under the false impression that because the lesion is small and seemingly unimportant he is wasting the surgeon's time, and may expect that a small lesion will receive minor treatment leaving minimal scarring. When the diagnosis is malignant disease, the resulting deformity may be considerable because cure of the lesion takes precedence over the cosmetic result. This must be explained to the patient, because unexpected scarring may be a major cause of patient dissatisfaction. When the proposed surgery is for diagnostic purposes or for treatment of a disfiguring benign lesion, different priorities apply. It is extremely important that the patient is not left worse off, with a more disfiguring scar. In some cases it will be better to advise against surgery for benign conditions.

Keloid scars A previous history of abnormal scar formation is a strong contra-indication to surgery, as recurrent keloid is very likely to occur. Special care is needed if the biopsy is to be performed on a benign dermal tumour that might itself be a keloid scar. Recurrence is inevitable and, if any biopsy is done, either intra-lesional biopsy or biopsy at an inconspicuous place is preferable (Fig. 12.1).

Surgical expertise   If a surgeon who is about to embark on such surgery is not confident in his knowledge or ability to cope, it is extremely important not to proceed but to seek help and refer the patient appropriately. In difficult cases, a team approach is called for and combined clinics provide a suitable forum for multi-disciplinary consultation. Suitable facilities are essential for surgical treatment, including sterile theatre conditions with good lighting and experienced assistants.

Prevention of complications

Every care should be taken to eliminate and treat all factors that might produce delayed healing and unsightly scar formation.

Pre-operative assessment   Unless the lesion is assessed correctly, both for pathological diagnosis and extent of disease, treatment cannot be planned or discussed with the patient. In particular, the presence of malignant disease must be suspected pre-operatively. A painless lump of the skin that is increasing in size is suspicious, especially if there is spontaneous bleeding or ulceration.

Figure 12.1
An injudicious biopsy was performed in this patient with keloid scars following chicken pox. The conspicious area over the shoulder should have been avoided and a biopsy near the bra strap line was preferable.

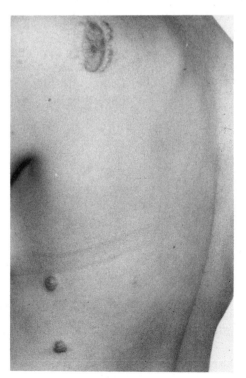

Patient consent   Matters discussed should include the likely extent of the resection, damage to deep structures that might arise during
excision, for example, facial nerve palsy if the lesion is near the
parotid, the likely method of reconstruction, and the scars that
will be left.

The treatment plan must include alternative strategies for
dealing with possible difficulties that may be encountered. In
particular, it must be pointed out that it may not be possible to
complete the operation in one stage, particularly if there is
doubt about the diagnosis and frozen-section biopsy is involved.
If radiotherapy or other treatment is to be used, the appropriate
specialist should give the patient advice and obtain consent to
the relevant parts of the treatment.

Recurrence of the lesion

The most serious complication in treatment of skin tumours is
recurrence. Recurrence implies that the lesion has been incompletely excised or inadequately treated.

Predisposing factors

Tumour type   The distinction between benign and malignant tumours is of
outstanding practical importance and the treatment required is
greatly affected by it.

Benign lesions

There is no tendency for a benign lesion to invade the local
tissue, but the outline may be irregular making resection difficult. A false capsule may be present and the whole capsule plus
contents must be excised. Cystic lesions must be excised *in toto*
as any remnant of cyst wall may give rise to recurrence.

Malignant lesions

There is potential for all malignant tumours to spread and they
do so to varying degrees depending on the histological type.
Direct invasion of the surrounding tissues can make local
excision difficult if the extent of tumour is not appreciated.
Permeation of lymphatics or perineural spread is a common
cause of local recurrence. If the lesion has already spread
beyond the surgical field, as in lymphatic spread to the lymph
nodes or by blood from metastases, excision of the primary
lesion is inevitably incomplete and additional local, nodal or
systemic therapy is needed.

Tumour behaviour   Tumours vary in their rate of growth and potential for metastasis. The speed of growth correlates with the degree of differ-
entiation of the primary tumour. A well-differentiated tumour
closely resembles the tissue of the origin, grows slowly and
metastasizes less readily. Poorly differentiated (anaplastic)
tumours grow rapidly, spread vigorously and have a much

poorer prognosis because of their capacity for recurrence and metastasis.

The clinicopathological diagnosis determines the pattern of tumour behaviour. Basal-cell carcinomas rarely metastasize but are locally invasive. The squamous-cell carcinoma has variable behaviour but is both locally malignant and develops secondary metastases. Malignant melanoma is highly malignant and has a large potential for metastatic spread.

Surgical techniques

Tumours, benign or malignant, can be seeded in the surgical field causing recurrence. Malignant lesions can also, theoretically, be disseminated widely if handled roughly or squeezed. Gentle, no-touch technique is essential. If a tourniquet is applied, exsanguination by an Esmark bandage should be avoided as the tumour may be traumatized and spread by blood or lymphatics. Once the tumour is removed, the wound should be irrigated to remove loose cells.

The flap or graft donor site should be cleaned separately and kept covered until the resection is complete. If a split-skin graft is required it should, preferably, be taken from another limb.

Prevention of complications

Pre-operative assessment

Diagnosis. Tumour identification is usually based on the clinical features. If there is any doubt it is essential to perform a diagnostic biopsy before proceeding.

Extent of lesion. The anatomical site of the tumour must be determined. A mobile lesion is unlikely to be deeply invasive. Examination under anaesthetic can be performed at the same time as diagnostic biopsy in difficult cases.

X-ray examination, including CT scans, may also be useful, especially in the head and neck region. The true extent of the primary can sometimes be fully evaluated only after histological examination of the excised specimen.

Clinical staging. Gauging the extent of the primary tumour and any metastatic spread is essential if a malignant tumour is to be treated. Full clinical examination should include assessment of the draining lymph nodes. Chest X-ray, full blood count and liver function tests should be performed. Scanning by isotopes for bone and brain metastases can also be included with CT scans as necessary, if there is cause to suspect disseminated spread.

Plan the treatment

Once a full assessment and diagnosis has been made, the treatment priorities can be established to treat the disease in the context of the whole patient.

● Early primary disease is best treated by surgery.

- If the tumour is anaplastic, radiotherapy can be added either before or after surgery or as a split treatment before and after.
- In some circumstances, if the patient is not fit for surgery or anaesthesia, or if surgery would mean sacrificing vital structures, radiotherapy alone can be used. There is little place for prophylatic chemotherapy in skin cancer.
- If the primary disease is extensive and near important structures, combined consultation at the planning stage with the appropriate specialist will help to avoid unexpected results with change of treatment that may upset the patient and relatives, who might suspect that the line of treatment is uncertain.
- When the disease is widely disseminated and the chance of cure has gone, different priorities apply. There is no justification for the radical surgical *'tour de force'* just because the technology is available, although palliative resection may be indicated to prevent fungation. If the disease is sensitive, systemic chemotherapy would be more logical, but severe side-effects may outweigh the benefits of treatment.
- Reconstruction of the defect to be left by extirpation of the tumour must also be planned in advance. If possible, primary reconstruction is carried out to improve the patient's quality of life and avoid multiple operations with greater risk of complication. Alternative plans for unexpected problems must always be considered, particularly if the tumour proves to be inoperable. If reconstruction is very difficult, for example after nose, ear or orbital resection, a well-made prosthesis may save countless operations and donor scars and give a much more aesthetic result (Fig. 1.5).

Surgical techniques

Anaesthesia   Local or general anaesthetic can be used depending on the size and site of the lesion and the personality of the patient. Local anaesthetic with an added vasoconstrictor such as adrenaline gives the advantage of a bloodless field. It is extremely important that the local anaesthetic is not injected directly into the lesion. A local field or regional block should be used (Fig. 12.2).

Biopsy   If there is any doubt about the clinical diagnosis, a biopsy should be performed, but care should be taken to see that nothing is done to make the treatment more difficult.

Type of biopsy
For superficial lesions, a shave biopsy may be suitable. A punch or curettage biopsy is also possible but does not give a true picture of the whole lesion or the edge of the lesion. In many cases it is the edge of the lesion that gives important diagnostic

Figure 12.2
Field block local
anaesthetic technique.
The needle should
never be inserted
directly into the lesion,
to avoid possible
spread of infection or
tumour, or disruption
of the specimen, which
interferes with the
pathology.

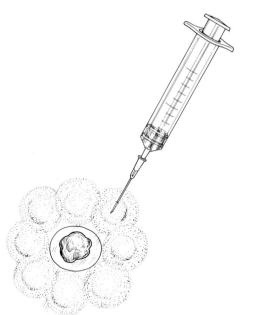

clues to the pathologist. Cytology is not sufficiently accurate in most instances and additional biopsy is required.

Excision biopsy is ideal for small lesions (Fig. 12.3). Incisional biopsy should remove a representative piece of the lesion that includes a small area of adjacent normal skin.

In treating malignant disease, the surgical biopsy wound must also be excised. Therefore, care is essential, in placing the biopsy, not to enlarge the defect, or to transgress into or open up deep tissue planes (Fig. 12.4). For this reason, the biopsy is best done by or under the supervision of the surgeon who will be responsible for the definitive treatment.

Care of the specimen
The specimen must be handled gently and not crushed with instruments as this will break up the architecture and cause cellular distortion. It must be labelled adequately to identify it and if necessary marked with a suture to help the pathologist to orientate it. *All* specimens must be sent for histological examination. Shave biopsy or thin, fragile specimens should be placed on card before fixing so as to aid orientation and handling by the pathologist. Frozen-section examination, if available, may speed up the process of treatment and allow excision and reconstruction in one operation, thereby minimizing complications. But it may not be possible to get a firm diagnosis, in which case paraffin sections will be required. If it is possible it is most convenient to arrange the biopsy under local anaesthetic with the patient starved and prepared for general anaesthesia. If

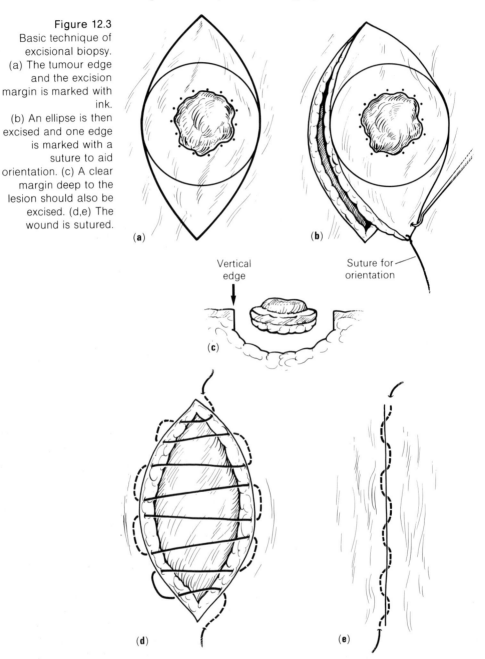

Figure 12.3
Basic technique of
excisional biopsy.
(a) The tumour edge
and the excision
margin is marked with
ink.
(b) An ellipse is then
excised and one edge
is marked with a
suture to aid
orientation. (c) A clear
margin deep to the
lesion should also be
excised. (d,e) The
wound is sutured.

(a)

(b)

Vertical
edge

Suture for
orientation

(c)

(d)

(e)

the frozen-section biopsy is positive, appropriate treatment can
then proceed without delay under general anaesthesia if necessary. This shortens the anaesthesia time. If the result is uncertain, the wound can be dressed or sutured and the patient is
returned to the ward to await the result of paraffin sections.

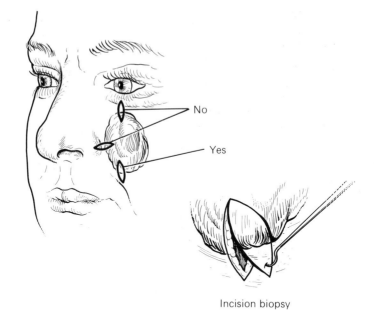

Figure 12.4
Incision biopsy. A
section of normal
surrounding skin
should be included in
the specimen to aid
the pathologist. The
direction of the biopsy
should not transgress
anatomical zones if
possible.

No

Yes

Incision biopsy

Marking the tumour

The tumour should be inspected under a good strong operating light and its margins marked. The use of magnification such as operating loupes may be very helpful.

Tumour edge
It is usually quite easy to identify the tumour edge. In the case of the basal cell carcinoma, skin infiltration may be missed (Fig. 12.5) and a useful technique for seeing the full extent is to spread the skin gently. The tumour will blanch more than the surrounding skin, to reveal the characteristic pearly appearance (Fig. 12.6a,b,c). Gentle palpation will usually give a good guide to subcutaneous infiltration by tumour. Pre-operative investigations such as CT scans can also help to determine the tumour margin. The infiltrating basal cell carcinoma is notoriously difficult to treat and the full extent of tumour can easily be missed by the inexperienced or unsuspecting surgeon (Fig. 12.7).

Vascular lesions are best marked without any tension on the skin, as they may be blanched by pressure. It is also essential in the case of pink lesions such as Bowen's disease or Paget's disease that the margin of the lesion is marked *before* infiltration with local anaesthetic, particularly if a vasoconstrictor is used.

Margin of excision
This will vary with the type of lesion that is being treated and should be marked on the skin around the lesion (Table 12.1). Because in many cases the exact histology including type and grade of tumour cannot be readily confirmed until after excision

Figure 12.5
Diagram to illustrate the difficulty in determining the edge of a basal-cell carcinoma depending on the morphological type of tumour.

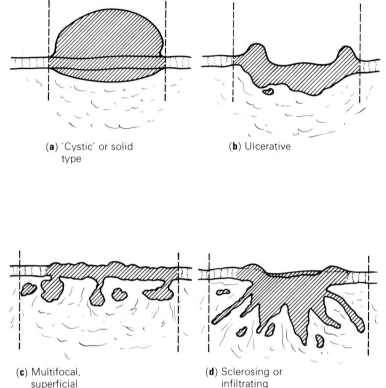

(**a**) 'Cystic' or solid type

(**b**) Ulcerative

(**c**) Multifocal, superficial

(**d**) Sclerosing or infiltrating

of the complete lesion and its pathological examination, frozen-section biopsy or a staged excision may be indicated. The deep margin of excision is generally similar to that marked on the skin but it is not always possible to plan this until the excision gets under way.

Excision   Adequate excision of the tumour, both in surface area and depth, is an essential prerequisite for repair and reconstruction. Careful, sharp dissection of the excised specimen is required with a gentle no-touch and non-crush technique to prevent seeding and contamination of the surgical field. This is particularly important in ulcerated or fungating lesions to prevent contamination of the wound with mitotic cells or pathogenic organisms.

The excision of the tumour must not be compromised to make the repair easy. Any doubts about completeness of excision must be resolved at the time of operation. If tumour is cut at the edge of the specimen, a further width or depth must be excised as necessary. Frozen-section examination can be used to assess the completeness of excision. Hypotensive anaesthesia and a skilled assistant using a fine suction to produce a bloodless field will help to minimize errors.

Figure 12.6
The tumour edge is not the ulcer edge (a). Gentle compression of this ulcerative basal-cell carcinoma shows a zone of blanching (b), which is dotted in with ink (c). (d) The excision margin is then marked and also the flap to be used based on an aesthetic unit, the cheek. The final result at operation (e), and on follow up at ten years (f).

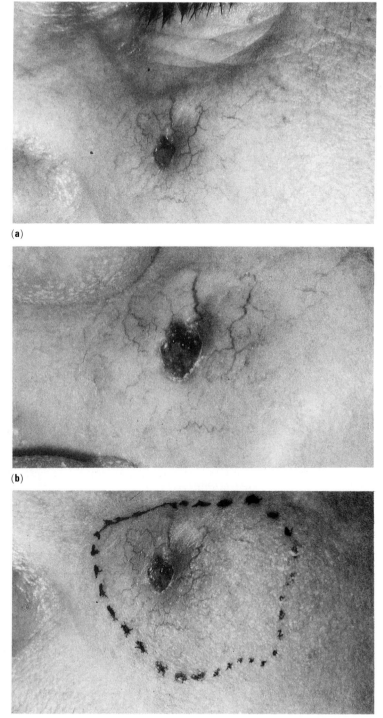

(a)

(b)

(c)

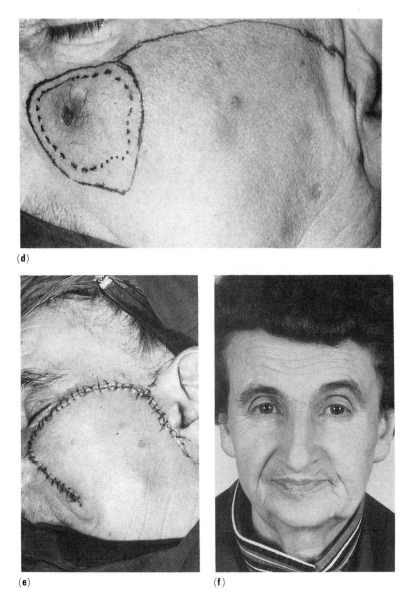

(d)

(e)   (f)

Assessment of
excised specimen
This is an essential part of treatment. The specimen must be inspected by the surgeon at the time of excision to ensure that the tumour has been completely excised. To aid the pathologist, an orientation mark such as a suture should be made and the clearly labelled specimen must be sent for histology. The histology report must contain details of the morphological type of tumour, level of penetration, vascular lymphatic or nerve infiltration and completeness of excision.

Figure 12.7
The infiltrating basal-cell carcinoma is notoriously difficult to diagnose. This patient had radiotherapy and excision and flap repair for this tumour of the inner canthus 20 years previously. Watering of the eye was her only complaint, but the displacement of the globe (a) and the pearly induration (b) are an indication of extensive infiltration, which required exenteration of the orbit.

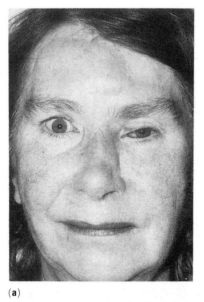

(**a**)

(**b**)

Table 12.1
Suggested excision margins for skin tumours

Benign lesions	0.1 cm sufficient to excise lesion completely
Benign subcutaneous lesions	No routine skin excision necessary
Premalignant skin lesions	0.1–0.5 cm all round and deep
Basal-cell carcinoma	0.2–1.0 cm all round and deep
	Small margins for tumours less than 1 cm diameter
	Larger margins for tumours more than 1 cm diameter
Squamous-cell carcinoma	1.0–2.0 cm all round and deep
Malignant melanoma	1.0 cm skin margin per millimetre of thickness
	Depth to deep fascia only
	See Chapter 13
Sarcoma	1.0–2.0 cm

Reconstruction   When a flap repair is to be used, it is vital that the lesion be completely excised. If confirmation of this is not available, a temporary repair using a split-skin graft is preferable, this acting as a 'window' through which a recurrence can be more easily detected. This graft may prove satisfactory but can always be excised later and reconstructed. Flap repair over an incompletely excised tumour is a disaster, because further excision carried out later will usually entail sacrifice of the reconstruction.

Follow-up and postoperative care   The basic principles of postoperative care of wounds is covered in Chapters 2, 3 and 4. After wound healing has been obtained, the most important measure is to arrange long-term follow-up of the patient if malignant disease has been treated. The patient with a squamous-cell lesion should be seen for follow-up every two or three months initially, increasing the intervals to six months later. At each visit the patient should be asked if anything new has occurred. Follow-up can usually be discontinued after five years. Examination should include a search for local recurrence and examination of draining lymph nodes. After excision of a basal cell carcinoma, follow-up should be for one or two years unless the lesion has been incompletely excised or if it is at the inner canthus, side of the nose or near the ear.

Lymph node dissection   Elective lymph node dissection is not usually required for skin tumours. Therapeutic lymph node dissection is performed as necessary. The complications of lymph node dissection are discussed in Chapter 13.

Management of incomplete excision

Unexpected malignancy shown by histopathology   If the margin of excision is found to be adequate on histology, even though the diagnosis of malignancy is unexpected, an expectant policy can be adopted with careful follow-up. However, if there is any doubt about the excision margins, re-excision or referral for other treatment such as radiotherapy is essential.

Excision inadequate on histology   The tumour may be found at the margin of excision or within one high-power field. This does not mean that recurrence is inevitable but the chances of recurrence are much higher. A basal cell carcinoma at special sites such as the inner canthus, ala of nose or ear, a squamous-cell carcinoma, or a sarcoma should be re-excised. Basal-cell carcinoma elsewhere need not be re-excised but should be followed up carefully.

Alternatively, the patient can be referred for radiotherapy. Another important finding that suggests incomplete local excision is perineural spread. Re-excision is usually recommended, but a decision will depend on the type of tumour. Vascular or lymphatic invasion by tumour is also a bad sign and careful follow-up is required, paying particular attention to draining lymph-node areas. Prophylactic chemotherapy is rarely indicated in the treatment of skin malignancy.

Tumour not resectable It may be found on exploration that the tumour is too extensive to excise as it involves vital structures. The operation then becomes palliative and the main aim should be to debulk the tumour, avoiding any surgical damage that would unnecessarily increase postoperative morbidity. A decision may be made to cover the defect with a flap to aid hygiene and patient comfort. Radiotherapy and chemotherapy can be used as necessary postoperatively.

Recurrence The incidence and site of recurrence depends on the type of tumour being treated. Squamous-cell carcinoma is more likely to spread to nodes. Basal-cell carcinoma will spread locally if it recurs. Forty per cent of patients with a basal-cell carcinoma develop a second lesion on follow-up within five years. The treatment of recurrent disease is similar in principle to the treatment of primary malignancy but there is a different balance of factors to be taken into account. Particularly important is a search for widespread secondary disease.

- For isolated local recurrence re-excision or radiotherapy is indicated.
- After radiotherapy has been used previously, repetition of it would give rise to radionecrosis and the treatment of choice is surgical. If possible, the area of radiotherapy-treated skin should also be excised and flap reconstruction is required because skin-graft take will be poor.
- When there is widespread disease or, if the tumour is unresectable, palliative treatment is indicated. The emphasis is on relieving symptoms to keep the patient comfortable. Radiotherapy, chemotherapy or surgical resection of selected areas should be considered. In general, removal is desirable of the primary or any skin secondary lesion that is likely to fungate.
- Pain relief is very important by analgesics or nerve blocks as necessary.

Complications of benign lesions

When the skin lesion is benign, particularly if it is to be removed for cosmetic reasons, it is essential to consider the degree of scarring that will result from the operation. Alternative treatment such as skin camouflage to disguise a flat blemish may be preferable to surgery. The patient must have no illusions about the degree of scars that will result and full consent is essential.

Keratoacanthoma The diagnosis must be made with extreme caution and the lesion must be treated with respect. The most important complication is mistaken diagnosis. The problem is that a rapidly advancing lesion with the features of a keratoacanthoma may be a squamous-cell carcinoma (Fig. 12.8). If it is a squamous-cell carcinoma, the rapid growth means that the rate of spread will be rapid and the prognosis poor. It is therefore preferable with any suspected keratoacanthoma to perform excision biopsy, if practicable. It will result in a better scar and afford the chance of full histological examination of the lesion.

Pyogenic granuloma
Mistaken diagnosis is a dangerous complication. It is essential to send all curettings for histological examination to exclude malignant disease. Such a lesion on the hand should be X-rayed

Figure 12.8
(a) A 'typical keratoacanthoma'. (b) A similar lesion of the left outer canthus. Both proved to be squamous-cell carcinomata on excision biopsy. Any lesion that grows progressively should be treated as suspicious and biopsied.

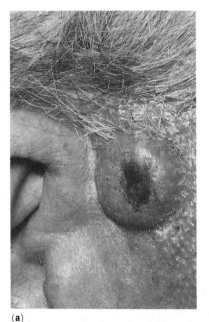

(a)

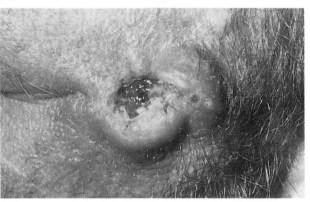

(b)

pre-operatively and inspected at operation for the presence of underlying foreign body.

Cysts A large variety of cysts occur in the skin. Special care must be taken at special sites such as the outer canthus, pre-auricular, midline of the nose, midline of the neck or lateral neck to exclude congenital developmental dermoid cysts. There may be deep extensions and careful exploration and excision is required. Simple enucleation may not be adequate treatment and the whole cyst plus any capsule and attached track must be excised completely, otherwise recurrence is inevitable.

Infected cysts should be drained to allow the infection to settle before excision is attempted. Chronic discharging sinuses must be adequately investigated before excision is attempted. Such lesions in the cheeks or over the lower jaw may be derived

Figure 12.9
Multiple neurofibromata (a) are most easily treated by excision using cutting diathermy to limit blood loss (b).

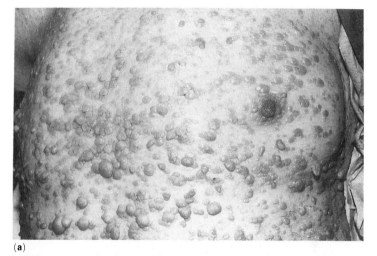

(a)

(b)

from deep sepsis (for example, a retained tooth root) and X-ray examination of the jaw is indicated. Removal of the retained root will cure the sinus.

Neurofibroma Most neurofibromata are small and usually multiple and may be excised for diagnostic or cosmetic reasons (Fig 12.9). Large tumours can give rise to pain and pressure on nerve trunks, depending on their site. A common complication of excising the larger ones is haemorrhage, which may be catastrophic, and it is essential to prepare for loss by having a drip running and cross-matched blood available for transfusion prior to the operation. Hypotensive anaesthesia is useful for diminishing blood loss.

The most serious complication is malignant change. Treatment is by wide resection with a clear margin of several centimetres, followed by radiotherapy.

Persisting controversies

- The use of frozen section pathology in surgical treatment of skin tumours.
- The 'safe' margin of excision for malignant tumours.
- The indications for and value of, follow-up consultations.

Further reading

Emmett, A.J.J. & O'Rourke, M.G.E. (Eds) (1982) *Malignant Skin Tumours*. Edinburgh: Churchill Livingstone.

Mandel, M.A. (Ed) (1980) Skin Tumours. *Clinics in Plastic Surgery*. Philadelphia: Saunders.

13 Pigmented Lesions

The pigment melanin is produced by melanocytes, cells of neuroectodermal origin found chiefly in the basal cell layer of the epidermis but also in the choroid of the eye and mucosal surfaces around the mouth, paranasal sinuses and the perineum. Melanin is chiefly responsible for the colour of the skin, although skin thickness, vascularity and other factors play a role. The physiological role of melanin is to protect the body from excessive exposure to ultraviolet light. In dark-skinned races and tanned individuals, the concentration of melanin in the skin is increased. Pigmented skin lesions are usually caused by a localized increase in the numbers of melanocytes. The management of skin pigmentation caused by extraneous pigment such as tattooing is discussed in Chapter 5.

Benign pigmented lesions

The vast majority of benign pigmented lesions are moles (or naevi). Congenital naevi are present at birth; acquired naevi, which develop later in childhood and early adult life, are probably present but invisible at birth. They reveal themselves by growing or becoming pigmented later. The general complications of treatment of naevi are similar to those for removal of other benign skin lesions discussed in Chapter 12. In addition, there are several specific complications that can arise.

Malignant change

Malignant change can present in several ways, as a primary lesion or by secondary metastasis (Fig. 13.1). Unfortunately, many lay people and some medical practitioners believe, erroneously, that a mole should never be removed because trauma to a mole might induce malignant transformation. In practice, however, when a pigmented lesion bothers a patient it usually means that a malignant change *has already developed* and excision or biopsy is *not* the cause of change. Local recurrence or secondary spread after excision of a supposedly benign naevus indicates that the original lesion was already malignant but unrecognized as such at the initial excision. (Fig. 13.2).

Prevention Approximately one-third of malignant melanomas develop in pre-existing pigmented lesions. However, the chance of any one particular naevus becoming malignant is very slight. The aver-

Figure 13.1
(a) Biopsy of an enlarged node in the neck revealed metastatic melanoma. The primary is visible at the right inner canthus (b). After initially increasing in size, the primary had been getting smaller for several weeks and this spontaneous regression makes diagnosis very difficult.

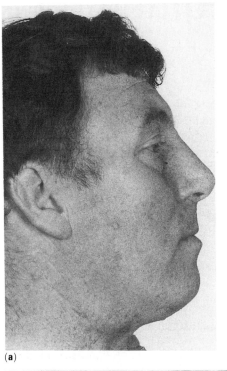

(a)

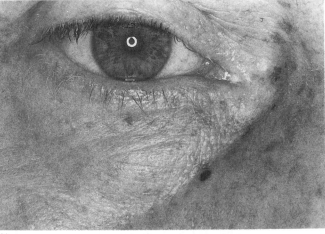

(b)

age white person has about 40 moles. Prophylactic excision of benign moles is therefore not an appropriate or realistic proposition except in rare cases of the dysplastic naevus syndrome or the giant hairy naevus, when there is an appreciable risk of malignant change.

Uncertainty about the diagnosis of malignancy can be prevented in two ways.

Figure 13.2
This patient with
recurrence at a biopsy
site presented with
enlarged nodes in the
neck. Six months
previously an
enlarging, itchy,
bleeding mole on the
back of the scalp had
been removed but not
sent for histological
examination. This
history suggested that
at the time of the
biopsy the lesion was
already a malignant
melanoma.

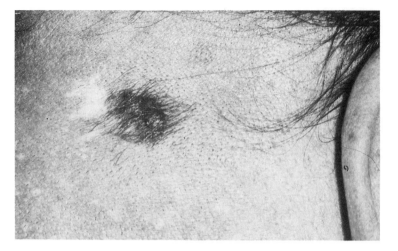

1 Maintain a high index of suspicion that any pigmented lesion that has changed its size, shape or colour or, on examination, has an irregular colour pattern, surface or edge, may be malignant and must be treated appropriately.
2 It is a sound policy to send all lesions, especially pigmented lesions, that are excised for histopathological examination (Fig. 13.2).

Incomplete excision
Prevention of complication due to incomplete excision is a matter of technical expertise. Lateral incomplete excision can arise if the edge of the naevus is indistinct or pale (Fig. 13.3) and careful marking in a good light is essential before excision. The other main problem is incomplete excision in depth, particularly in hairy naevi when recurrent hair growth in the scar may cause a problem.

Management   If the lesion is benign it is not essential to re-excise the lesion, but if there is any junctional activity in the biopsy specimen, then follow-up is indicated. If there is recurrence, excision should be carried out. Hair growth can be treated by ensuring that the re-excision extends below the depth of the hair follicles that are deep to the skin.

Giant hairy naevi

Giant pigmented naevi are variably defined by several authorities as, for example, those lesions that involve an area greater than 144 square inches or cover the major portion of the face or a hand. They can, for practical purposes, be taken to be any

Figure 13.3
(a,b) Incomplete
excision caused
recurrent pigmentation
in this scar following
removal of a benign
pigmented lesion.
(c) The result of
further excision seen
one year later.

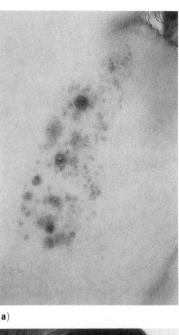

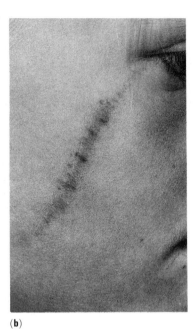

(a)

(b)

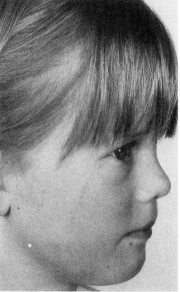

(c)

pigmented hairy lesion occupying more than 1% of the total
body surface. Some may be gigantic, occupying up to 50% of the
body surface. Prophylactic excision of these lesions is important
as there is an increased chance of malignant change developing
in the lifetime of the patient. A policy of observing the lesions
and treating them expectantly is difficult because they have a

variegated appearance (see Fig. 13.4) that makes malignant change difficult to diagnose, and because rapid spread is common, once malignancy develops. They also present a severe cosmetic disability and treatment is indicated for this reason alone.

Surgical technique

By virtue of their size, direct closure of the defect after excision of a giant naevus will be impossible. Graft or skin-flap repair must be planned in advance and discussed with the patient, if the patient is old enough to understand, and with the parents. Donor sites for skin grafts may be limited, in which case mesh grafts can be used. If there are multiple moles on the prospective donor site, they should be excised on a prior occasion, as skin grafts with moles in them give a most ugly cosmetic appearance.

If the giant naevus is particularly large, excision will present a major task with the appreciable risks of a long operation and blood loss. In these cases, serial partial excision is indicated.

Dermabrasion   Early, deep dermabrasion in the neonatal period before the child has reached the age of 4 weeks has been advocated as a way of

Figure 13.4
Giant hairy naevus.
The typical variegated
appearance makes
follow-up with
detection of change
very difficult.

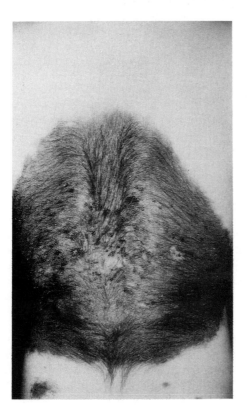

removing giant naevi. The outer pigmented layer is easily removed and the skin heals with a pale colour. However, recurrence of pigmentation is a problem and, if the naevi are treated after the age of 3 months, recurrence is inevitable.

Dermabrasion for treatment of pigmented lesions has several complications, the chief of which is the chance of scarring if the dermabrasion is too deep, or if infection occurs, giving rise to a deep wound that heals slowly.

Chemical peeling is not indicated for pigmented moles. Skin-bleach treatment may mask malignant change and delay treatment.

Camouflage   In appropriate cases, skin camouflage therapy is an alternative to be considered, particularly in the large pigmented lesions that are flat and non-hairy, for which excision and grafting would give rise to more noticeable scarring.

Malignant melanoma

The incidence of malignant melanoma is increasing worldwide and is doubling in incidence approximately every ten years. It used to be thought that the prognosis was poor, but if it is diagnosed and treated at an early stage it is a curable form of cancer. The major problem in treating the disease is establishing the diagnosis at *an early stage*. Unfortunately, many melanomas are missed until a late stage because they seem innocuous at first. The clear-cut symptoms and signs that alert the patient and are easily recognized, such as bleeding, ulceration and satellite formation, are signs of late disease. If diagnosis is late, recurrence or extension and spread of the disease is more likely.

Predisposing factors

Missed melanoma

Errors of diagnosis   Diagnosis of the type and extent of disease is essential before treatment is performed. The differential diagnosis of malignant melanomas is very wide and there are several recognized difficult diagnostic situations in which a melanoma can be overlooked. A melanoma in the hair line or on an unexposed surface may not be seen. Subungual melanomas, particularly amelanotic lesions, are notoriously difficult to diagnose and a specimen must be sent for histology (Fig. 13.5).

Inadequate excision   As with all malignant lesions, incomplete excision usually leads to local recurrence of disease. Malignant melanoma has a tendency to spread locally in the dermal lymphatics and recurrence is more likely unless appropriately wide excision is performed.

Figure 13.5
(a) Subungual
melanoma.
(b) Amelanotic
melanoma. Both
lesions are easily
misdiagnosed as
infected granulation
tissue. This error can
be prevented by
maintaining a high
index of suspicion and
sending a biopsy of all
such lesions for
pathological
examination.

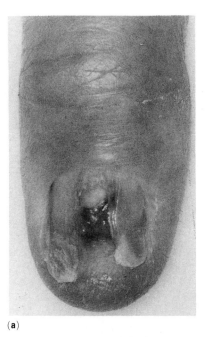

(a)

(b)

Figure 13.5 (a) Subungual melanoma. (b) Amelanotic melanoma. Both lesions are easily misdiagnosed as infected granulation tissue. This error can be prevented by maintaining a high index of suspicion and sending a biopsy of all such lesions for pathological examination.

Prevention of complications

Early diagnosis and treatment

Avoiding delay in treatment by efficient early diagnosis can improve the prognosis of malignant melanoma. Experience and a thorough knowledge of the clinical features of melanoma will help to avoid errors (Fig. 13.6). Patient and doctor education campaigns are required to alert patients with early lesions to attend for treatment (Fig. 13.6c).

Biopsy to confirm the diagnosis

All suspicious lesions should be biopsed. Excision biopsy is the method of choice because it allows a full histological assessment of the whole lesion for diagnosis of morphological type, level of

Figure 13.6
The clinical features of
melanoma can be
quite variable.
Contrast these more
easily recognised
melanomas with those
in Fig. 13.5.
(a) Superficial
spreading melanoma
with a nodule 1 cm in
diameter at the lower
edge. (b) Nodular
melanoma 1 cm
diameter. (c) Early
superficial spreading
melanoma. (d) lentigo
maligma melanoma of
left cheek.

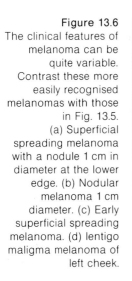

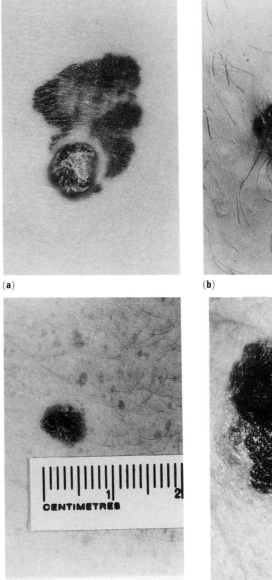

(a)

(b)

(c)

invasion and tumour thickness, allowing prognostic evaluation. Frozen sections can be obtained if there are trained staff available. Alternatively, paraffin sections can be obtained within 48 hours.

The excision biopsy should preferably be performed by, or under the direction of, the surgeon responsible for definitive treatment, with a gentle no-touch technique to avoid the theoretical risk of seeding or spreading the tumour by handling it. The biopsy should include a small margin of normal skin (0.5–1.0 cm) around the lesion and adequate subcutaneous tissue to excise the lesion in depth.

Incision biopsy is permissible but must be followed by immediate definitive treatment. If melanoma is present, the prognostic factors can only be determined fully if the whole lesion is examined histologically.

Assess the patient   All patients should be fully examined clinically to check for other primary or secondary lesions. Chest radiography should be performed. Bone, brain, or liver scans and CAT scans can be performed, if necessary, to search for secondary spread if the history or clinical examination have suggested any abnormalities. Having determined the stage of the disease (Table 13.1) and the histological diagnosis, appropriate treatment can be planned and discussed with the patient.

Primary tumour

Adequate treatment   Complete excision of the primary melanoma with a margin of surrounding normal skin is the treatment of choice (Fig. 13.7). Each lesion requires individual evaluation according to the prognostic features. The most accurate prognostic indicator is the tumour thickness measured under the microscope on the fixed specimen (Breslow thickness, Table 13.2). The surrounding margin of skin is removed because it may contain micrometastases. The width of the excision margin is controversial but a balance must be struck between adequate excision and the avoidance of unnecessarily wide disfiguring scars (Table 13.3).

Table 13.1
Clinical staging of
malignant melonoma

I	Local
II	Nodal disease
III	Widespread disseminated disease

Table 13.2
Prognosis of
malignant melanoma

Tumour Breslow thickness (mm)	Prognosis	Approximate 5-year survival
<0.75	Good	>95%
0.76–1.49	Intermediate	90%
1.5–3.0	Poor	50%
>3.0	Very poor	<40%

Table 13.3
Suggested excision margin of primary malignant melanoma

Breslow thickness (mm)	Excision margin (cm)*
<0.75	1
0.76–1.49	1–2
>1.5	2–5

*Margin wider if ulceration or regression in primary. Margin narrower on head and face, wider on trunk.

Lymph nodes

In Stage II disease, therapeutic lymph-node dissection is indicated. Prophylactic dissection may be performed in poor-prognosis cases, but only if the draining lymph node area can be defined with certainty. If a tumour is sited over or near to a lymphatic drainage site, it may be convenient to include a node dissection in continuity with the excision of the primary. In very poor-prognosis patients, there is a high chance of blood-borne metastases developing and prophylactic lymph-node dissection is not indicated.

Advanced disease

For Stage III disease, excision of the primary tumour is usually performed because it may help to prevent the unfortunate

Figure 13.7
(a,b) The excision margin required for treatment of a malignant melanoma should be marked around the edge of the total lesion, not the edge of the nodular area.

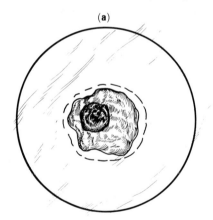

(a)

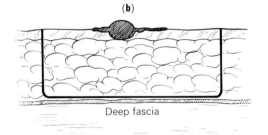

(b)

Deep fascia

complication of fungating local disease. Similarly, isolated secondaries can also be treated surgically. If the disease is confined to a limb, isolated hyperthermic perfusion using chemotherapeutic agents, such as melphelan, can be very helpful in symptomatic relief and in preventing or delaying fungation. For widespread disease, treatment by systemic chemotherapy should be considered, but the complication rate is high.

Surgical technique

Once a diagnosis has been confirmed, the margin to be excised must be planned and marked at operation. If a skin graft is to be required, it must be harvested before the melanoma is excised and must be taken from another limb. This is to prevent the possible spread of blood-borne or lymphatic secondaries to the donor site.

The specimen excised must include a disc of full-thickness skin and subcutaneous fat down to the deep fascia. It is not necessary to remove the deep fascia routinely, since it makes no difference to the prognosis unless the tumour involves the deep fascia, in which case a deeper excision is required.

Direct closure or flap repair will help to minimize the resulting scar, but a skin graft will be necessary when the defect is large. The size of the cosmetic defect can be reduced by undercutting the margin of excision into the surrounding subcutaneous fat and advancing and suturing the wound margin to the deep fascia with an absorbable suture. This has the added advantage of aiding haemotasis and stabilizing the bed to aid graft take (Fig. 13.8).

(a)

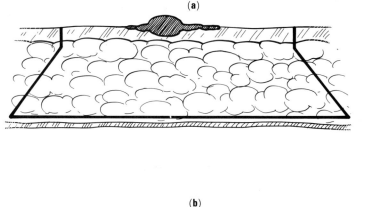

Figure 13.8
A method of excision used in attempting to avoid the punched-out appearance of the defect after removal of a melanoma (a). The dermis of the wound margin is sutured down to the deep fascia before the skin graft is applied (b).

(b)

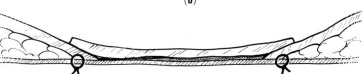

Postoperative care and follow up

Particularly in the lower limb, rest and support is required to assist graft healing and minimize oedema that can be caused by excision of a large skin area with its lymphatics. Elastic support will be needed for at least 2 months. If oedema can be prevented in the early postoperative phase, it rarely causes problems.

Early detection and treatment of local recurrent or lymph-node spread will improve the prognosis. Frequent follow-up examination is indicated every 2 months for 18 months and then 3-monthly up to 3 years. After 3 years the incidence of recurrence declines and follow-up at 6-monthly intervals is usually sufficient but the patient must be warned to return immediately if he suspects any recurrence rather than waiting until the next follow-up visit.

Management of complications

Recurrent disease The most appropriate treatment must be carefully planned after full evaluation of the individual patient. The choice available will depend on such factors as the patient's age and general fitness, the stage of the disease, the degree of spread and the presence or absence of symptoms. Local recurrence can be re-excised widely. Involved lymph nodes should be excised by block dissection. There is a place for palliative treatment by further excision of other lesions to prevent fungation. Radiotherapy is useful for palliation. Chemotherapy is the most appropriate treatment for widely disseminated disease, but if the patient is asymptomatic it may be better to withhold treatment because complications such as vomiting, anorexia, neuropathy and alopecia are common and there is as yet no really effective chemotherapeutic agent for melanoma.

Unsightly scar The extent of excision to remove all the subcutaneous fat causes an unsightly, punched out, depressed scar, particularly on the limbs in females, where there is a greater proportion of subcutaneous fat. It has been found that if the patient is carefully counselled pre-operatively about the true extent of the defect and, if necessary, shown photographs of representative results, acceptance of the scar is much better and causes less distress.

Once the scar has healed and softened, there are several possible alternative strategies.

1 Serial excision of the scar, advancing local tissue to fill the defect.
2 Tissue expansion followed by advancement of local skin.
3 Excision of the graft and flap repair.
4 In carefully selected cases, the surrounding fat can be thinned. Suction lipectomy of the subcutaneous fat is a useful technique for doing this easily and efficiently to smooth off the contours.

5 A soft, flesh-coloured custom-made silastic prosthesis worn under stockings will fill out the defect (Fig. 13.9).

6 Camouflage treatment with cosmetics is relatively ineffective but can be used to disguise the colour change that sometimes develops in the grafted area. Ultraviolet sun-block cream is also advisable to stop the relatively greater tanning of a grafted area.

Complications of lymph-node dissection

Predisposing factors

Anaesthesia Full general anaesthetic is essential to allow adequate access and exposure. Hypotensive anaesthesia, by reducing bleeding, makes node dissection easier and safer, particularly in the neck.

Surgical expertise The surgeon must be familiar with the anatomy of the region and suitably experienced to perform the surgery. Careful tissue handling with meticulous dissection to avoid injury to major nerves and vessels is required. If the thoracic duct is damaged it must be ligated, if possible, to prevent a chylous fistula.

Wound healing All the general problems of wound healing occur in block dissections. In addition, the main object of a block dissection is to remove all the soft tissue from groin, axilla or neck. Wide flaps are cut to give adequate exposure and some of the blood supply to them is then removed as part of the excision, giving

Figure 13.9 (a,b) A custom made silastic prosthesis worn to disguise a depressed scar following excision of a melanoma.

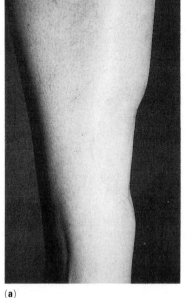

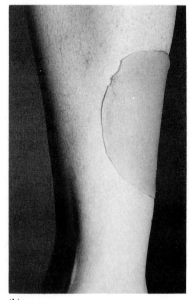

(a)   (b)

rise to an increased chance of flap necrosis. If the dissection is performed after radiotherapy, there is a greater chance of flap necrosis, which puts the great vessels at risk.

Prevention

The incision The incision should give good exposure and easy access without increased risk of necrosis. Simple oblique or S-shaped incisions are safer in axilla or groin than complex incisions that require several flaps. Before closure, the skin flaps should be examined for ischaemic damage and non-viable areas should be excised at the time. If major vessels are then exposed, a muscle-flap transposition should be used covered by a split-thickness graft, e.g. sartorius, to cover the femoral vessels.

Wound drainage Suction drainage is essential after block dissection to remove haematoma and lymph and allow the flaps to drape into the defect to eliminate dead space. Lymph drainage may be prolonged and the drain should be left in place for at least five days.

Postoperative Early, controlled mobilization is encouraged. However, block-dissection wounds cross joint crease lines and movements that would cause shearing by compression of the flaps must be avoided in the early stages. In-patient care for a week to ten days is essential. Any infection must be treated with antibiotics and haematoma must be evacuated. Compression bandaging must be applied to the arm or leg to prevent lymphoedema. Exercise will increase the flow of lymph and, therefore, very strenuous exercise should be avoided for a week or two after surgery.

Postoperative complications

Haematoma Haematoma formation and seroma formation are common after block dissection. There is wide undermining of tissues and division of many vessels and lymphatics. Closed suction drainage must be maintained to keep the skin flaps in apposition to the bed. Drainage usually declines after five days and drains can be removed shortly thereafter. Large haematomas should be drained surgically to prevent infection and wound dehiscence.

Lymph fistula All block-dissection wounds drain lymph for a few days. If the wound drainage persists in large quantities, particularly in neck dissection, and if the discharge is milky, a chylous fistula is present. Most leakage slows with compression dressing and rest. A fat-free diet helps lymphatic-duct fistula. Large doses of citrus fruits may also help.

   If the drains have already been removed before the lymph accumulation develops, aspiration should be repeated as necessary and compression dressings may be applied.

Delayed healing Some degree of marginal wound necrosis is common after block dissection. The sutures must be left in longer than usual. If major necrosis occurs that might risk wound disruption and major vessel blow-out, early excision and repair using muscle-flap-covered graft or skin flaps must be considered.

Recurrence Recurrent disease after block dissection is an extremely unpleasant complication, often leading to fungation. A discrete isolated recurrence can be excised but resection is often impossible and palliative radiotherapy is probably the treatment of choice for the more extensive recurrence.

Lymphoedema

The lymphoedema occurring after block dissection is the acquired or secondary variety. It is more likely if there has been previous radiotherapy. In the leg, oedema occurs more frequently when the iliac and inguinal nodes are both removed (Fig. 13.10).

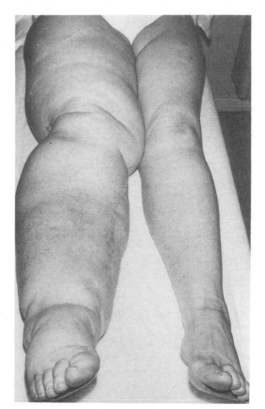

Figure 13.10
Severe lymphoedema after radical groin dissection removing the inguinal and iliac nodes.

Prevention   Vigorous prophylactic measures are important because it is difficult to reverse the oedema once it develops. The lower limb is the most frequently affected area and rest, elevation and elastic support begun immediately postoperatively are effective in the majority of cases.

Streptococcal or staphylococcal infections causing cellulitis exacerbate oedema, and antibiotics should be given as necessary to treat infection.

Lifelong co-operation from the patient is essential to treat lymphoedema if it develops and the patient should be counselled carefully about the need for prevention.

Conservative   Gravity tends to keep lymph in the limb that is dependant.
treatment   Simple elevation is effective in increasing venous and lymphatic return. Time spent standing should be kept to a minimum and when the patient is seated the leg should be elevated at least to the horizontal.

Compression using elastic support stockings, blue line bandages or external pressure devices is very effective in reducing oedema, particularly in the early stages before fibrosis develops. The compression must be continued indefinitely to prevent recurrence (Fig. 13.11).

Diuretics can be useful in the short term, for example, postoperatively but are ineffective in prolonged use.

Surgical   *'Physiological' operations* to increase lymph drainage can be
treatment   effective in acquired lymphoedema, in which the peripheral lymphatic system is usually intact. Lymphaticovenous anastomosis by microsurgery has been used with benefit. In unilateral acquired lymphoedema of the leg, a transposed flap (for example contralateral groin flap or inferior epigastric flaps turned across to cover the groin can give rise to considerable reduction in oedema.

Excisional operations remove as much of the swollen subcutaneous tissue as possible. They are most useful in idiopathic lymphoedema when the lymphatics are deficient or absent. The Sistrunk operation removes skin and fat.

The Kondoleon method involves removing a wide strip of deep fascia in an attempt to promote lymph drainage to the deep lymphatics. In the Thompson operation, a de-epithelialized strip of dermis is tucked into the deep fascia and a wedge of skin and fat is excised.

These operations do not seem to work any better than the Sistrunk simple excision. The radical Charles operation requires the removal of all skin and subcutaneous tissue. The skin is defatted and returned as a full-thickness graft. The degree of scarring and deformity is severe.

In all excisional surgical procedures, careful post-operative management is the key to success. Continued elastic support is

Figure 13.11
Idiopathic
lymphoedema (a)
treated conservatively
by compression with
blue-line and Tubigrip
support (b). Once the
oedema has been
removed, the condition
is maintained by
wearing elastic
stockings thereafter.
(c) One year later.

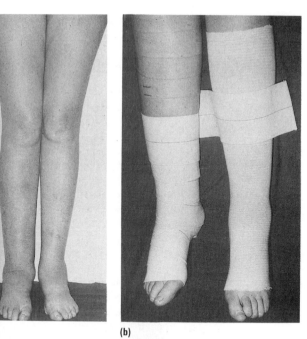

(a) (b)

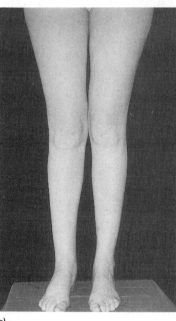

(c)

essential permanently if recurrence of lymphoedema is to be prevented.

Complications of surgical treatment

Recurrence is inevitable if long-term support is neglected. Rest and elevation of the limb is essential in the acute phase because exercise makes the oedema worse. Intermittent external compression at night using a suitable pump can be carried out at home.

Infection is a common complication of treatment and of the lymphoedema *per se*. Antibiotics may be needed in the long term. Penicillin is the treatment of choice to prevent streptococcal cellulities, or an equivalent drug in a sensitive individual.

Scars are inevitable but usually heal well with time. The radical Charles operation carries many more severe complications because failure of the full thickness graft to heal is a problem; unstable scarred areas leading to hyperkeratosis, papillomatosis and weeping. There is also characteristic 'plus four' deformity of the legs treated by this method.

Persisting controversies

- Early detection and diagnosis of malignant melanomas.
- Extent and depth of excision required for primary treatment of malignant melanoma.
- Is elective lymph node dissection indicated in malignant melanoma?
- The surgical techniques for treatment of lymphoedema.

Further reading
Balch, C.M. & Milton, G.W. (Eds) (1985) *Cutaneous Melanoma. Clinical Management and Treatment Results Worldwide*. Philadelphia: J.B. Lippincott.
Roses, D.F., Harris, M.N. & Aclerman, A.B. (Eds) (1983) *Diagnosis and Management of Cutaneous Malignant Melanoma*. Major Problems in Clinical Surgery. Philadelphia: Saunders.

14 Birthmarks

Haemangioma

Haemangioma, lymphangioma and arteriovenous malformations fall into the category of congenital endothelial hamartomata and are the commonest type of cutaneous tumour seen in plastic-surgery paediatric practice. Some of these lesions are very extensive and are situated in prominent parts of the body, in particular the face, giving rise to considerable disfigurement and associated embarrassment to the patient. Many different forms of therapy have been tried for these patients, particularly those with port-wine stains, none of which are entirely successful.

It is important to differentiate the types of haemangioma because the natural history is quite different for different types of lesion, some resolving spontaneously and others not. In the former group, inappropriate surgical intervention will result in unnecessary and often extensive scarring. Other lesions are extremely vascular, with large feeding vessels. Surgery here may be catastrophic; occasionally however, it may be essential and even life-saving, and pre-operative planning and investigation will be all-important.

Classification   The terminology of these lesions is confusing. A classification based on the clinical appearance of the lesion is probably that most widely used, using terms such as strawberry naevus, port-wine stain, salmon patch, etc. More recently, a classification based on the endothelial features of these lesions has been proposed. Using this method, a more accurate prognosis can be made. There are two major categories in this method. Firstly, haemangiomas—vascular tumours with increased endothelial turnover during the proliferative phase—and secondly, malformations—vascular anomalies with a normal endothelial cell cycle. There is evidence to support the validity of this classification, in that mast cells are increased in proliferative-phase haemangiomas: they fall to normal levels with involution. Mast cells are not elevated in vascular malformation tissue. *In vitro* studies have also shown that endothelium derived from young haemangiomas grows easily in tissue culture and forms capillary tubules, whereas endothelium from malformation tissue cannot easily be cultured and does not form tubules.

A more commonly used clinical classification will, however, be used here for the basis of describing these birthmarks:

1 Capillary haemangioma—port-wine stain, strawberry haemangioma, salmon patch.
2 Capillary cavernous haemangioma.
3 Cavernous haemangioma.
4 Lymphangioma.
5 Lymphangiohaemangioma.
6 Arteriovenous malformation.
7 Vascular gigantism.

These will be considered individually, together with their complications and their management, but individual lesions may be
composed of a combination of different types of haemangioma.

Capillary haemangioma

This is the commonest group of these lesions. They usually lie in
the dermis or, more rarely, immediately under the dermis. They
discolour the skin without actually distorting it. The colour
varies from a pale pink (salmon patch) to the deep red or purple
colour characteristic of the port-wine stain (naevus flammeus).
This latter lesion tends to darken with increasing age and in
adulthood may become raised, with areas of thickening developing. Their distribution may be small, covering only a very small
area of the body, or much more extensive and covering large
areas of the body surface.

Port-wine stain

The appearance of these has already been described. It presents
at the time of birth and tends to be located on the face and neck
but can cover other areas of the body as well. These lesions
persist throughout life and show no sign of spontaneous regression. When very extensive areas of skin are involved, haemangiomatous tissue may also be found in deeper structures in
the body. Unless they are very small, these lesions give rise to
considerable embarrassment to most patients.

Complications of the condition

Sturge–Weber syndrome
In Sturge–Weber syndrome the choroid and pia mater tissues are
also involved with haemangiomatous tissue. It most commonly
involves the fronto-temporal lobes. Clinically, the distribution
of the cutaneous haemangioma covers the areas supplied by the
ophthalmic and maxillary divisions of the trigeminal nerve. The
patient presents with a port-wine stain associated with epileptic
attacks. Eventually a spastic hemiparesis develops on the
contralateral side. Later in the disease 'tram line' calcification
is characteristically seen on the skull X-ray. Mental retardation

usually develops and progresses. Glaucoma may also develop and require surgical intervention.

Prevention of complications. The management of Sturge–Weber syndrome is control of the epileptic attacks as far as possible. Many different techniques have been devised, however, to try and reduce the psychological consequences of the cosmetic disability of these lesions. To be most effective in preventing this developing, effective treatment would ideally be carried out before the patient's peers highlight the deformity, i.e. preferably before school age. However, methods currently available all fall short of this goal and all are associated with their own complications.

Mafucci's syndrome
In Mafucci's syndrome there is a combination of haemangiomas with dyschondroplasia.

Cosmesis
The appearance of these lesions can, of course, lead to considerable psychological trauma, as they persist throughout life. This can sometimes have a profound effect on a patient's personality.

Prevention of complications

Treatment
Many different methods have been used to treat these types of haemangiomata but none are entirely successful.

Cosmetic creams (Fig. 14.1) Because these haemangiomata are flat lesions they can often be very satisfactorily disguised by masking cosmetic creams. A combination of these to achieve the best colour match for the normal skin can be applied over the haemangioma. However, in practice patients often do not persist with them, complaining about the consistency of the cream, and so on. They tend, therefore, to be most useful for particular occasions rather than for continuous use.

Complications
Patients' compliance is the main complication of this form of treatment. The cosmetic creams used tend to be of very thick consistency and patients often dislike having to put them on. For lighter-coloured haemangiomas, however, it is usually much easier to find a lighter cream to apply. Very young and elderly patients often lack the skill to use these.

Excision Smaller lesions can be excised and the defect directly closed. Serial excision may also be successful. These will, of course, leave a scar but, if this is sited correctly, the end result should be a noticeable improvement. Larger haemangiomata may be

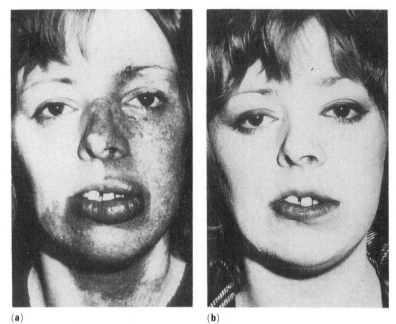

(a)   (b)

excised and the defect skin grafted. Full-thickness grafts or
thick split-skin grafts should be used and if meticulous attention
is paid to haemostasis, etc., so that an almost perfect take of the
graft is achieved, then excellent results can be obtained.

Complications

1 *Scar.* A scar is inevitable following excision, though much
can be done in the planning stage to reduce the effect of this,
e.g. alignment in or parallel to a crease line, avoidance of
undue tension, etc. All the other complications of scars
(discussed in Chapter 5) are potentially possible as well and
these should be given careful consideration and discussed
with the patient, balancing them against the disfigurement of
the lesion before deciding on the right course of action. Where
a graft is used, then the donor site 'scar' must also be
considered. Where a full-thickness skin graft is used, the
donor site will almost certainly need to be grafted. Therefore,
it must be taken from an inconspicuous site such as the
buttock.

2 *Colour match.* This can be a real problem when a graft is
used. As mentioned, the donor site, particularly where a large
graft is required, must be taken from an inconspicuous site
such as buttock, where the colour match may be far from
ideal. The overall benefit, therefore, particularly if the haemangioma is pale, may not be as great as hoped for.

3 *Growth deformity.* When simple excision and direct closure
or graft is carried out in childhood, distortion of the treated

area may result as the child grows, with possible contracture formation. Further secondary surgery may be required, therefore, and close follow-up during the growing years is important.

Tissue expansion More recently, the concept of tissue expansion has been used for this condition, whereby an expander is placed in the adjacent normal tissue and inflated over several weeks, thus producing more skin available for rotating or advancing into the defect following excision of the haemangioma. This will obviously give a much better quality of skin since it comes from the area immediately adjacent to the lesion. Texture, colour, etc., are all therefore bound to be better than those of a graft or distant flap. This method should enable quite large haemangiomas to be removed; for very extensive lesions, the expander may be re-inflated after the first advancement of tissue.

Complications
The complications of tissue expanders have been outlined in a previous chapter, viz. infection, extrusion, discomfort following expansion, temporary deformity associated with the expanded balloon, etc., and all of these apply in the context of this condition. Of particular concern, however, is a tendency for the scar (at the junction of the expanded skin and 'normal' tissue) to stretch over the months following the procedure. A further potential problem is that if expansion is carried out too rapidly, there may appear in the expanded skin 'stretch marks' that may persist.

Tattooing The technique of tattooing pigment into the skin to camouflage the lesion was introduced in the 1940s. A variety of pigments have been used, white titanium dioxide being one of the commonest. Haemangiomas lying predominantly in the deep dermal and subdermal layers are those for which this form of therapy is best suited. The pigment is introduced using a special needle.

Complications
It is important not to tattoo pigment beyond the haemangioma—even a small amount will give a 'halo' effect. To avoid this, the margin of the lesion should be clearly delineated prior to commencing treatment. Once treatment has started, it is sometimes difficult accurately to define margin. This can be done either by marking it with methylene blue ink or using tape of some sort. A further problem may be the introduction of excess pigment, giving a rather irregular pattern. The major problem, however, is the gradual loss of the pigment from the tissues. This is particularly seen in the subepidermal variety. This 'fading out' of the pigment does seem to be less marked in adult patients than in children. Although a perfect colour match may not be obtained with the normal surrounding skin, it may enable the

use of lighter and more acceptable cosmetic creams to be used by the patient.

Laser therapy   An argon laser beam will coagulate the small vessels in the dermal and subdermal layers associated with port-wine stains without causing necrosis and subsequent scarring at the site of treatment. This would sound an ideal method, therefore, for treating these lesions and in many patients significantly better results than from other methods have been achieved. At the present time, lesions that give the best results are those slightly dark in colour, particularly where small papules or raised areas within the haemangioma have developed. This is most commonly seen in older patients. However, scarring may develop if the technique is incorrectly used. The other major disadvantage is that, with the tiny beam from the laser, treatment can take a considerable time, the actual process being extremely tedious and time-consuming to administer. Attempts are being made to computerize and automate the technique. As mentioned, the darker lesions tend to respond better than the lighter coloured lesions and therefore have proved more useful in the older age group. Attempts are also being made to 'tune' the laser to different colours. Despite the problems with this technique, it does hold great promise for the future and may well develop as the treatment of choice in the years to come.

Prevention of complications associated with laser therapy   In order to reduce the risk of complications in this form of therapy, a test patch should be treated initially in an inconspicuous area of the haemangioma. Pre- and post-treatment photographs should be taken and a period of three months should be allowed to elapse before assessment of the area to ascertain (i) the response and (ii) the scarring, if any, produced. Further treatment can then be carried out on the basis of this assessment, if indicated and following full discussion with the patient.

Complications

Scarring. Hypertrophic scarring is a potential complication, particularly if a high dosage is used.

Hyperpigmentation. This has been found to be a problem, though often resolving spontaneously after a few months. If the area is exposed to strong sunlight, then protective cream should be used.

Atrophy. Atrophic changes in the superficial layers of the skin has been reported, giving the treated area a 'depressed' appearance compared with the adjacent normal skin. This is seldom severe and can be treated with dermabrasion.

Variable response

Not all haemangiomata respond to laser treatment equally effectively. Most published series have shown that therapy is most effective in the more purple-coloured lesions in adults. The various complications associated with scarring appear much more prevalent in younger people with pale lesions.

Treatment time

At present (owing to the small size of the laser beam) treatment times are lengthy even for small lesions. This is particularly a problem in children, when several sessions of treatment may be required to cover the whole lesion.

Danger to staff

Staff administering the treatment must be protected from reflection of the laser beam and should wear protective glasses.

Cryotherapy   Cryotherapy has also been used, but with only partial success and has not been widely adopted as a method for treating these lesions.

Infrared   Several authors have reported using the infrared coagulator to
coagulation   treat vascular naevi of various sorts. Good results have been reported using a sapphire end-piece. The instrument is still under investigation, but it is considerably cheaper and more portable than a laser.

Strawberry haemangioma

Strawberry haemangioma is present at or shortly after birth. It tends to grow rapidly over the first few weeks or months of life and then slowly regresses over several years, being largely resolved by the age of 7 or 8 years (Fig. 14.2). Its growth can be alarming and distressing to the mother and reassurance must be given as to its likely course. The rapid growth of these lesions results in invasion and replacement of the skin (Fig. 14.3). The reason for this is obscure but there is some evidence to suggest that it may be hormonal. The colour may vary from bright red to purple. At the end of the growth phase, small grey patches appear in the haemangioma heralding the start of regression. If the lesion becomes ulcerated and/or infected, this will tend to speed up the process of resolution. At the end of the period of resolution, there may be surplus skin that requires trimming but generally the scar resulting will be very much less than that resulting from early excision and almost certainly than by that from skin grafting. This type of haemangioma may develop in any part of the body and is usually confined to the skin only. Some, however, have a significant amount lying deep to the dermis.

Figure 14.2
Spontaneous
resolution of
strawberry
haemangioma. (a) 6
months; (b) 5 years.

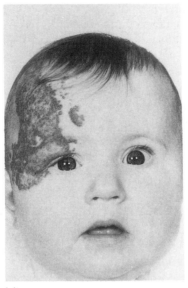 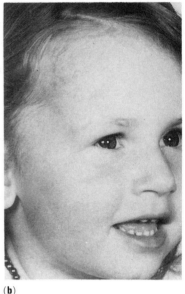

(a) (b)

Complications

Kassabach–Merritt syndrome

Kassabach–Merritt syndrome is a rare complication, sometimes referred to as 'platelet trapping' (Fig. 14.4). The platelets would appear to be destroyed in the vascular spaces of the haemangioma and, when the haemangioma is extensive, may lead to thrombocytopenia and disseminated intravascular coagulopathy.

Ulceration

Mild repeated trauma may result in surface breakdown or ulceration, which may become infected (Fig. 14.5). Treatment here is to dress with the appropriate cleansing agent, such as tulle gras impregnated with an antibacterial agent, and possibly systemic antibiotics if the infection is severe. As healing occurs, the haemangioma will tend to scar at the site of ulceration and this will often accelerate regression. Ulceration is particularly seen if the child is constantly rubbing at the lesion or if it is a site such as the perineum where it is being repeatedly soiled. Where lesions are small and excision and repair are easily carried out, then this should be done.

Occasionally, a more aggressive form of ulceration develops, the so-called 'wild fire' or pseudomalignant ulceration, which may even cause infarction of the underlying tissue. This again may require surgical intervention if it cannot readily be controlled with topical dressings and antibiotics.

Figure 14.3
Surplus skin for
trimming (pre- and
post-resolution).
(a) 6 weeks; (b) 5
months; (c) 18 months;
(d) 9 years.

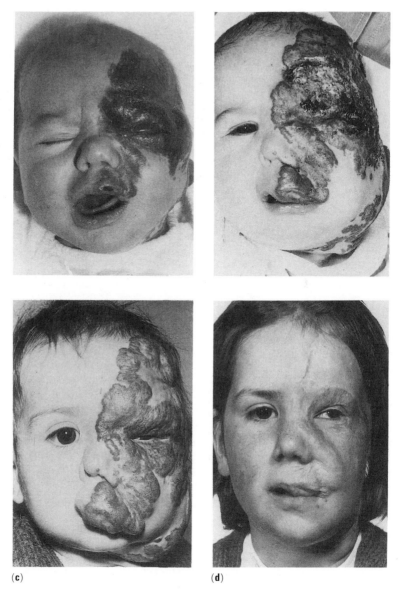

(c) (d)

Haemorrhage

Haemorrhage is obviously more likely to occur than in normal tissue following even quite minor trauma. The application of direct pressure to the haemangioma will usually control the problem temporarily. In more extensive lesions, however, with severe trauma, considerable haemorrhage may occur and may result in a disseminated intravascular coagulopathy. This is also occasionally seen following surgery of these lesions, particularly if only part of the haemangioma has been removed.

Figure 14.4
Platelet trapping (abdominal haemangioma).

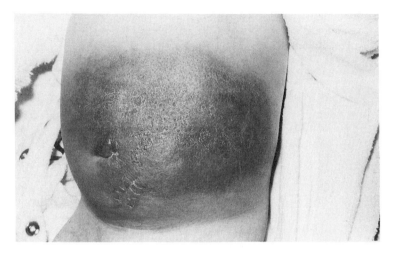

Figure 14.5
Ulcerated haemangioma (secondary to infection).

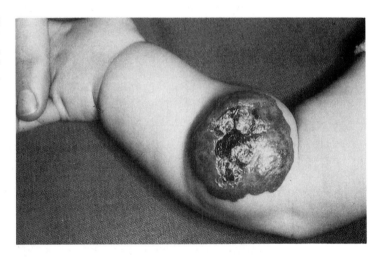

Visual obstruction
When the haemangioma lies in the region of the eyelids and/or orbit, and when vision becomes obstructed as the haemangioma enlarges, then a deprivation amblyopia may occur (Fig. 14.6). Close follow-up of lesions in this area must be maintained with an ophthalmologist so that this can be detected at an early stage.

Cosmesis
Although these lesions are self-limiting they can cause great distress, to the parents in particular. They often commence as areas of slightly deeper pink but rapidly grow over several weeks to become grossly disfiguring.

Figure 14.6
Obstructing eye.

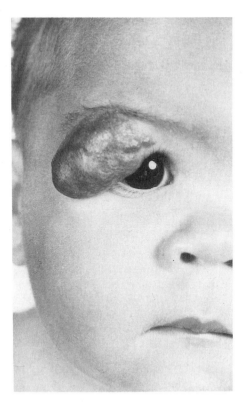

Prevention of complications

Conservative The typical clinical course of a strawberry naevus is unique when compared with other simple tumours, in that it generally appears within a few days of birth, growing rapidly over the following few weeks or months and then regressing spontaneously over several years until the child is about 7 or 8 years old. The colour also changes over this period of time, becoming paler. The vast majority of these tumours behave in this way and the correct management is, therefore, careful observation with frequent follow-up clinic visits, at which photographs should be taken for comparison at subsequent visits. The parents need a lot of reassurance and support, particularly in the early weeks and months. When surgery is carried out at an early stage, considerable scarring may be incurred that may be unnecessary. Occasionally, a small excision of redundant tissue may be required at the end of resolution. Protect the area to avoid ulceration, if possible, as this, together with surgery, will leave areas that have permanent scars.

Complications
1 *Incorrect diagnosis.* Before embarking on conservative

management, reassuring the parents, etc., one must be as sure as possible that this is not a port-wine stain type lesion, in which no significant improvement is seen after many years' observation. The time of appearance of the lesion is the best aid to this diagnosis, together with its activity over the first two months, but an accurate diagnosis can be difficult at the time of first presentation.

2 *Deprivation amblyopia.*   Failure to watch these lesions closely in the region of the eye can result in reduced vision. These children must be reviewed every four weeks, with photographs taken regularly over the first twelve months in particular. There is no place for conservative management once the visual field has been occluded.

Treatment

Compression   Compression bandaging can be useful in reducing the size of these lesions and may, therefore, accelerate the rate of regression. Ideal sites are on the limbs, where circumferential pressure can readily be applied with an elastic stocking type of dressing.

Complications
1 *Excessive pressure.*   The bandage or stocking may become too tight, particularly in a growing child. This needs to be checked every few weeks and a larger size used if indicated.
2 *Friction.*   The bandage or stocking may cause rubbing against the lesion, with resulting bleeding, ulceration and secondary infection: it should then be abandoned until healing has occurred.

Steroid therapy   Recent papers have shown that a dramatic reduction in the size of these lesions can sometimes be achieved with the use of high-dose steroids, either prednisolone or dexamethasone being used. These have been administered both systemically and directly into the lesion. This form of therapy is particularly useful in the small lesions surrounding the eye, where a good cosmetic result from surgery is difficult to achieve, or in very extensive lesions, again including the eye (where systemic administration of the drug is more appropriate). Other groups have been using steroids in combination with surgery. When marked fibrosis is induced by the steroid injection into the haemangioma, surgery is likely to be safer and less extensive, and should reduce the risk of coagulopathy.

Complications
These drugs are given in high dosage but for a short period of time and therefore should avoid the long-term complications of osteoporosis, growth retardation, etc.

Surgery   Surgery can be used in conjunction with steroid therapy. The indications for surgical intervention are very few and have already been mentioned. After resolution of a very extensive haemangioma, trimming of the redundant skin may be indicated. Due consideration must be given to the advantages gained measured against the resultant scar. Following excision of large lesions, skin grafting may have to be carried out.

Complications
1 Unnecessarily extensive scarring will result if this self-limiting lesion is excised without indication, i.e. for purely cosmetic considerations. Distortion of the surrounding structures is likely as the child grows.
2 *Haemorrhage.* Large feeding vessels may be present, making serious haemorrhage a problem. Injection before surgery of the lesion or feeding vessels with a sclerosant or embolization can minimize this risk. This itself, however, may be hazardous, leading to necrosis of surrounding tissue or even worse if extension to intracranial structures results. It needs to be carried out under careful radiological control.

Radiation   Radiation has been used in the past but is rarely, if ever, indicated today.

Cryotherapy   Cryotherapy has also been used to a relatively small extent and has little value in the management of this lesion.

Laser therapy   This has been more widely used in the management of port-wine stains than in that of strawberry naevi. It may be effective, however, particularly in small flat lesions. The complications of laser treatment were discussed earlier in the chapter.

Dermabrasion   Dermabrasion has been advocated as a possible treatment. However, as most of the abnormal vessels in this type of haemangioma lie in the deep dermis or subdermal layer, these areas so treated will at best heal as a deep dermal burn.

Complications
Hypertrophic scarring is a likely complication of dermabrasion, as the dermabrasion will of necessity need to be carried out into the deeper layers of the skin.

Sclerosant embolization   This may be used on its own or in conjunction with surgery. If it is correctly placed, the major feeding vessels can be thrombosed and the lesion will regress and fibrose. The vessels need to be cannulated under radiological control before injection of the sclerosant.

Complications
These have been covered above under complications of surgery (point 2).

Cavernous haemangioma

Cavernous haemangiomata present clinically as deep-blue, diffuse swellings, often in the limbs. There is great variation in their size. Many of these (at least 60–70%) will resolve spontaneously, though this may take several years (up to the age of 8 years or so). Regression may not be complete, however. Various complications are associated with these lesions, some of which have been mentioned earlier.

Complications

Haemorrhage
These lesions initially contain large endothelial filled cavities, fed predominantly by the venous system. Any trauma may, therefore, result in fairly considerable bleeding.

Thrombocytopenia
These lesions may also cause a platelet-trapping type of phenomenon with a tendency to haemorrhage.

Gigantism
Gigantism may involve local soft tissues or skeletal tissue. For example, a large lesion of the lower lip may result in enlargement of the mandible as well as the soft tissues of the lip (Fig. 14.7). In the peripheries, finger enlargement may result.

These lesions may remain quiescent for many years and then start to enlarge, seemingly invading surrounding tissues. This is often the time when surgical excision or other form of treatment is indicated.

Figure 14.7
Gigantism of lower lip associated with haemangioma.

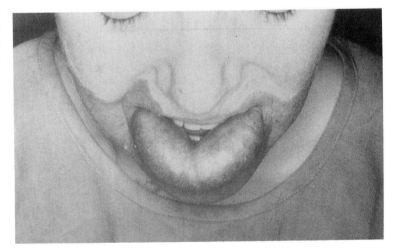

Treatment

Conservative As mentioned, many of these lesions will regress spontaneously. A conservative approach is especially indicated in sites where it would be difficult to achieve a good scar if the lesion were to be excised. This is particularly true of the particular type of cavernous haemangioma found at the tip of the nose—often described as a 'Cyrano' nose. A series comparing operative and conservative management of these lesions has shown significantly better long-term results with the conservative approach.

Complications
1 *Unexpected growth.* Although it is usual for these to spontaneously regress, this is not inevitable and they may start to increase in size. Conservative management may then have to be abandoned, depending on the site and rate of growth.
2 *Surplus skin.* After regression has taken place, the resulting skin may have a patulous appearance and be disfiguring. Excision of this will often improve the appearance.

Sclerosant injection Sclerosant injection may be intralesional or intravascular. This should only be attempted under very careful radiological control after an arteriogram has been carried out, when a suitable feeding vessel is seen and cannulated. In these cases, some regression in the size of the lesion may be achieved; it may also help as a pre-operative method of reducing blood loss.

Complications
Extension of the necrosis beyond the designated area may occur. In the head and neck this is particularly dangerous. Careful analysis of the arteriogram must be carried out first and this treatment should be avoided if there is significant arteriovenous malformation.

Surgery For smaller lesions on which surgery can readily be carried out and when an inconspicuous scar can be achieved, excision may be the treatment of choice, particularly when spontaneous regression has not taken place. More limited surgery involving ligating of feeding vessels can be carried out around the periphery of the lesion in an attempt to cause ischaemia and regression in size. This occasionally can result in some reduction in size.

Complications
1 *Haemorrhage.* This is particularly likely to be a complication when excision of larger lesions is undertaken. On a limb, excision can be carried out under tourniquet control, though this does cause some 'collapse' of the lesion, making it difficult to delineate.

2 *Recurrence.* Some shrinking in the size of the lesion can often be achieved by ligating and/or dividing the feeding vessels. However, new vessels tend to enlarge over subsequent months and the angioma starts to increase in size once more.

3 *Disseminated intravascular coagulopathy.* This may result where excessive blood loss occurs.

Steroids The use of these in strawberry haemangiomas has already been mentioned. Short courses of even quite large doses can occasionally have a dramatic effect on these lesions. Direct injection into the lesion itself can also be useful. This is particularly the case in fairly small lesions that it is desirable to remove although this will result in significant scarring if surgical intervention is carried out; an example is a lesion obstructing vision in a very young baby when there is a risk of deprivation amblyopia occurring.

Complications

Fluid retention, growth retardation and osteoporosis can result from long-term administration of steroids. This should, therefore, be avoided but short courses of high-dose steroids have been shown to be of benefit without these complications. They should, however, only be administered in conjunction with a paediatrician and with extreme care in very young children.

Capillary/cavernous haemangioma

Capillary/cavernous haemangiomata involve characteristics of both the capillary and cavernous types of haemangioma.

Arteriovenous fistula

This is the most serious of all the haemangiomata. Often fed by large vessels, they can be a very large size and tend to be warm to palpation and may pulsate. Gigantism is a common complication of the surrounding tissues and trauma can lead to catastrophic haemorrhage. Other complications that can occur in association with these lesions include the Kasabach–Merritt syndrome and obstruction to surrounding tissues, e.g. trachea when in the neck. When significant arteriovenous shunting is occurring, cardiac failure may be precipitated. The management of these lesions is extremely difficult. Feeding vessels may be ligated surgically but, although in the short term a certain amount of growth or even involution may occur, other vessels tend to enlarge and the lesions start growing again. An arteriogram is essential as a first step to identify the main vessels. Embolization under radiological control, either on its own or as an adjunct to surgery, may be helpful but is not without its complications if emboli escape into the general circulation.

Different materials have been used as emboli, including microspheres and small particles of muscle. Some people have found treatment with steroids and radiotherapy helpful, though these have not been widely accepted as treatment modalities in this condition.

Lymphangiomas

This is a relatively avascular congenital lesion that is usually classified according to its structure. Capillary lymphangiomas, seen in the lip and tongue, give rise to local gigantism in the form of macrocheilia and macroglossia, respectively. Elsewhere, these may be encountered in the skin, mucous membranes, neck, axilla and groins and are usually cavernous and called cystic hygromas. They may contain only a few large cystic spaces and are multiloculated. They tend to permeate between the vessels and nerves, making dissection hazardous. The capillary type of lymphangioma rarely causes a serious problem but cystic hygromas, on the other hand, can be associated with several potentially very serious complications.

Clinically, most cystic hygromas appear in the posterior triangle of the neck, including the supraclavicular fossa. They may, however, extend deep into the structures of the mouth and tongue or into the neck (trachea, oseophagus, etc.). The overlapping skin is usually normal in texture, though a slight bluish tinge may be seen due to the fluid content of the lesion. It is characteristically soft and cystic on palpation and transluminates brightly (unless there has been haemorrhage or infection into it). There is controversy whether these lesions regress spontaneously. It has been stated that they are virtually never seen in adulthood, suggesting that spontaneous resolution does occur fairly frequently. It would appear that a small percentage of pure cystic hygromas will involute provided there is no haemangiomatous component within the lesion. However, treatment is often carried out owing to the presence of complications in these lesions before time can be allowed for spontaneous resolution to take place.

Complications

Compression
This may present at birth with obstructed labour. It may, on the other hand, cause compression of surrounding structures, most seriously in the neck, the trachea often being displaced from its normal position. This can be shown on soft tissue X-ray of the neck or using a CT scan. This may present as an emergency when rapid decompression of the cystic hygroma or tracheostomy may have to be carried out.

Infection

These patients may develop infection in the cystic spaces of the hygroma, leading to a lymphangitis. This must be actively treated with antibiotics. Recurrent infection tends to lead to fibrosis and will make a surgical removal significantly more difficult. Surgical intervention should, therefore, be carried out to avoid recurrent infection.

Haemorrhage

Haemorrhage may occur into a hygroma, particularly if there is a haemangiomatous component to the lesion. This may result in a rapid increase in size of the swelling, with secondary obstructive consequences (Fig. 14.8). Urgent decompression may be required. Along with an increase in size, the consistency will be noted to change, becoming much firmer on palpation.

Cosmesis

The presence of a large cystic swelling in the region of the neck is understandably a distressing thing for a mother to have to live with. The head may be held in a lateral flexed position. The larger the lesion, the more difficult it is to make the decision to wait and see if spontaneous regression is going to take place.

Malignancy

There is a very small chance of malignancy developing in very large lesions, in the form of a lymphangiosarcoma. This is, however, extremely rare.

Treatment

Conservative   For small lesions a conservative policy should be adopted initially. For larger lesions the decision is much more difficult.

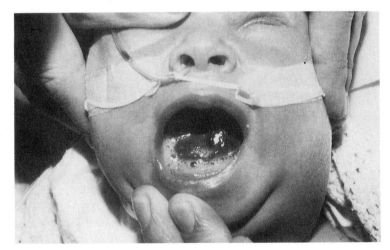

Figure 14.8
Haemorrhage into cystic hygroma.

Prevention of complications
Very careful monitoring of its size and direction of extension is important and evidence of complications developing should be promptly recorded and treatment, where necessary, should be commenced.

Complications
Rapid increase in size, resulting in compression of vital structures, is always a risk when a conservative policy is adopted. This is more likely if there is a significant component of the hygroma lying deeply in the neck.

Treatment
Treatment surgically is indicated if acute compression supervenes.

Surgery   In the vast majority of these lesions, surgical excision will eventually have to be carried out. As mentioned previously, these lesions are no respecters of tissue planes, and, with many important anatomical structures lying in close proximity in the head and neck, the potential for significant operative morbidity is high. Dissection is particularly difficult when the hygroma consists of multiple small cysts. Sometimes, when a few large cysts only are encountered, the lesion shells out relatively easily. As much of the hygroma as possible should be removed and suction drainage in the postoperative period is important. Aspiration and/or marsupialization may be indicated, particularly in the case of acute obstruction of the airway, but this is rarely a satisfactory long-term procedure unless the lesion consists of one or two large cysts only.

Prevention of complications
1 *Investigations.* As full a knowledge as possible of the size and distribution of the lesion should be obtained prior to commencing surgery, e.g. by soft tissue X-rays, CT scans and dye studies.
2 *Anatomy.* A thorough knowledge and understanding of the normal anatomy is vital. The normal tissue planes are often unhelpful in the dissection and the unwary surgeon is likely to damage important nerves. In particular, this type of surgery should only be undertaken by an experienced head and neck surgeon (for cystic hygromas in this region).
3 Use of a nerve stimulator is very helpful to identify nerves during surgery.

Complications
1 *Nerve damage.* The nerves at risk will obviously depend on the site of the lesion. In the upper neck and lower face region the facial nerve is most at risk and this can leave a most disfiguring facial weakness if it is not recognized and repair is

not carried out. The accessory nerve in the upper neck is also at risk.

2 *Haemorrhage.* With many large arteries and veins in this area, significant haemorrhage is always a risk. Blood should always be available, with the patient grouped and cross-matched pre-operatively.

3 *Incomplete excision.* It is often impossible completely to remove these lesions. This is particularly the case when surgery has to be carried out as an emergency to decompress a vital structure.

Treatment
Damaged nerves should be repaired at the time of surgery, i.e. primarily. Identifying nerves in scar tissue at a later stage is extremely difficult and often unrewarding. Further surgery may need to be carried out if the lesion has been incompletely excised, particularly if further increase in size occurs.

Sclerosant injection Incision and drainage followed by sclerosant injection may be indicated in small lesions but in large multicystic hygromas it is unlikely to do much more than slightly reduce the overall size of the lesion, and may cause temporary catastrophic increase in swelling.

Prevention of complications
The exact distribution of the hygroma should be known before sclerosant injection. Inadvertent intravascular injection may result.

Complications
1 *Vascular.* Thrombosis following injection into vital vessels, particularly in multicystic lesions.

2 *Poor response.* When the sclerosing agent may only act in a small part of the lesion, a disappointing result may be obtained.

3 *Fibrosis.* The agent may induce considerable fibrosis, making subsequent surgery more difficult.

Radiation This has no place in the management of lymphangiomas, though it is often mentioned as being of help.

Present controversies
- The role of steroids in haemangioma management
- Conservative management of cystic hygromas

Further reading
Mulliken, J.B. & Glowacki, J. (1982) Haemangiomas and vascular malformations in infants and children: A classification based on endothelial characteristics. *Plast. Reconstr. Surg.* 69, 412–420.

Colver, G.B., Cherry, G.W., Dawber, R.P.R. & Ryan, T.J. (1986) The treatment of cutaneous vascular lesions with the infra-red coagulator: A preliminary report. *Br. J. Plast. Surg. 39*, 131–135.

Ryan, T.J. & Cherry, G.W. (1987) *Vascular Birthmarks, Pathogenesis and Management*. Oxford: Oxford University Press.

15 Complications of Plastic Surgery of the Eyelid

Introduction

Close examination of the normal eyelid reveals a finely developed and adapted structure able to perform its functions of protecting the eye against injury, glare, invasion of foreign bodies and drying of the cornea. This last function requires complete coverage of the eye when closed, as in sleep. The cornea requires a moist environment for it to remain healthy and this is provided by the secretions of the lacrimal gland, which bathe the cornea during the reflex blinking movements of the eyelids. An efficient drainage system at the medial side of the eyelids avoids epiphora. The puncta are placed at a particular angle to the eye and the pumping mechanism of the lacrimal sac is assisted by the action of the superficial and deep pretarsal muscles during blinking. The lacrimal duct system allows the drainage of the secretions into the nasal cavity. The function of the eyelashes is to act as a sort of filter, preventing airborne foreign particles entering the eye.

The upper lid is responsible for 90% of the opening of the eye and is obviously essential for the normal functioning of the eye as a visual organ. Several factors in its anatomy assist in this function, including its overall thinness (the skin of the upper eyelid is the thinnest in the body), the smoothness with which its conjunctival surface glides over the cornea, and the co-ordinated functions of its musculature. Opening of the eye by elevation of the upper lid requires the simultaneous contraction of the levator palpebrae superioris muscle (innervated by the oculomotor nerve) and of Muller's muscle (innervated by the sympathetic nerves). Closure is carried out by contraction of the orbicularis oculi muscle (innervated by the facial nerve) in combination with relaxation of the levator muscles. The degree of opening, therefore, depends upon the co-ordinated action of these groups of muscles.

Conversely, the lower lid is designed for support with a much more rigid structure.

An understanding of these mechanisms and, in particular, the anatomical features necessary for their specialized activities is essential when reconstruction following trauma, cancer surgery, etc., is required to prevent complications. Other factors should also be borne in mind, such as colour match, skin thickness, and so on, as the position of the eyelids means they are always exposed to the gaze of others.

Plastic and reconstructive surgery of the eyelids involves four main categories of conditions:

1 Trauma (including burns injuries).
2 Neoplasia (including various benign and malignant skin tumours).
3 Ectropion/Entropion which can arise from a variety of causes.
4 Cosmetic—blepharoplasty.

Less commonly, surgery is undertaken for congenital causes, including anomalies of the palpebral fissure (such as in Down's Syndrome), displacement of the canthi, ankyloblepharon (fusion of the eyelids to varying degrees) and blepharophimosis (diminution in size of the palpebral fissure). The latter conditions will not be discussed in detail.

Prevention of complications—general principles

Several simple principles form the basis of all methods of reconstruction of the eyelids, whether the cause is trauma, cancer, congenital defects, etc. An understanding of these is essential to reduce the risk of complications in this form of surgery.

1 Replace what is missing with similar tissue, as far as possible, i.e. use skin for skin loss, mucous membrane for conjunctiva, cartilage for tarsus.
2 Normal function should be restored, i.e. palpebral occlusion and corneal coverage. This necessitates a thin, mobile upper lid, since it is the upper eyelid, as already mentioned, that supplies the major part of these functions. It also includes patent lacrimal passages where possible.
3 Obstruction to vision should be kept to a minimum during the reconstruction—avoid lengthy tarsorrhaphy wherever possible.
4 Whereas the lower lid may be used to reconstruct upper-lid defects, one should think long and hard before using the upper lid for lower-lid reconstruction. The function of the upper lid has already been mentioned, being more important for corneal coverage than the lower lid. In experienced hands, deformity of the upper lid is rare following its use in lower lid reconstruction, but when it does occur it may be very difficult to correct.

Specific conditions

Trauma

Trauma to the eyelids is common in association with facial injuries in general. Severe blunt injuries may be associated with fractures of the orbit, injuries caused by sharp objects, such as glass or knives are more likely to be associated with injuries to the globe itself.

When discussing the complications of these injuries and their management, it is important firstly to consider the associated complications of eyelid injuries themselves: these should be looked for during the initial assessment of the patient's eyelids. A brief description of the methods of repair will be outlined and then the longer-term complications of these injuries, including the methods of repair, will be discussed together with their correction.

Complications of eyelid injuries

Injured eye This may not at first be apparent. The patient may have sustained a head injury and be unable to give the examiner an accurate account of the vision present or absent in the eye. It may be due to haematoma formation in the surrounding damaged soft tissue or to oedema, causing the lids to close. It is sometimes extremely difficult to see the globe in this situation and the patient is often unco-operative when the examiner tries to open the lids to get a better view. Yet damage may have occured, and it is important, in order possibly to save the vision in the eye, to seek an urgent ophthalmological opinion. The commonest error is to miss a foreign body. Following a road-traffic accident there may be particles of glass present in and around the damaged eyelids. These may have penetrated the eye. Careful removal is imperative as injudicious removal may in itself damage the eye. It is better to irrigate the eye in saline to get a better view; this will also assist in washing out any foreign material that may be present. Another hazard here is to remove blood clot from the injured area if it is adherent to the globe— this may be associated with a penetrating injury and iris tissue may be adherent to the clot.

Orbital fracture Particularly when the injuring force has been severe, the orbit is likely to be fractured. This again may be difficult to diagnose owing to swelling and haematoma in the region, but localized bony tenderness, obvious deformity and mobility of the bony anatomy in the region of the injury will all give clues to this complication. A blow-out fracture, a particular type of fracture of the orbital floor, characteristically presents with diplopia and enophthalmos. This type of fracture results from a sudden increase in intraorbital pressure from an external force applied to the soft tissue of the orbit, e.g. by a squash ball (Fig. 15.1). The orbital contents are forced back and exert pressure on the thin orbital floor or medial wall causing it to fracture. This may result in entrapment of the inferior rectus and inferior oblique muscles with their surrounding fat and connective tissue, resulting in vertical muscle imbalance and diplopia. The enophthalmos results either from prolapse of tissue from the orbital cavity or from enlargement of the cavity itself (later on it may be due to fat atrophy or contracting necrotic muscles).

Fractures of the facial bones may also occur and careful physical examination, X-rays and a CT scan will help to define accurately the extent of the bony injury.

Intracranial injury As the upper wall or roof of the orbit is very thin, separating the orbital contents from the anterior cranial fossa, a penetrating injury, particularly of the upper eyelids, may penetrate this,

Figure 15.1
Blow-out fracture caused by squash ball.

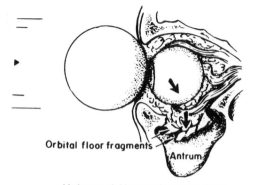

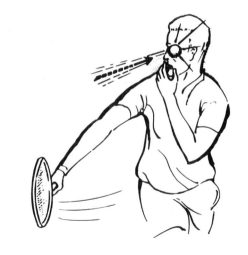

Orbital floor fragments

Antrum

Mechanism of "blow-out" fracture of orbital floor.

with a resulting potential intracranial injury complicating the eyelid injury.

Nerve injury The most serious nerve injury is to the optic nerve. This will tend to be associated with severe injury to the globe or with head injury, making initial assessment difficult. The pupil will usually be fixed and unreactive.

When the injury to the eyelid extends deeply laterally, the ophthalmic branch of the facial nerve may be injured. This will have serious implications when it comes to restoration of normal functioning. The supraorbital nerve may also be damaged. Although of little functional significance, this can lead to considerable discomfort for the patient, both due to the sensory loss over its distribution in the forehead and anterior scalp, but also due to the very painful neuroma frequently associated with this nerve injury at the site of damage, which is difficult to treat later.

Ectropion This may develop as a late complication and will be discussed in detail later on. However, in a severe burn injury affecting the eyelids, it may develop very rapidly as soon as the swelling has subsided. Emergency management by covering the eye with ointment, watch glass or polythene should be started as soon as possible. The patient is unable to close the eyes and will require early release of the ectropion, usually with full-thickness grafts. This may have to be repeated again after several weeks when the overall condition of the patient has improved. Failure to recognize this complication may result in corneal damage.

Infection Eyelid infection is fairly rare—unless a contaminated wound is left without being cleaned or repaired—owing to the excellent blood supply to the area. However, infection here is serious owing to the connections between the draining veins at the medial margin of the orbit and the intracranial venous sinuses. Aggressive treatment with antibiotics and drainage of pus must be carried out and more formal repair of the damaged tissues carried out as a secondary procedure.

Prevention of complications in eyelid injuries
As in so much of reconstructive surgery, accurate knowledge of the normal anatomy and careful assessment of exactly what the damage is, particularly of whether tissue is lost or just lacerated, is necessary to achieve the optimum result following corrective surgery and to minimize the risk of complication.

General points 1 *Debridement.* It is extremely important to carry out a meticulous debridement of these wounds; use of magnifying loupes is helpful. Even small amounts of foreign material can contribute to long-term problems associated with scarring, infection, and tattooing.

2 *Fracture reduction.* The bony anatomy of the orbit and face forms the foundations of any repair or reconstruction of the eyelids. Therefore, any fractures in this region should be reduced and fixed before soft-tissue repair is undertaken. This will prevent later reopening of carefully sutured wounds, but, more importantly, may alter the landmarks upon which the correct relationships of the reconstructed soft tissues have been based.

3 *Emergency measures.* Emergency measures to prevent further damage to the eye and eyelid tissues should be instituted as soon as possible. The eye should be irrigated with saline and a moist dressing applied and replaced as necessary to prevent desiccation of the tissues and globe.

Specific conditions

1. Lid laceration

These may be superficial or deep. Superficial injuries may be parallel to the lid margin and these can readily be sutured, smaller ones may not even require a suture. Lacerations vertical to the lid margin need accurate suturing, care being taken to align the grey line (Fig. 15.2). Lacerations of the muscle layer should be repaired with fine absorbable sutures. Deep lacerations involving the full thickness of the lid require careful examination to exclude damage to underlying structures. These should be repaired wherever possible within the first 24 hours as prolonged gaping will eventually cause fibrosis and contracture of the muscles and thickening and retraction of the tarsal plate. Repair should be in layers, fine absorbable sutures being used to

Figure 15.2
Suturing lid
(importance of
aligning the grey line).

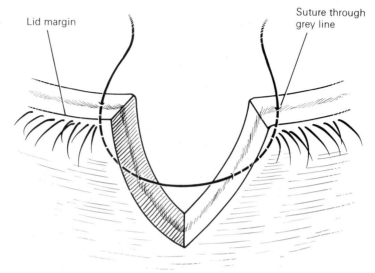

Lid margin

Suture through
grey line

close the conjunctiva, a pull-out nylon suture for the tarsal plate and a pull-out continuous suture for the skin. It is often helpful also to have a single interrupted suture on the grey line to align this correctly.

Complications and their management

1 *Notching.* Failure to align the structures correctly will result in some notching along the lid margin.

Identification of the grey line and inserting the first suture through this on either side of the laceration should ensure that correct alignment is achieved here.

2 *Corneal irritation.* This will result if too-heavy sutures are used to repair the conjunctiva and/or the knots are placed on the surface of the conjunctiva next to the globe. This is particularly a problem in upper-eyelid injuries owing to the greater excursion of movement of the upper eyelid. It may also result if the margins of the wound are not correctly aligned, resulting in the lashes being inverted (entropion).

Careful placing of the sutures will help to avoid the problem, viz. away from the conjunctival surface.

3 *Ectropion.* This may result if the tissues in the lower lid are not correctly aligned. More commonly it occurs owing to injuries just below the eyelid, particularly when a transverse scar results and there is associated tissue loss.

This complication can be prevented by careful alignment of the tissues and accurate suturing of each of the layers divided. Unrecognized tissue loss is another reason for ectropion, and primary reconstruction of the defect should be by either a graft or a flap.

Urgent treatment of upper-lid ectropion is indicated if the cornea is exposed when the eyes are 'closed'. Release of the scar and suturing carefully in layers should be carried out. Sometimes inserting a Z-plasty in the scar will help prevent any recurrence. Where there is significant tissue loss, reconstruction with grafts and flaps will have to be undertaken.

2. Lid defect

It is important to determine whether the injury has resulted in simple laceration or whether there is associated loss of lid tissue. Owing to the excellent blood supply, very small flaps of tissue in this area will heal well and there is no place for aggressive excision of tissue during debridement without first carefully examining the tissue for viability. On the other hand leaving non-viable tissue, or simply suturing the wound margins together without recognizing the loss of tissue, will lead to complications that are often difficult to correct at a later stage.

Defects may be partial-thickness or full-thickness, full-thickness implying either vertical or horizontal loss of tissue and affecting upper, lower or both eyelids.

Partial thickness loss

Grafting. Full-thickness or split-skin grafts can be used on either lid. Split-skin grafts have the benefit of being thin and thus mobile (of benefit in the upper lid) but tend to contract significantly (and therefore to be of little use in the lower lid, where ectropion will result). Full-thickness grafts do not contract but have the disadvantage of being too thick and may interfere with normal lid movement. Therefore, they are more appropriate in the lower lid rather than for upper lid defects.

When reconstructing an upper-lid defect with a split-skin graft, a large graft should be used in anticipation of some degree of contraction. A tie-over dressing is useful, particularly when a full-thickness graft is being used—this should be left in place for 4–5 days. The split-skin graft may be taken from the arm or leg (or postauricular region). A full-thickness graft is most conveniently taken from the pre- or postauricular region or the neck, the secondary defect being sutured. Occasionally, particularly in older patients in whom there is a surplus of skin in the upper lid, the graft may be taken from there. However, this is ill-advised if the defect is large, if there is any damage of the upper lid, or if there is little surplus skin present.

Flap reconstruction. Flap reconstruction will be discussed in more detail under 'Neoplasia'. Deep (partial-thickness) losses, i.e. skin, subcutaneous tissue, tarsal plate, should be reconstructed with skin flaps. Except on very rare occasions, when massive tissue loss is present, local flaps can be used. Flaps in general result in a better cosmetic appearance than do grafts and when designed correctly, the problem of contraction should not occur. Lower-lid and cheek defects are usually well reconstructed using lateral cheek rotation flaps. Flaps advanced from below the eyelid (lower-eyelid defects) tend to contract and often result in ectropion. Medially based flaps have a similar tendency to do this. Forehead flaps for large defects may be used for both upper and lower lid defects. The more limited Frické forehead flap is another method, though this has limited size, tends to pull the eyebrow upwards and usually requires a two-stage revision of the pedicle.

Full-thickness loss
The principles governing reconstruction of full-thickness defects are as follows.

1 Reconstruct cover, support and lining.
2 Use lower lid to reconstruct upper but use other tissues to reconstruct the lower (in full-thickness defects).
3 The reconstruction of a stable lid margin is all important and lack of this is the greatest single weakness of reconstructed eyelids.

4 Types of reconstruction:
  (a) Cover (flap) + lining (graft).
  (b) Cover (graft) + lining (flap).
  (c) Cover + lining (flap) + cartilage for support.
  (d) Defects of one-quarter of the eyelid, upper or lower, can be sutured directly or, if slightly greater, release of the lateral canthal ligament can be carried out (lateral canthotomy). Larger defects will cause excessive tightness and alternative methods will be required.

Lower lid. For defects of a quarter to a half, a lateral advancement flap can be used for skin—a chondromucosal graft if the defect is greater than 6–7 mm, for support. Defects of greater than half of the lid can be reconstructed using a chondromucosal graft and cheek rotation flap. Horizontal loss of the lower lid can be reconstructed using a chondromucosal graft in combination with a bipedicled upper-lid musculocutaneous flap. Several other methods for lower lid reconstruction have been described (for skin cover), e.g. Frické flap, central forehead flap and nasolabial flap (superiorly based). The Kollner lid-sharing method can be used for small defects; this can be associated with significant complications, which will be discussed later.

Upper lid. Defects of a quarter to a half of the upper lid can be reconstructed using a 'lid-switch' procedure (using a quarter of the lower lid; the secondary defect can therefore be closed by direct suture). Defects of a half to the whole of the upper lid can be reconstructed by transfer of up to three-quarters of the lower to the upper lid; reconstructing the lower-lid secondary defect has already been described.

Horizontal loss of the upper lid can be reconstructed using a bipedicled lower-lid musculocutaneous flap and chondromucosal graft with full thickness skin graft reconstruction of the secondary lower lid defect. Other methods of upper lid (skin) reconstruction include lid sharing by advancement flaps and the lateral advancement flap of McGregor. Several important points should be noted when using these various techniques for upper lid reconstruction. Firstly, the lower lid pedicled vessels are usually 3 mm from the lid margin and lie on the anterior border of the tarsus. This is important when raising the flap at its base. Secondly, elevation of the upper lateral fornix conjunctiva needs to be done carefully so as not to sever the tiny lacrimal ductules. Thirdly, the skin of the reconstructed upper lid must be attached to the tarsus, otherwise the lid skin will hang down. Fourthly, it is important that the levator muscle should be attached into the reconstructed segment, particularly in large defects.

Both lids. It is rare for both lids to be lost and the globe to be intact. Reconstruction of the lids in this situation can be carried out by covering the eye with conjunctiva then covering the whole with a midline forehead flap and then, at a second stage, creating two lids; obviously, lid mobility is likely to be severely limited.

Complications of eyelid reconstruction and their management

The greater the defect, the higher the potential risk of developing some complications, because the more sophisticated the reconstruction has to be. Complications such as haematoma and infection can be avoided if careful debridement and haemostasis are carried out before the reconstruction is performed. Complications of repair include the following.

Failure of graft take
Grafts will normally take well in the eyelids because of excellent blood supply.

Prevention. Adequate debridement must be carried out and non-viable tissue excised, otherwise graft failure is inevitable. The graft also may be inadequately immobilized and the use of a few interrupted sutures around the margin of the graft and a tie-over bolus over the graft will help to reduce this mobility. This is particularly important for full-thickness grafts in the lower lid.

Treatment. If total failure occurs, reconstruction by further grafting when conditions are favourable or local flap repair should be carried out.

Care must be taken to avoid the cornea being exposed and a temporary tarsorrhaphy will be required if indicated.

Ectropion
Prevention. Split-skin grafts to reconstruct lower lid defects should be avoided as ectropion is certain to follow as the graft contracts. In the upper lid, split-skin grafts are preferred as they are thin and will allow adequate mobility of the upper lid.

Treatment. Correction by release of the ectropion and reconstruction of the skin defect with a full-thickness graft or flap is the treatment of choice. If there is considerable scarring around the lower lid, then a flap is a better choice than a graft. The choice of flap will depend on the size of defect, etc. Lateral cheek flaps or a Tripier flap from the upper lid are two such flaps that may be used. It is important also to determine the degree of cartilaginous support; the tarsal plate may also be damaged and reconstruction needed.

Unstable lid margin
Lower eyelid
Failure to achieve a permanently stable margin may result in sagging or even ectropion. This is usually a complication of full-thickness defects, especially when grafts have been used. It may result from inadequate support from the orbicularis muscle

(owing to poor repair or nerve injury), or it may result from poor support of the cartilaginous graft.

Prevention. Three important points should be observed. Firstly, when using a chondromucosal graft, a large graft (for the lower lids) sufficient for it to rest on the bony orbital rim should be taken. This greatly adds to its support—its extra size in the lower lid is important in relation to restricting lid movement. Secondly, sufficient mucosa should be taken with the cartilage graft to bring this over the superior surface of the graft for suturing to the margin of the skin flap. Thirdly, the graft should be taken from that part of the nasal septum that is slightly curved, and this curvature (convex side outwards) should be used to achieve greater apposition of the reconstructed lid to the globe. Many people prefer to take the graft using the upper lateral cartilage of the nose together with its overlying mucosa. An alternative method is to cross-hatch the cartilage.

Upper eyelid
An unstable lid margin in the upper lid may also occur, with possible resulting entropion and corneal irritation. One cause is inadequate or deficient cartilaginous support. This may be from the injury or as a result of using the upper-lid tissue in lower-lid reconstruction. The method of Kollner has been associated with this problem.

Prevention. The problem may be reduced by making the inferior incision of the tarsoconjunctival flap form the upper lid, a distance of 3 or 4 mm from the lid margin rather than 2 mm. The length of this flap should be equivalent to the length of the defect minus one quarter. It is therefore necessary to limit the indications for this procedure and not to try to adapt it to defects extending the entire length of the eyelid.

Cosmesis An unsatisfactory cosmetic result to the repair or donor site may be due to several causes, including poor healing, the wrong choice of repair method for the defect, or simply the unpredictable effects of scarring.

Colour
When a skin graft from, for example, the thigh is used, the colour may be different from that of the tissue around the recipient site and so may be very conspicuous.

Prevention. When a graft is used, skin from the face region will generally give a better colour match. Full-thickness grafts from the postauricular area or neck generally match well in the eyelid region. In many cases, pre-auricular skin grafts (when sufficient amount of tissue is available to achieve the direct closure of the secondary defect) gives an even better colour match.

Bulky flaps

One great disadvantage of the Tripier flap is its tendency to become tubular with the passage of time (Fig. 15.3). This can lead to a very bulky appearance of the lower-lid region. Midline forehead flaps or smaller glabellar flaps (used for inner canthal area reconstruction) can also be bulky. Similarly temporal flaps are often too bulky.

Prevention.   One method of helping to minimize the tubular effect of the Tripier flap is to use a tie-over bolus dressing which should be left in place for 7–10 days.

Treatment.   Bulky flaps can be raised at a later date and be thinned to improve their appearance. Extensive thinning should not be carried out at the time of division of a pedicled flap as this may compromise the blood supply.

Figure 15.3
Tubular reformity
associated with Tripier
flap.

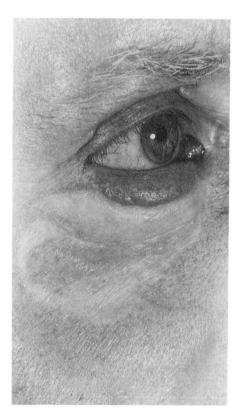

Donor-site scarring
Use of temporal flaps often requires skin grafts for the secondary defect. Use of upper lid skin for grafts for lower lid defects (where there is little spare skin available) can lead to imbalance between the normal and donor site upper lids—the sulcus being considerably more pronounced on the donor side. If a large cheek rotation flap is planned, the scars usually settle in well.

Prevention
1 It is important to design the flap to ensure that the scars lie in as close alignment as possible with the crease lines.
2 The actual size of the scar can be reduced in the cheek rotation flap by McGregor's Z-plasty modification, placed just lateral to the outer canthal area (Fig. 15.4). This will often give sufficient extra mobility to the flap and has the added advantage of repositioning the scar in a direction closer to the natural crease line in this area and thus improving the overall alignment of the scar.

Treatment. When the position of the defect being reconstructed does not facilitate an optimum design of flap scar, secondary revisionary surgery, e.g. insertion of Z-plasties, may be indicated.

Epiphora Where the medial ends of the lids are damaged there is the risk that the normal drainage mechanism for the tears may be disrupted. This may be evident at the time of the initial assessment and must always be examined for. It may, on the other hand, present late owing to scarring around the canaliculi or deep in the tear sac or nasolacrimal duct region.

Prevention. Initial management to repair the canaliculi (both upper and lower) should be carried out. This will have to be done

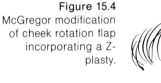

Figure 15.4
McGregor modification of cheek rotation flap incorporating a Z-plasty.

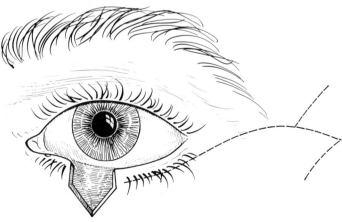

under magnification using 9-0 or 10-0 nylon sutures. A small silastic tube can be used as a step to ensure patency of the reconstructed duct. Alternatively a 3-0 or 4-0 nylon suture will usefully serve the same purpose—it can be fed down into the nose and tied as a loop for several days until healing is completed.

Treatment. When the condition presents late, a dacryocysto-rhinostomy will usually have to be carried out.

Eyelid burns

The majority of patients who sustain extensive burns to the face will have involvement of the eyelids as well. Several important principles in the assessment and management of these injuries are as follows.

Careful assessment The presence of singed eyelashes and brows can be an important sign suggestive of an extensive burn injury.

Visual acuity The possibility of visual impairment must be clarified at an early stage.

Conjunctival and corneal injury A careful examination of conjunctival and corneal injuries is imperative. Foreign bodies may be present (particularly if there has been an explosive element to the burn injury). Fluoroscein staining of the cornea to show any obvious abrasion is also necessary. The finding of chemosis or diffuse swelling of the conjunctiva strongly suggests an injury of the conjunctiva, though factors such as administration of excessive fluids during the course of the initial resuscitation may be the cause of oedema. An early ophthalmological opinion should be sought if there is any evidence of eye injury before swelling obscures the globe.

Cause of the burn It is important to ascertain the cause of the burn as this may influence the initial management.

Flash and flame burns
Flash and flame cause the majority of burns to the eyelids. Exposure of the eyes and eyelids to the heat in a flash burn is of short duration and the resulting injury usually superficial. Once injury to the eye itself is excluded, management consists of the application of antibiotic ointments and healing is usually uncomplicated. Flame burns may be deeper. The real danger in the initial phase, having excluded acute damage to the eye itself, is complications arising from exposure of the cornea. This is more likely to occur if the burns involve the full thickness of an eyelid skin. Management consists of protection of the exposed cornea with artificial tears, ointments or external exclusive dressings, or a combination of these. In severe cases, particu-

larly when the exposure of the cornea persists following resolution of the initial swelling, a more aggressive approach is indicated—release of the contracture and grafting with or without tarsorrhaphy.

Chemical burns
Immediate irrigation of the eye and eyelids with water or saline should be carried out. With acid burns, the injury is usually superficial unless the contact with the acid is prolonged, the acid is very strong, or the commencement of irrigation is delayed significantly. Alkaline fluid, however, can result in significant complications and an urgent ophthalmological opinion should be obtained. Tissue damage tends to be much more extensive. The extent of damage may be further aggravated by collagenases liberated from the epithelium and infiltrating leucocytes. Extensive fibrosis of the eye and surrounding structures may result.

Prevention of eyelid burns and their complications
The use of properly fitting goggles or masks can reduce the incidence of these serious injuries and should be worn by those at greatest risk, e.g. those working with welding apparatus or in the chemicals industry (Fig. 15.5). Where molten metal etc. has become adherent to the lid, it should be removed as quickly as possible. In chemical burns to the eyelids, copious irrigation using saline should be instigated as soon as possible.

Full-thickness burns of the eyelids are complicated most frequently by ectropion, but the effects of this can be partially prevented in the early post-burn period by using eye ointments, artificial tears and blinking exercises.

Long-term complications and their management

Lid ectropion This is the commonest complication of eyelid burns. The management of ectropion in the early post-burn period should be conservative as far as possible, using ointments, blinking exercises, etc. When the problem is not controlled by these, a temporary tarsorrhaphy should be carried out, followed if necessary by a full surgical release and graft. Where this is necessary in the early post-burn phase, a full-thickness graft should be used in the lower eyelid and a split-skin graft in the upper; this may have to be repeated after several weeks. In the late presentation, a full-thickness graft should be used for lower-lid release and a split-skin graft for upper-lid release.

Treatment
The releasing incisions are made a few millimetres above or below the affected lid ciliary margin. The incision should be extended from medial to lateral canthal regions and in the lower lid it may need to be extended for a further centimetre or so in a

Figure 15.5
(a) Burn caused by
molten metal.
(b) Goggles prevented
eyelid and eye injury.

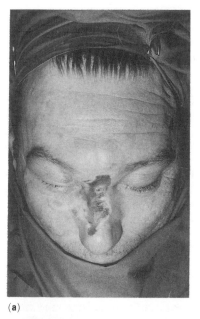

(a)

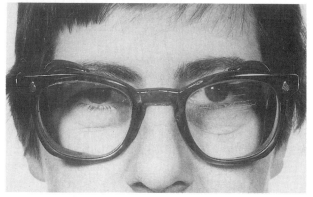

(b)

Figure 15.5 (a) Burn caused by molten metal. (b) Goggles prevented eyelid and eye injury.

slightly upward direction from the outer canthus. Excision of the scar itself need not be carried out. The graft should be taken and sutured into place in the usual way with a tie-over bolus for the lower-lid full-thickness graft. Extensive loss of the full thickness of the lid will require a chondromucosal graft and flap, as already discussed in the previous section. Some people have found a temporary tarsorrhaphy a helpful adjunct to this surgery during the immediate postoperative period. When not being carried out in the acute situation, release of the ectropion is probably best left for at least 6–9 months or longer if possible so as to allow the scars to reach their maximum contracture, otherwise the need for a further release operation will be inevitable.

Palpebral fissure stenosis

This may result from full-thickness burns of the eyelids when adhesion of the tarsal margins occurs, resulting in spherical contraction of the eyelid margins, or 'porthole' deformity. Management is surgical to correct the deformity.

Treatment

It is important to estimate the extent of tissue loss or deficit in both upper and lower eyelids and this must be corrected before attempting to widen the palpebral fissure. Release is fairly straightforward, dividing the bridge between the eyelids and suturing the skin and conjunctival edges of the individual lids together. However, the release must be adequate to allow repositioning of the medial canthus. It may be further complicated by ectropion and epiphora (from canalicular obstruction). It is particularly important to correct the ectropion before the stenosis is corrected, otherwise an eversion deformity of the tarsal margin can result.

Canalicular obstruction

This is usually only seen in very extensive burns with considerable scarring around the eyelids and surrounding structures. The canalicular openings may be partially or completely obliterated with resulting epiphora. This is not always troublesome for the patient but, where it is, surgical intervention is indicated.

Treatment

Probing of the canaliculus should first be carried out to determine the extent of the obstruction. It may be due to foreign material and not to scar tissue, and it may be possible to clear the passages. If not, a new drainage route is created. One method of doing this is to raise a medially based conjunctival flap from the lower conjunctival sulcus and tunnel this through the nasal bone into the nose. A small silicone-rubber catheter may be placed along the path of the flap and should stay in place for several months.

Eyebrow deformities

Some hair follicles will remain in the eyebrow region in most cases, but in a severe burn there is total loss. In female patients, particularly when there is only loss of eyebrow hair, the use of an 'eyebrow pencil' is very effective in disguising this defect. In male patients, or in females when there is total loss, two main techniques of reconstruction can be used.

Treatment

Free hair grafts. It is important that a donor site is selected so that the hair is pointing in the right direction. A further complication is, of course, failure of all or part of the graft. This may result from the following.

(a) Poor haemostasis at the recipient site.

(b) Inadequate preparation of the graft. Excessive fat in the base of the graft should be trimmed but excessive trimming may destroy some of the hair follicles.

(c) The recipient site or base may be too scarred to be able to sustain the skin graft.

(d) The graft may be too large. Preferably a narrow strip (of the desired length of eyebrow) not more than 0.5 cm in width should be used.

Scalp is the donor site most commonly used.

Hair-bearing island pedicle flap. This is based on the superficial temporal artery and vein. A strip of hair-bearing skin based on this pedicle is raised, the pedicle is dissected back, and the vascularized flap is tunnelled into the required position in the eyebrow. The donor defect is then closed directly. This usually results in a very bushy eyebrow that needs to be frequently trimmed, as one might expect. In female patients, the thickness of the hair is often unacceptable. Its main advantages are that it gives an immediate result and that it can be used in very scarred areas since, being a pedicled flap, it is not dependent on the base for nutrition.

Neoplasia of the eyelids

Squamous-cell carcinoma of the eyelids is rare, but basal-cell carcinomas are common. The principles that govern the reconstruction of the eyelid following excision of these lesions have been described, together with the different flaps and their limitations and complications.

Specific complications encountered with eyelid malignancy

Notching of the lid margin   A traumatic defect cannot, as it were, be 'controlled' (i.e. the shape or position of the defect). When excision, for example of a basal cell carcinoma, is carried out the excision should at first be vertical to the lid margin, continuing into a V (Fig. 15.6). This will avoid notching along the limb margin. The same rules apply to suturing of the wound (or of the graft into place) using pull-out fine nylon sutures for the tarsal plate and skin layers and correctly aligning the grey line.

Recurrence   Adequate clearance of the tumour is obviously of paramount importance. The method of reconstruction should never compromise an adequate cancer excision.

Donor-site morbidity   When a cartilage graft is required for tarsal plate reconstruction, the nasal septum is best avoided in elderly patients,

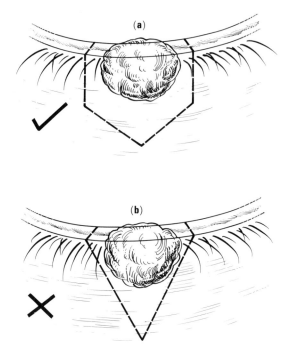

Figure 15.6
Correct incision lines
for wedge excision
involving lid margin to
help prevent notching.

particularly if they are hypertensive, as troublesome bleeding from the donor site can often result. It is better either to use upper lateral nasal cartilage or to take a graft from the pinna of the ear.

Ectropion

Ectropion has already been mentioned as a complication of various operative techniques around the eyelids. Most of these will result in what is usually defined as a cicatricial ectropion. However, ectropion may also occur secondary to other disease processes and two other main groups are usually described viz. senile ectropion, in which the lower lid is horizontally elongated from partial or complete disinsertion of the canthal tendons, the orbicularis attachments to the pretarsal tissues are compromised, and the orbicularis muscle is hypertonic and has probably migrated inferiorly to some extent. Paralytic ectropion results from facial nerve palsy.

Predisposing factors

Cicatricial ectropion This occurs as a result of vertical shortening of the external layers of an eyelid. This may result following chemical and thermal burns, tumours in the region adjacent to the lids, collagen diseases that tighten the skin, radiation to the lids or orbital region or poor repair of eyelid lacerations. Longstanding senile ectropion may also be a cause.

Treatment
This consists of releasing the contracture and skin grafting the resulting defect. For the lower lid, as already mentioned, this should also be done using full-thickness skin grafts, usually of postauricular skin. Several points in the technique should be stressed as recurrence of the deformity may result from in-adequate surgery.

1 Any subcuticular scars and bands should be excised rather than simply released.
2 The eyelid should be in the normal position at the end of the release procedure prior to repair of the defect with a skin graft. Any deformity at this stage will persist and almost certainly result in a recurrence of the ectropion when the area is healed.
3 Meticulous technique should be observed when preparing the bed and graft. In particular, there should be no bleeding from the bed, as this will interfere with graft take.
4 The graft should be cut slightly larger than the defect. It should be sutured into place with some traction on the eyelid. A tie-over bolus dressing should be used and this should be left for 4–5 days.

Senile ectropion This results from a weakening and atony of the fibres of the orbicularis and, on the other hand, to a relaxation and disten-sion of all the tissues of the lower eyelid and a subsequent elongation of the free margins of the lid. This may be associated with hypertrophy and keratinization of the conjunctiva, and the tarsus itself may become thickened and encourage it to 'bend outwards'. In senile ectropion, the eversion is usually most marked at the medial end with eversion of the lacrimal puncta, which may result in blocking of the lacrimal passages; episodes of recurrent blepharitis may occur.

Treatment
In order to achieve a full correction of this and avoid the main complication of inadequate correction, all the features present in a senile ectropion must be recognized as outlined above. The correct procedure should therefore:

1 reduce the cutaneous distension by skin excision;
2 shorten the tarsoconjunctival layer and free margin by a resection;
3 reinforce the muscular tone by shortening of the muscle.

Although several techniques have been described, the modified Kuhnt–Szymanowski procedure fulfils all these criteria and has been found to work well in practice (Fig. 15.7). This method combines a tarsoconjunctival and cutaneous resection. An incision is made along the free edge near the ciliary margin, and the skin undermined, more extensively at the lateral extent of the incision. The incision is extended laterally and superiorly towards the lateral extent of the eyebrow. Next, an excision of a superiorly based tarsoconjunctival triangle is carried out near the lacrimal punctum, the size depending upon the amount of distension (the larger, the greater the excision). This is sutured with a running tarsoconjunctival suture. The orbicularis is then sutured and a triangle of skin is excised at the lateral margin of the dissection, as much as required. Several points need to be stressed.

Figure 15.7
Modified
Kuhnt–Szymanowski
procedure.

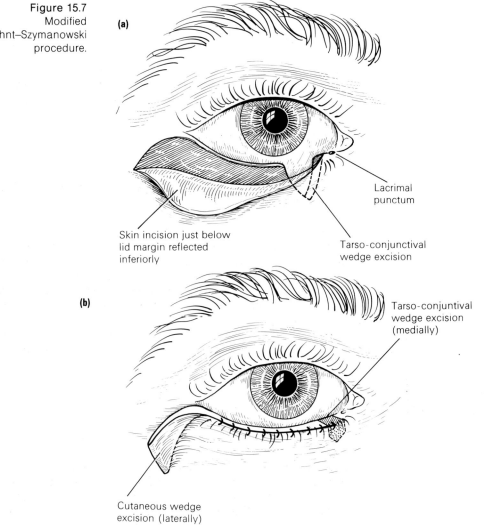

(a)

Lacrimal
punctum

Skin incision just below
lid margin reflected
inferiorly

Tarso-conjunctival
wedge excision

(b)

Tarso-conjuntival
wedge excision
(medially)

Cutaneous wedge
excision (laterally)

1 The tarsoconjunctival resection should be carried out as close to the lacrimal punctum as possible to avoid damage to the motor branches of the facial nerve.
2 To avoid a lowering of the lateral commissure, the skin incision is carried beyond the outer canthus.
3 Where thickening of the conjunctiva, due to keratinization, occurs, a thin horizontal strip of conjunctiva may be excised. Otherwise, full correction may not be achieved.

Paralytic ectropion   Paralytic ectropion results from facial nerve paralysis and its severity (and subsequently the correct management) may vary. In mild cases, a simple tarsorrhaphy may be all that is required. In the more severe cases, the procedure described for senile ectropion treatment can be used.

Blepharoplasty

This operation aims to correct the 'baggy' appearance of the upper and/or lower eyelids that may be due to lax or excess skin and/or fat in the subcutaneous tissue (which originates from the orbital fat). The aims of the operation are:

1 to excise the excess skin;
2 to remove the fat hernias;
3 to reduce the wrinkles of the crowsfeet.

The surgery may be carried out under local or general anaesthetic.

Prevention of complications
Careful assessment pre-operatively of these patients is all-important. For example, brow ptosis may be the predominant problem rather than baggy eyelids (which may at first sight appear the dominant problem); surgery to the eyelid only might therefore accentuate the problem rather than improve and correct it.
Meticulous surgical technique will also help prevent many of the complications, in particular, haematoma formation.

Complications and their treatment

Undercorrection   Undercorrection is the easiest complication to rectify, whether it is insufficient skin or fat that has been removed. The treatment is the additional excision of tissue as required.

Haematoma   Haematoma may occur superficially in the wound or form deeply in the orbit. The former can readily be released by removing a few sutures. The latter is one of the disastrous complications, as it can lead to blindness. It is usually associated with sudden severe pain. The eye must be examined immediately and the haematoma evacuated, decompressing the orbit. If this is unsuccessful, canthotomy with release of the canthal tendons may be necessary. Visual acuity should be determined and the fundus examined. If there is any doubt, an urgent ophthalmological opinion should be sought (reports have shown that with paracentesis of the anterior chamber, patients have gone from no light perception to good visual function when this has been performed promptly).

Infection Infection is rare but active treatment with the appropriate antibiotic is indicated.

Muscle imbalance Muscle imbalance may lead to diplopia. This complication, though rare, usually clears without surgical intervention. Surgery should be deferred as long as improvement is taking place.

Hypertrophic scars Hypertrophic scars are again a rare complication and is probably best treated with triamcinolone injection if there has been no improvement over the normal scar-maturation period.

Brow complications One of the commonest mistakes is a failure to recognize and correct brow ptosis, which results in fullness of the upper eyelid. Trying to correct this with a blepharoplasty alone will result in a poor cosmetic result.

Corneal exposure

Complications specific to the upper eyelid This will result from incomplete closure of the upper eyelid and may be caused by either excess skin excision or incorporation of the orbital septum in a low-placed scar. Waiting for the scar to mature is often all that is required. Attempts at trying to stretch the lid may correct this, but surgical exploration to release the scar and replace deficient skin with a skin graft may have to be carried out if these measures fail. The cornea should be protected until this time, e.g. using artificial tears.

Complications specific to the lower lid The most common complication involving the lower lid is retraction of the lid inferiorly, the free border no longer covering the inferior limbus. True ectropion occurs more rarely.

Predisposing factors
The main cause for these complications is excessive resection of the skin, but it may be due to retraction of the septum owing to poor placing of the incision, or palpebral atony.

Prevention of complications
1 Carry out a fairly wide skin undermining before carrying out the skin resection.
2 Avoid excess skin resection. One advantage of carrying out the operation under local anaesthetic is that the patient can

be asked to open their mouth; this tightens the cheek and will enable the surgeon more accurately to assess the amount of skin he can safely resect.

3 Do not suture the septum to avoid its retraction.

4 Use careful haemostasis.

5 Use of steristrips to 'suspend' the eyelid (which also gives good localized compression on the wound).

6 Surgery should be avoided on those patients who have a tendency to atonic ectropion, i.e. careful selection of patients.

7 Finally, the experience of the surgeon performing the operation is also an important factor in determining how much tissue to remove in order to achieve the optimal aesthetic improvement without risking complication.

Treatment
Where the surgeon is fairly confident that excess skin has not been removed, then massaging the scar and a conservative approach should be adopted. After several weeks the lid retraction should improve. If excess skin has been taken, tightening of the lower lid by resection of a small segment of the lid at its lateral end may be sufficient on its own, but if a larger amount of excess skin has been removed, then this is corrected with a full-thickness graft to the defect of the lower lid following release of the ectropion.

Persisting controversies
- Techniques that utilize upper-lid tissue to reconstruct lower-lid defects.
- The optimum flap for lower-lid reconstruction.

Further reading
Tessier, P., Rougier, J., Hervouet, F., Woillez, M., Lekieffre, M. & Derome, P. (1981) *Plastic Surgery of the Orbit and Eyelids*. New York: Masson Publishing.

Macomber, W.B. (1978) Orbital and Eyelid Surgery. *Clinics in Plastic Surgery*, Vol. 5:4. London: Saunders.

Mustarde, J.C. (1966) *Repair and Reconstruction in the Orbital Region*. Edinburgh: Churchill Livingstone.

Collins, J.R. (1983) *A Manual of Systematic English Surgery*. Edinburgh: Churchill Livingstone.

16 Complications of Operations on the Nose

Historically, reconstruction of the nose has been a focal point in the development of plastic surgery. The vulnerability of the nose to injury and the custom of punitive amputation of the nose have presented ample challenge for treatment. Virtually every reconstructive technique has been used, including split- and full-thickness skin grafts, local, distant or free microvascular flaps. The general complications of these methods are discussed in other chapters, but the specific complications as applied to surgery of the nose will be discussed here.

Treatment of nasal trauma

While nasal injury is rarely life-threatening, the prominent position of the nose, as a principal feature of the face, makes correct treatment of damage vitally important if the patient is not to suffer long-term distressing disfigurement.

Predisposing factors

The chief cause of complications of treatment of nasal trauma is failure to diagnose or assess the condition correctly. When the patient is suffering from severe, life-threatening injuries, the nasal injury may go unnoticed. Associated injuries of the face or skull may also distract attention from the fractured nose. The degree of swelling in these cases may obscure the extent of nasal injury. It is important to examine the nose correctly and (especially if the patient is under general anaesthesia with a nasotracheal tube, which can mask injury) palpation must not be omitted. Associated injuries including naso-ethmoid fracture, orbital fracture and septal trauma may also be missed.

In all cases, if diagnosis is delayed, treatment will be delayed; late repair will be very much more difficult if not impossible, since facial bones become 'sticky' and fixed in the displaced position in a few days. Failure to consult with and refer to an appropriate specialist in the early stages is a potent cause of unsatisfactory results.

Prevention of complications

Assess the patient Fracture of the nose may occur as part of a more severe multiple injury and is frequently associated with damage to other facial bones. Thorough physical examination must include examination of the whole patient, paying particular attention to the skull, middle third, mandible and dentition. Fractures of the ethmoids, and eye damage, must also be detected at the preliminary stage. In severe blunt trauma to the head, X-ray of the facial bones and skull is essential. In children, fracture of the nose is less common, but more difficult to diagnose because of the small size of the nasal bones. (Fig. 16.1).

Assess the nose A full routine examination of the nose should be made externally and internally to check the airway and septum. In severe trauma or when the patient is seen late, it is often difficult to make an accurate assessment because of the severe bruising and swelling that develops. The diagnosis of a fractured nose is usually based on clinical findings. As the skeletal support of the nose is mostly cartilage, X-ray examination is frequently not helpful. It may, therefore, be necessary to

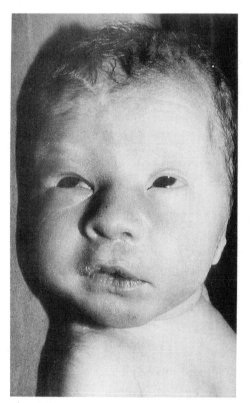

Figure 16.1
Deviation of the nose in a newborn child caused by obstetric forceps. X-ray examination is unhelpful and diagnosis rests on clinical examination.

re-examine the patient 48 hours later, once the swelling is subsiding, to see whether there is any deformity of the nose. The degree and extent of injury should be determined, making a careful note of damage and loss of tissue, as well as asymmetry. Clinical photographs make an important record for future reference and it is useful to obtain a pre-injury photograph of the patient.

Plan the treatment　Once the full extent of the injury has been determined, the nasal injury can be allocated a priority and treatment can be planned accordingly. It may be convenient to continue treatment of the nose under the same anaesthetic administered for other treatment. Ideally, nasal fracture reduction should be performed before the swelling occurs; if it is seen late, it would be better to delay until the oedema subsides, allowing more accurate judgement of the reduction achieved. When there are open wounds, early treatment affords the opportunity of exploring fractures through the wounds to assess the accuracy of the reduction and perform internal fixation if necessary.

Operative treatment　Basic principles of the repair of trauma apply. Repair must begin from a solid foundation and other facial bone fractures must be reduced and fixed internally or externally, if necessary. The nasal bones are then reduced and if they are unstable some form of mechanical stabilization must be applied. Once the skeletal framework is correct, the soft tissue is repaired in layers, suturing lining and cover separately.

Post-operative care　This depends very largely on the nature and extent of other injuries. The patient should be sitting upright as soon as possible, in order to reduce any swelling and bruising. External splints must be maintained in place to hold the position and the patient must be encouraged to rest for a few days. Bending down and straining are discouraged and nose blowing must be forbidden, as there is a risk of surgical emphysema and soft-tissue infection developing. Internal nose packs that obstruct the airway should be removed early, if possible within 48 hours; if there is a CSF leak, appropriate antibiotic prophylaxis must be given. If the leak does not stop within a few days after reduction and fixation of facial fractures, a neurosurgeon's opinion should be sought. When fractured nose has been treated in a child, there may be later deviation with growth: careful follow-up is indicated.

Management of complications

Haemorrhage　A severe nose-bleed is a rare complication of nasal fracture or elective nasal surgery. Full blood-clotting studies should be performed and any deficiencies corrected. The nose should be examined carefully to try to identify a bleeding point. An easily accessible anterior bleeder can be cauterized. If none is found and haemorrhage persists, the patient should be admitted for bed rest and sedation. An intravenous line should be set up and blood should be cross-matched.

Local measures. Anterior packing may suffice but posterior packing may be needed in addition. A softly inflated Foley catheter held forward under slight traction is a useful method for compressing a bleeding point posteriorly.

If haemorrhage is not controlled and persists in any great volume, ligation of the supplying arteries should be considered—for example, the anterior ethmoidal artery or transantral ligation of the maxillary artery.

Septal haematoma This is potentially a very severe complication, as it may lead to infection and necrosis of the septal cartilage, with subsequent nasal collapse, or to impaired nasal growth in a child. Organization of the haematoma and new cartilage formation will cause widening of the septum with airway obstruction. Inspection of the nose internally is essential and immediate draining of any haematoma must be performed together with packing of the nostrils to prevent recurrence.

Septal cartilage injury This is the commonest cause of persisting or recurrent nasal deviation. Treatment depends on the time at which it is discovered.

Early deviation. If initial reduction is not satisfactorily achieved or tends to relapse immediately, the septum should be inspected carefully for evidence of a tear. If necessary, a submucous resection of partially damaged or torn cartilage should be performed to allow full correction.

Late deviation may present as recurrent deformity with poor airway in an adult in the months after injury, or, if the fracture has occurred in childhood, growth defects or nasal obstruction may develop gradually years later. The septal cartilage can be removed by submucous resection or a septoplasty can be used with trimming or cross-hatching as necessary to straighten the deflected septum, carefully preserving the mucosa and sparing sufficient cartilage to maintain tip support (Fig. 16.2).

Naso-ethmoid complex injuries Early detection, if necessary by open exploration, is essential in treating this severe complication of nasal fractures. The late repair of such fractures is extremely difficult and results are very poor. Early management must concentrate on diagnosis and reducing deformity (Fig. 16.3).

Comminuted fractures. The principal deformity is broadening of the nasal base and separation of the canthi. Internal wiring to

Figure 16.2
(a,b) Collapse of the nose caused by excessive removal of deviated septal cartilage. A dorsal strut of septum should have been left to support the bridge-line.

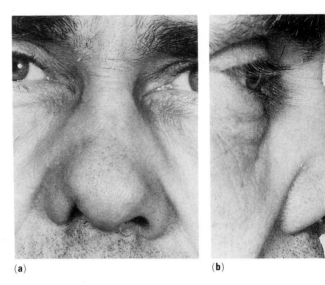

(**a**)   (**b**)

Figure 16.3
Compound fracture of the naso-ethmoid area that was not diagnosed initially when the skin wound was sutured (a). On exploration two days later, the centre of the nose is filled with blood clot (b). (c) The separation of the canthi is treated by transverse wiring. (d) The result three months later shows the reduction maintained. The senile ectropion may have confused the surgeon who first saw the patient.

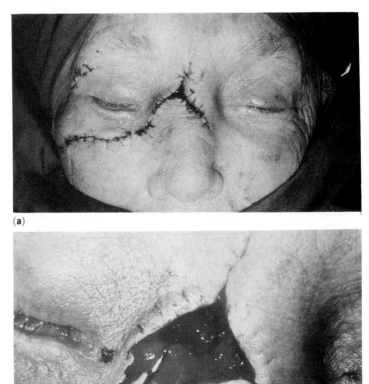

(**a**)

(**b**)

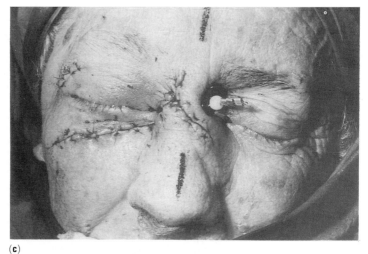

(c)

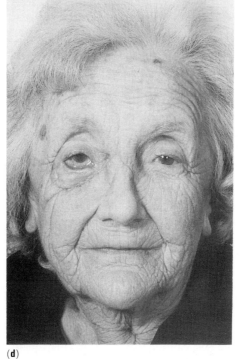

(d)

narrow the canthi gives the best results. Forward traction may
also be required.

Lacrimal injury.   Reduction of the fractures to an anatomical
position will usually prevent obstruction. Later, lacrimal drainage operation may be required.

Depressed fractures. The nasal bones may be impacted as a single block or as part of severe comminuted fractures. Elevation may be possible at operation, but forward traction will be required. This is best applied by wiring forward on to a T-piece supported from a halo or supraorbital pins. Elastic traction can also be used.

Nasal reconstruction

Predisposing factors

Failure to eradicate the underlying cause of damage to the nose, whether infection or tumour, makes nasal reconstruction not only unsuccessful but disastrous, in that the repair itself may be destroyed or have to be resected. Poor assessment, so that the full anatomical extent of loss is not determined, will give rise to unsatisfactory results. For example, if the lining is inadequate, no amount of skeletal support will keep the nose in good shape.

Inappropriate assessment and patient counselling may give rise to exaggerated patient expectation and lead to disappointment. Inelegant surgical technique or needlessly visible donor scars may also mar the final result.

Prevention of complications

Pre-operative assessment

In the treatment of tumours of the nose, the true extent of the nasal defect may not be evident until the primary lesion has been resected; but before reconstruction can be planned, the extent of loss, both quantitative and qualitative, must be diagnosed. There are four fundamental elements to be considered, any or all of which might be involved:

1 foundation;
2 lining;
3 cover;
4 support.

Planning

Once an accurate assessment has been made, planning of the repair must be performed in addition to seeking informed consent from the patient.

Foundation

The basis of all reconstructive procedures is to start with a stable, sound foundation, which, in the case of the nose, a midline structure, must be symmetrical. If the bone foundation of the maxilla is not suitable, it must be reconstructed or adjusted first.

Lining

Good-quality lining is an essential component of the nose. Deficiency causes shrinking, collapse and deformity, even if the skeletal support and cover are adequate, by allowing chronic infection and fibrosis to develop. Free grafts of skin or mucosa are only suitable for small defects because of the inherent tendency of free grafts to shrink. Local flaps of skin, either from the edge of the defect or nasolabial flaps from non-hair-bearing areas, give much more satisfactory results. Mucosal flaps from the lip are ideal lining for reconstruction of the tip of the nose and septum or columella. Thick flaps such as forehead skin are not suitable for lining, as they give the nose a bulky appearance that is difficult to thin without damage to the blood supply. Free flaps are better reserved for cover when there is a large defect to be repaired.

Cover   The texture of nose skin is unique and attention must be given to replacing it with the next-best available alternative, but minimizing the donor defect. The forehead flap of the Indian rhinoplasty gives adequate quantities of ideal skin, but the donor site can be conspicuous. Local flaps from the nasolabial area, if non-hair-bearing, are suitable for smaller defects and give a good colour match. Distant flaps are less suitable because the colour and texture are very different, but the donor sites can often be placed inconspicuously. For small defects, free full-thickness skin grafts from pre- or postauricular skin or the neck settle in very well, particularly in older patients. Composite grafts from the ear are a convenient method of repairing small defects of the rim or columella.

An important technique for disguising repairs so that they fit into the face unobtrusively is to pay particular attention to the aesthetic units and subunits of the face. The nose is an aesthetic unit in itself and it is divided into readily identified subunits (Fig. 16.4). If a repair is to be performed, better results are usually obtained if the margin of the defect and reconstruction correspond to the subunits (Fig. 16.5).

For larger defects, the skin flap size must provide a generous extra margin to allow for the curve required in forming a nose (Fig. 16.6).

Support   One-stage reconstruction of all four elements of nose construction can be performed. Alternatively, the support can be inserted once adequate lining and cover have been provided, but, if the support is not provided early, there is a danger of collapse developing. It is equally important not to rely on a skeletal support jacking up inadequate soft tissue, as the implant or graft may ulcerate and extrude, become infected and be lost. Support for the bridge line can be provided with bone, cartilage or silastic. Bone grafts may resorb, but if they take and unite soundly to the bridge line the nose can be unnaturally hard or easily fractured. Cartilage grafts give better support with flexibility, but all autografts except ear cartilage leave visible donor scars. Fresh cartilage from a donor carries risk of transmitted disease but processed sterilized bovine cartilage avoids these

Figure 16.4
Diagrammatic
representation of the
aesthetic subunits of
the nasal skin.

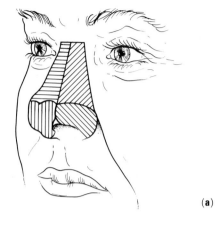

(**a**)

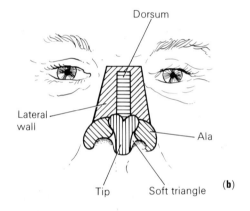

Dorsum

Lateral
wall

Ala

Tip　　Soft triangle　(**b**)

risks. Silastic support has the advantage of ready availability
with no donor defect. Ready-made implants are available but if
they are trimmed and modified the cut edge must be smoothed
carefully to avoid sharp edges or points that can penetrate the
soft tissues and allow movement or extrusion. Tip or alar
support is most conveniently provided by auricular cartilage
grafts (Fig. 16.7).

Timing.　While immediate reconstruction of a defect can give
great help to a patient in avoiding deformity and morbidity,
there are several factors which would make delay desirable.

Malignant disease.　After ablation or malignant disease, if
there is any doubt about the completeness of excision it is better
to delay the reconstruction. A temporary external prostheses
can be supplied. These prostheses may form the basis of a
permanent solution and the patient may be satisfied with the
result, avoiding the need for further reconstruction altogether.

Figure 16.5 Reconstruction of a defect caused by excision of a lesion of the ala of the nose. (a) The excision margin is enlarged to the size of the aesthetic subunit, and an appropriate flap is sutured in place (b). The bridge is divided and the flap inset two weeks later (c).

Figure 16.6 The size of flap cover for the nose must allow a generous extra margin to allow for the curvature of the dorsum.

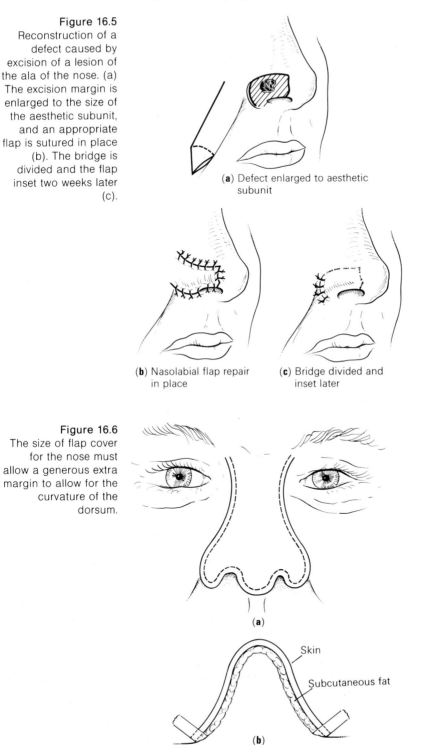

(**a**) Defect enlarged to aesthetic subunit

(**b**) Nasolabial flap repair in place

(**c**) Bridge divided and inset later

(**a**)

Skin

Subcutaneous fat

(**b**)

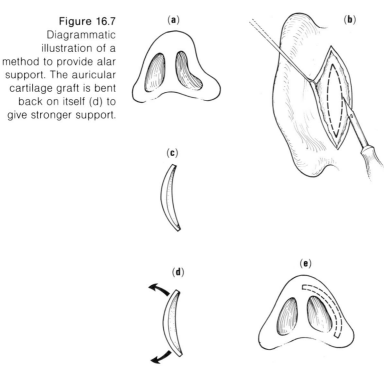

Figure 16.7
Diagrammatic illustration of a method to provide alar support. The auricular cartilage graft is bent back on itself (d) to give stronger support.

Infection and swelling. Any local infection must be cleared before reconstruction is performed. After infection or local trauma, there will inevitably be swelling and oedema. If this is not allowed to settle the viability of flaps may be compromised, and if the reconstruction is planned on a swollen base it will collapse as the swelling subsides.

Management of complications

Flap necrosis Complete necrosis of the flap is a disaster that should be prevented by careful planning. If the circulation of a forehead flap is compromised, judicious suture removal to reduce tension is indicated and any haematoma must be released. Infection must be treated vigorously with antibiotics. If the necrosis is substantial, slough must be removed and the viable tissue allowed to heal, if necessary with split-skin grafts, so that a repeat repair can be carried out later. A partial prosthesis to mask the defect can be used as a temporary or permanent solution. Soft silicone prostheses glued to the defect can be very satisfactory.

Donor scars The chief problem is the scar from a forehead flap. This defect can be minimized in several ways.

1 Use a midline symmetrical donor site if possible, so that the scar will be less conspicuous.
2 An inner upper-arm split-skin graft applied to the secondary defect is less likely to develop hyperpigmentation than is a thigh graft.
3 Direct closure of the defect immediately, or later removal of the skin graft with the help of tissue expansion, can provide a very great improvement of the donor scar.
4 Linear vertical donor scars can be improved by Z-plasty.

Loss of support If the support framework fails to take and is absorbed, it should be replaced. Temporary support with a moulded stent worn inside the nostrils may help to maintain the shape until a new support is fitted. If the support is too big and tight, it should ideally be trimmed electively before it becomes exposed, thus risking loss.

Colour A forehead flap usually gives excellent colour match and texture but may need to be protected from excessive sun exposure. If an Italian, upper-arm flap rhinoplasty, or distant free-flap repair has been performed, high-factor sunscreen cream or a brimmed hat to decrease actinic damage is essential to stop hyperpigmentation. Camouflage make-up can disguise the defect. Dermabrasion may help the colour match. Excision of the covering skin with overgrafting of suitable full-thickness graft, for example from supraclavicular or postauricular areas, is a useful method for giving a better colour.

Columella loss Support at the columella is vital to secure stability and durability of the nasal reconstruction. The original flap cover must be designed to allow for a columella. If loss occurs, small island flaps of lip or nasolabial skin can be used.

Cosmetic rhinoplasty

The complications of cosmetic rhinoplasty are legion and full discussion is outside the scope of this chapter. However, they fall into three basic categories.

1 Complications of patient selection for cosmetic surgery. The principles of presentation and management of these complications has been discussed in Chapter 1.
2 Complications of treatment selection. It is vital that the surgeon should know what the patient wants and expects and should gain the full understanding and consent of the patient, so that the patient is not dissatisfied with a technically satisfactory result.
3 Technical problems when the desired end result is not achieved, either owing to complications developing or by

deformities being produced. Rhinoplasty surgery is a difficult art, there is a variability of technique and wound healing that can produce variable results. The patient must be told of these factors and the prudent surgeon will advise the patient that in a small proportion of cases a second operation may be required.

Predisposing factors

General.   The factors common to all operations can give rise to complications. In particular, disorders of the blood-clotting mechanism, from specific coagulation defects or secondary to drug therapy, will predispose to haemorrhage.

Local factors.   Acute upper respiratory tract infection is a contra-indication to rhinoplasty. Care should be taken to ensure that the patient is free of acute or chronic infection of the tissues of the nose or the skin of the face, prior to treatment.

Surgical skill and experience.   Rhinoplasty can be a very difficult operation and the surgeon must be sufficiently trained and skilled to perform the task. If there is any doubt, help should be sought from a senior colleague.

Prevention of complications

Pre-operative assessment   A full history must be taken and specific enquiry made about bleeding disorders or medication that might interfere with the blood-clotting mechanism, such as anticoagulants, aspirin or the contraceptive pill.
   Examination of the nose must include internal examination to assess the airway and septum, external examination and assessment of the nose relationships with the face, facial bones, chin, dentition, stature and body build. In particular, asymmetries of the nose and the rest of the face must be noted. An accurate record, both written and photographic, should be made and kept for future reference.

Pre-operative planning   The treatment must be tailored to the individual patient, taking into account his or her wishes to achieve a result harmonious with the face and general body build of the patient. In some cases, for example, although the patient complains of the nose, it may be that the chin is not in proportion to the face. In these cases, surgery to alter the chin or size of the lower jaw must be considered, as the nose may not be the source of the problem (Fig. 1.4).

Check the plan   When the patient is admitted for treatment, the planned procedure should be checked with the patient before any premedication is given. It may be difficult in some circumstances if the patient is nervous or agitated at this stage. If the patient has serious doubts about proceeding with the operation or is uncertain what he or she wants done, it might be better to postpone surgery for a time and arrange a further consultation.

Anaesthesia   General or local anaesthesia can be used. As the operation is elective, the patient must be in peak physical condition with all correctable predisposing factors avoided. In Great Britain, a general anaesthetic with hypotension is the usual choice, so that blood loss can be kept to a minimum. This allows a much better view of the operative field to the surgeon.

Surgical technique   Careful operation by a suitably experienced surgeon with gentle tissue handling is the key to gaining the optimum result. Care must be taken to avoid excessive removal of tissue. Accurate sharp dissection with removal of measured amounts of bone and cartilage is the aim. Lining must be preserved at all costs, keeping its excision to a minimum. If the nose is symmetrical before operation, a similar mirror-image procedure must be performed on each side. Only if there is asymmetry should different procedures be employed on each side.

Incision   External skin incisions leave permanent scars and should be avoided on the dorsum of the nose. Mucosal incisions are preferable because the scar is concealed. Circumferential nostril incisions must be avoided to prevent stenosis.

Operative technique

Skin marking   The planned procedure, marked out in Bonney's Blue on the skin of the nose before any local infiltration is inserted, acts as a useful aid in performing the stages of the operation.

Sequence   The precise sequence can be varied, but it is usually best to develop a basic routine order so that essential steps are not omitted.

1 Septal surgery should be performed first, if required, especially if asymmetry is to be corrected. This gives a symmetrical foundation on which to proceed.
2 Tip surgery conveniently follows next, so that accurate trimming can be done before the swelling and bleeding, which often begin as the hump is treated, obscure the surgical field.
3 The hump is next removed, followed by an infracture. The septal length must be checked after hump removal to see whether columellar reduction is required (Fig. 16.8).
4 Finally, soft-tissue excision at the alar base is performed if necessary.
5 Any skin incision is sutured but it is not always necessary to suture the mucosa. Septal incisions should be sutured in

Figure 16.8
Tip length adjustments
must not be made
until after hump
reduction. In this
patient (a) the tip was
already short and no
tissue was removed
from the septal tip or
lining to prevent
excessive tip-tilting of
the nose (b).

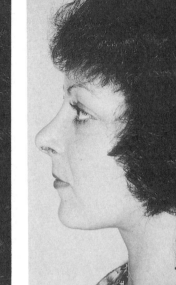

(a)   (b)

stepwise fashion on each side to prevent asymmetry developing.

Proceed one stage
at a time

After each stage of the operation has been performed, the result
must be checked and minor adjustment and trimming carried
out as necessary. Any removed cartilage or bone must be kept
moist in saline gauze. This aids checking for symmetry but also
allows replacement of a part as a free graft if too much has been
removed. For example, if an excess of hump has been removed, it
can be trimmed and replaced.

Use sharp
instruments

Particular care must be taken to ensure that clean, sharp cuts
are made in cartilage or bone. Blunt osteotomes can follow and
tear old fracture lines, particularly in previously comminuted
fractures, so that too much or too little is removed or jagged
areas are left. Rasping should be kept to a minimum in these
instances as it is very easy to remove too much of the softer,
friable bone. Cartilage should be incised cleanly to prevent
tears. Cartilage fragments that are still adherent must not be
pulled out blindly. The source of the tethering should be sought
and released.

Preserve tissue
attachments

It is important to keep the structures that are to be left in
anatomical continuity. This helps to avoid irregularities in
shape and will preserve blood supply. For example, periosteum
should only be elevated from bones that are removed (Fig. 16.9).
If the nose is 'skeletonized' and all the soft tissue attachments

Figure 16.9
Periosteal attachments
of the nasal bones
must be maintained
(b) to prevent
instability of the nasal
bone fragments which
could collapse into the
nasal cavity (a).

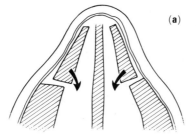

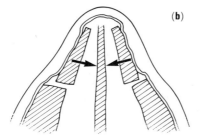

Figure 16.9
Periosteal attachments of the nasal bones must be maintained (b) to prevent instability of the nasal bone fragments which could collapse into the nasal cavity (a).

are removed, the bones can become unstable and may drop into the nasal cavity.

Avoid haematoma and infection Any haematoma or foreign body that could become a focus for infection must be removed at the time of operation. Bone or cartilage debris must be irrigated and sucked away (Fig. 16.10).

Post-operative care
After a reduction rhinoplasty, the skin will be excessive in size for the skeletal framework that is left. It is vital to prevent haematoma, oedema and fibrosis developing, which will prevent the skin from redraping, shrinking and taking up its new shape (Fig. 16.11). Internal packs and external support should be applied. Packs should be removed by 48 hours. The external support of tape, metal splint or Plaster of Paris should be left in place for at least a week to keep the reduced nasal bones in the desired shape. If there has been severe swelling, it may be better to replace the external splint for a further week.

Postoperative instructions must be firm and emphatic. The patient must not bend down or strain or blow the nose for one week postoperatively. It is best to sleep with extra pillows at night and to avoid lying flat for a week postoperatively. This helps to reduce the bruising and oedema. Gentle exercise, such as walking, is encouraged but strenuous activity should be avoided in the week or two following surgery. Contact sports must be avoided for at least six weeks.

Management of complications

Early complications The management of haemorrhage and haematoma has already been discussed.

Infection. An extremely rare but serious complication of rhinoplasty is meningitis via the cribriform plate. Severe headache and signs of meningism should alert the surgeon to the possibility of this complication; appropriate diagnostic measures should be taken and antibiotic treatment must be started.

Localized infection may occur at the infracture sites, especially when a saw has been used. Draining through a small stab incision will allow release of any pus and bone debris.

Figure 16.10 (a) Bone debris at the left inner canthus has caused new bone formation in the subcutaneous tissue. (b) View from above through a coronal incision, bone being removed. (c) External compression was maintained at night using an orthodontic head cap to prevent recurrence. (d) Six months later.

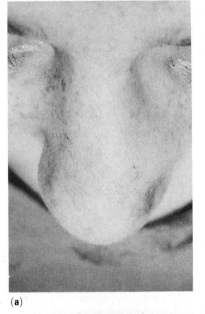

(a)

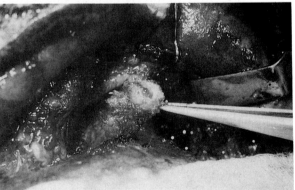

(b)

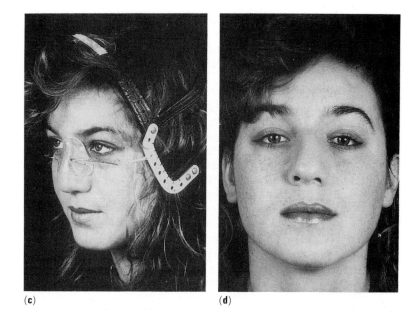

(c) (d)

Skin. Bruising and swelling inevitably occur but are usually transient lasting a few days. The application of tape usually causes small septic spots to develop, but these usually settle rapidly and spontaneously once the splint is removed.

Numbness. The patient should be warned that the tip of the nose will be numb or feel 'woody' for a few months. They must be

Figure 16.11 (a,b) The result of severe subcutaneous swelling caused by a badly applied external splint.

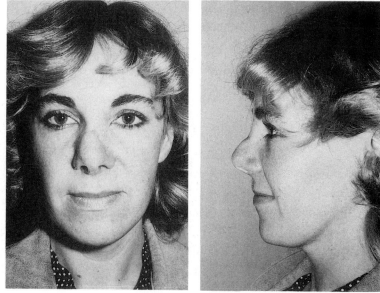

(a) (b)

instructed not to risk damaging the nasal skin by scratching it. This skin will be cold-sensitive and on really cold days care should be taken not to damage the tip, as chilblains or frost-bite may develop.

Late complications   The evaluation of late complications is very difficult. There will, inevitably, be swelling and oedema which may persist for months postoperatively. It is better to delay a decision about the need for reoperation for six months or a year rather than operate soon unless there is some obvious correctable deformity. Usually, if the surgeon has carried out careful reduction, the nose will slowly assume the desired shape. In the minority of cases, where a defect persists, the aim is to restore harmony to the shape of the nose, replacing tissue where an excess has been removed and trimming away where a surplus has been left.

Nasal tip.   Excessive removal of alar cartilage or mucosa is the commonest problem. An added auricular cartilage may suffice and build up or support the tip. Lining can be replaced using free skin or mucosal grafts or mucosal flaps from the upper lip.

Bridgeline.   A residial hump or irregularity of the bridge line can be smoothed by rasping to correct the deformity. A saddle deformity, where excess hump has been removed, can be corrected by a bone graft, cartilage graft or silastic implant.

Parrot's beak deformity.   This is a complication of excessive upper bridge line removal with bulbous swelling of the nasal tip. Correction is difficult. In some cases lining is required at the tip. Bridge line support can be inserted and supratip excess of septal cartilage can be trimmed.

Broadening of the bridge of the nose is a common problem. The relapse of the infracture may be early by loss of fixation or as a result of incomplete infracture. Repeat infracture must be performed thoroughly and good external fixation applied. The small glabellar, triangle of nasal bone should be cleared to allow a high infracture (Figs. 16.12, 16.13).

Deviation of the nose presents a very difficult problem. Sometimes, reference back to the notes and photographs will show that the deviation is not a complication of the procedure but a result of the pre-operative condition. The source of the deviation must be carefully analysed. If the septum is not straight, any further surgery must start with centralization of the septum, followed by repeat infractures and trimming as necessary. Caution should be exercised pre-operatively when the nose is deviated and no guarantee of complete correction of deviation should ever be made.

Figure 16.12
Two causes of a wide
nasal base post-
operatively.
(a) Insufficient removal
of the dorsal bone or
(b) oblique osteotomy
of the nasal process of
the maxilla.

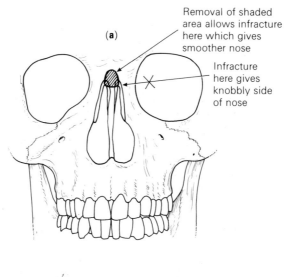

Removal of shaded
area allows infracture
here which gives
smoother nose

(a)

Infracture
here gives
knobbly side
of nose

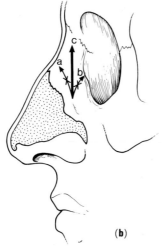

(b)

Airway problems. The nasal airway is slightly reduced after most reduction rhinoplasty operations, but symptoms of obstruction are not frequently complained of. The cause of the problem must be sought. A collapsing tip or alars needs septal support with an L-shaped graft. Collapsing alae can be helped with a small auricular cartilage graft acting as a spring support. Deviation of the septum must be corrected if possible. Nostril stenosis can be corrected by Z-plasty or graft of the lining.

Nasal implant. If a silastic implant is inserted via a columellar incision or through the buccal mucosa, it is less likely to cause

Figure 16.13
Failure of infracture
(a), was corrected by
removal of a small
fragment of nasal
bone at the dorsum
(see Fig. 16.12a) and
repeat infracture (b).

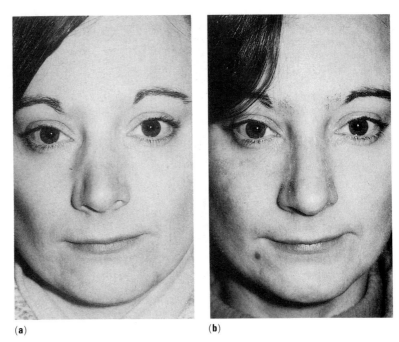

(a)   (b)

problems than if inserted via the nasal mucosa. If the implant becomes infected, it must be removed to allow the infection to settle. Unsatisfactory prostheses can be removed or adjusted as necessary. (Fig. 16.14)

Associated problems. In some cases, when rhinoplasty has been performed and the patient is not happy with the result, full reassessment must be made. A psychiatric problem may emerge and referral to a psychiatrist is indicated. If other problems, such as a small chin or malocclusion are marring the result, it will be better to correct these deformities if appropriate.

Conclusion

The nose is a principal feature of the face and its position makes imperfection, real or imagined, very important to the patient. The techniques of nasal reduction are many and varied. There is no substitute for experience and yet it is difficult for the beginner to gain experience. Attention to basic concepts, particularly the need to avoid excessive removal of tissue, will pay dividends. After all, it is usually easier to remove a little more at a second operation than to have to reconstruct the deficit. If the nose is symmetrical, similar procedures should be performed on each side.

Figure 16.14
Displacement of a silastic implant caused by trauma to the nose.

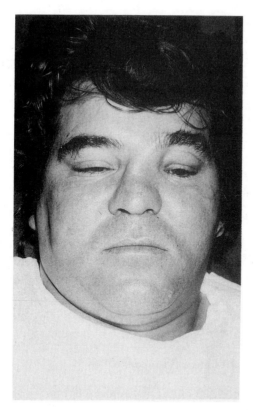

Persisting controversies

- Internal or external fixation in facial fractures?
- The place of submucous rhinoplasty.
- Correction of the deviated nose.
- Correction of the parrot's beak deformity.
- Which skeletal support for the collapsed nose or nasal reconstruction?

Further reading

Regnault, P.F. & Daniel, E.K. (Eds) (1984) *Aesthetic Plastic Surgery: Principles and Technique*. Boston: Little Brown.

Rowe, N.L. & Williams, J.L. (Eds) (1985) *Maxillo-facial Injuries*. Edinburgh: Churchill Livingstone.

17 Complications of Breast Surgery

The scope of breast surgery has increased dramatically since the development of the silastic prosthesis thirty years ago. The trend towards breast reconstruction following mastectomy and subcutaneous mastectomy with immediate reconstruction has increased the number of breast operations undertaken by an ever-expanding number of surgeons. There is a danger that dilution of surgical expertise will occur unless care is taken to understand and observe the basic principles. The occasional operator should beware of the problems and be prepared to consult with a specialist colleague sooner rather than later.

General complications of breast surgery

Predisposing factors

Age There is a changing anatomical and physiological pattern that alters breast shape and size from early puberty to old age.

- Before puberty, the breast bud is a small area immediately beneath the nipple. Damage to this small structure by excision, infection or a tumour may lead to complete or partial hypoplasia of the breast. Surgery and radiotherapy should be avoided if at all possible at this time (Fig. 17.1).
- During puberty, the breasts usually develop, but the full size and shape may not be established for several years. Initial development may be asymmetrical, but, unless the discrepancy is gross, early operative intervention is contra-indicated as there may be an equalization later.
- In pregnancy, there is usually an obvious enlargement of the breasts, with the development of striae. Surgery should be avoided at this time. Also, mastopexy operations should be postponed until after an expected pregnancy so as to avoid the overstretching of the skin that will cause the recurrent ptosis.
- With advancing years, at a variable rate, the breast tissue normally atrophies slowly and the breasts become ptotic. This is an inevitable process and the patient should be reminded of that if surgery is contemplated to correct unilateral hypoplasia. The lack of atrophy in a breast with an implant will give rise to increasing asymmetry with age.

Figure 17.1
Haemangioma of the right breast. Any treatment that injured the breast bud, such as radiotherapy or surgery, could cause breast development to fail at puberty.

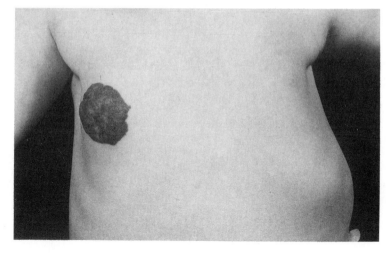

Obesity The breast is subject to extreme fluctuations in size and shape according to the obesity of the patient. There is variation between individuals, but breast size usually increases with weight gain. However, fat deposition varies and, in some patients, excess fat on the abdomen and hips alters the figure so dramatically that the breast size, while increasing in volume, may appear to become disproportionately small when compared to the general body shape.

Planning an operation in which volume change is needed—reduction, augmentation or reconstruction—is particularly difficult if the weight is fluctuating. Obese patients should diet pre-operatively to lose weight and maintain a steady level prior to surgery.

Blood supply Pre-existing scars affect the blood supply and incisions and flaps must be planned accordingly. If possible, the incisions used should incorporate pre-existing scars. Large inframammary incisions with undermining should be avoided if there are substantial scars over the centre of the breast. Radiotherapy impairs blood supply severely and can delay healing or cause skin necrosis.

Scar placement Some degree of scarring is inevitable. Several factors must be taken into account in placing the scar.

- The presternal area is particularly at risk of developing hypertrophic and keloid scars (see Chapter 5). Incisions in the upper anterior chest, between the breasts across the midline, should be avoided if at all possible (Fig. 17.2).
- Scars will be better tolerated if they are placed within the area usually covered by clothing (Fig. 17.3).

Figure 17.2
Preferred sites for
incisions in the breast.
The shaded area
should be avoided if at
all possible.

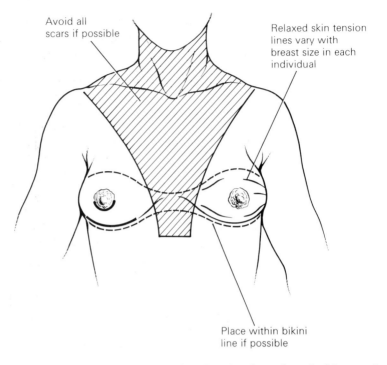

Avoid all
scars if possible

Relaxed skin tension
lines vary with
breast size in each
individual

Place within bikini
line if possible

- The scar should be placed either in the relaxed skin tension lines or at an anatomical interface, for example at the edge of the areola.
- The skin tension lines show considerable individual variation and depend to some extent on the body build, degree of subcutaneous fat and extent of breast development.

Haematoma   The nature of glandular breast tissue makes haematoma more common in breast surgery. If a small excision is made, the firm

Figure 17.3
This elective incision
for left thoracotomy
has left an extremely
disfiguring result. An
inframammary incision
would have been
preferable.

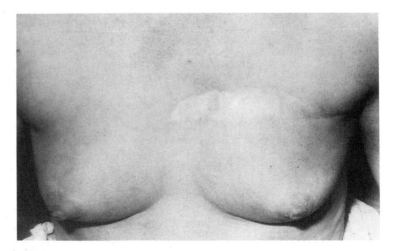

tissue cannot collapse to obliterate the cavity. Large flaps may not mould easily, leaving dead space. The blood vessels themselves retract into the tissue and haemostasis is difficult.

Foreign body   Haematoma predisposes to infection. In addition, in augmentation and reconstruction operations there is deliberate introduction of a foreign body, the implant. It is important when implants are used that haemostasis is complete and that further foreign body, such as suture material, is kept to a minimum.

Sensation   The nerve supply to the breast varies considerably in type and quantity. The nipple areolar complex has two basic types of sensation, normal somatic sensation present elsewhere on the body, and erotic sensation, which is extremely variable in different patients—some patients deny that they have any. Large breasts or breasts that have enlarged rapidly tend to have poor sensation. The nerve supply arises from supraclavicular nerves and intercostal perforators. The 4th lateral intercostal branch is important in supplying the nipple.

Infection   Breasts that have undergone operation are more likely to develop infection if the duct system is transected near the base of the nipple, as there is direct entry from the surface (Fig. 17.4).

Malignant disease   When the breast surgery is for, or follows, treatment of malignant disease, the possibility of recurrence must be borne in mind. If the nipple is preserved, recurrence may develop under it. Free grafts of nipple should not be 'banked' elsewhere on the body following mastectomy because, in rare instances, tumour has been implanted directly into the thigh or groin (Fig. 17.5).

Surgical expertise   Close attention to detail and artistic flair are required in planning and in handling tissues. There may be a need for the full repertoire of reconstructive surgical techniques. If the surgeon has insufficient expertise, he should seek help.

Postoperative care   There is an increasing tendency for surgery to be performed on a day-patient basis, or with early discharge home after surgery. It is vital that postoperative care is properly organized to help to prevent complications. The patient must not go home to inadequate care and be expected to look after children or relatives. Postoperative arm movements should be kept to a minimum for at least 48 hours. Vigorous use of the arm or lifting the arm above the horizontal must be avoided for at least two weeks. The patient should avoid sleeping prone for at least two weeks.

Prevention of complications

Pre-operative assessment   The essence of prophylaxis is recognition and correction, where possible, of predisposing factors. General examination should

Figure 17.4
(a,b) Infection in the left breast developed six months after bilateral mastectomy with immediate implants. The infection almost certainly gained entry via the nipple. If the implant had been placed deep to the pectoralis major muscle, the infection might have been prevented.

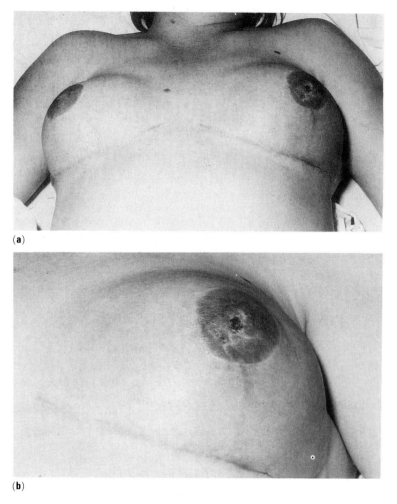

(a)

(b)

include assessment of the body build and degree of subcutaneous fat.

Symmetry   As the breast is a paired organ, particular attention must be paid pre-operatively to an accurate assessment of symmetry of the body in general, the chest wall, and the shape, size and position of the breast, and nipple areolar complex. Volumetric symmetry of the breasts is extremely rare pre-operatively. Good records, including frontal, oblique and lateral photographs are advisable.

Breast base   The thorax must be assessed. Spinal deformity, or irregularity of the rib cage or chest musculature can upset the balance of the foundation on which the breast is based (Fig. 17.6). Any pre-existing deformity such as pectus excavatum must be diagnosed

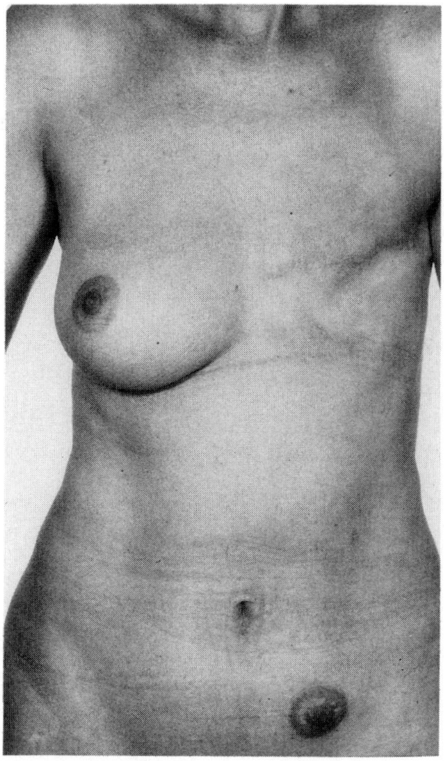

Figure 17.5
Nipple banking is not
only grossly unsightly,
but there is the risk of
implanting tumour
cells.

and pointed out to the patient, if necessary, in order to minimize postoperative dissatisfaction.

Breast shape   The degree of ptosis must be judged. A useful indicator is the position of the nipple in relation to the inframammary fold. The shape of the breast varies considerably with the position of the body. Assessment of ptosis must be made in the erect position with the arms symmetrically placed at the side.

Breast volume   There are three fundamental problems when measuring breast volume.

1 The breast is a subcutaneous organ and a large but variable part of its volume is fat. The axillary tail may be a very significant proportion of the volume and has to be included in any measurement.
2 The breast is mounted on a curved base and measurement is therefore difficult.
3 The breast volume can be considered as the amount that projects beyond the general skin surface, or as the total volume of soft tissue external to the chest wall within the

Figure 17.6
(a,b) In this patient
with muscular
dystrophy and
secondary scoliosis,
the slight asymmetry of
the breasts is grossly
exaggerated by the
underlying rib
deformity.

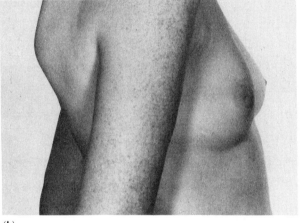

(a)

(b)

surface markings of the breast (Fig. 17.7). The apparent volume will depend on the technique used to measure it. For example, a mammometer with a larger base will show a bigger apparent volume because a larger area of subcutaneous fat is included. In order to get comparable results, it is essential that the same measuring device and the same technique be used each time.

In addition to actual volume measurement, the comparative size of the breast in relation to the chest wall must be measured. Conventionally, this is represented by 'cup size' for the breast and 'bra size' for the chest wall. It is important to understand that surgery altering the breast volume will only affect the cup size. If the patient wishes to alter her bra size she will have to alter the subcutaneous fat by putting on weight or slimming, or build up the chest musculature by exercises.

Figure 17.7
Diagrammatic
representation of
problems in breast
volumetry. The breast
volume is the same in
each case. (a) If the
breast volume is
measured as the
amount that projects
above the skin
surface, it is
apparently smaller
than the total volume
of breast and fat
included within the
surface confines of
the breast (b). Thus, if
a mammometer is
applied to the breast
without pressure (c) it
measures a smaller
volume than when it is
pushed into the
subcutaneous fat (d).
The apparent breast
volume therefore
varies depending on
the pressure applied to
the mammometer.
A small mammometer
(e) will give a smaller
apparent volume than
a large one (f).

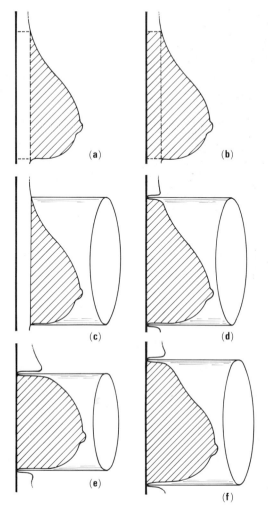

Breast tissue Lumps or cysts of the breast must be excluded by clinical examination prior to surgery. It is useful to repeat the examination the day before surgery, if possible, and certainly before premedication, so that any new or unexpected development can be evaluated before surgery. Pre-existing scars must be identified, as they give a guide to the quality of blood supply to the breast.

The nipple The position, shape and size of the nipple should be noted and sensation must be checked and recorded prior to surgery.

Patient selection The general cosmetic surgery considerations discussed in Chapter 1 apply. In addition, there are the particular problems of assessment and selection related to breast surgery. The chief problem giving rise to complications is the patient's having an unrealistic expectation and desire for change. For example, excessive augmentation can give rise to the undesirable side-effect of unbalancing the figure and can look rather grotesque. Assessment using external prosthesis inserted under a bra can help to illustrate to the patient the type of change that is desired. A patient with a large bust may wish unrealistic reduction of bra size, whereas only cup size can be decreased by mammoplasty.

Consent   After a discussion with the patient, including consideration of possible complications, consent should be obtained. It is particularly important to stress that, in any operation involving reconstruction of the breast, a second stage is likely to be required to adjust the breast volume or shape or the position of the nipple, or to trim the opposite breast.

Plan the operation   Careful planning is the key to successful breast surgery. Care must be taken not to compromise flap blood supply. The implant size and type must be carefully selected. Once the operation has been planned, the breast must be marked appropriately, prior to operation—before premedication is administered, since marking is better performed with the patient upright.

Keep accurate records   Good records, particularly with clinical photographs, are a good safeguard; used postoperatively to remind the patient of what she used to look like, they can sometimes defuse the situation and 'nip any complaint in the bud'.

Avoid haematoma   Careful atraumatic surgical technique with complete haemostasis is essential. Suction drains should be inserted if large tissue planes have been opened up. A closely applied dressing may also help, as will restricting arm movements postoperatively.

Postoperative care   A firm dressing or the patient's own brassiere gives good support. If a brassiere is used, and implants are in place, it is extremely important that the shoulder straps are not too tight, as the implants may be displaced upwards. Once the skin sutures are removed, tape support, for up to two months, can be used to try to limit the spread of scars. The patient's weight should be kept steady postoperatively. Weight gain may give recurrence of breast enlargement; weight loss causes ptosis.

Management of general complications

Haematoma   *Diagnosis* is usually straightforward. Severe onset of pain, with increase in size and tenseness of the breast, is diagnostic of large or expanding haematoma. A small haematoma may be silent and not suspected until later. If there is a suspicion of haematoma, it is essential to remove the dressings and inspect the skin to asses viability of the breast skin and nipple areolar complex (Fig. 17.8).

Surgical management by urgent release is mandatory for a large, tense haematoma in order to prevent skin necrosis, wound disruption or extrusion of the prosthesis. It is only rarely that a large bleeding point is found. After removal of haematoma and haemostasis, suction drains must be inserted before the wound is resutured or the implant re-inserted. Prophylactic antibiotic administration may be indicated to prevent infection. If the skin flaps are tense and viability is compromised, after release of haematoma it is probably best to leave any implant out to be re-inserted at a second stage.

Infection *Acute infection* presenting as a hot, tense breast with pyrexia demands urgent treatment. If there are localizing signs, sutures should be removed to release pus or haematoma and specimens should be sent for bacteriological investigation. Any implant should be removed. Systemic antibiotic treatment is indicated (Fig. 17.4).

Chronic infection may be localized to the suture line, in which case it should resolve with dressings, or it may be related to an implant. Systemic antibiotics can be used, but, if the infection does not clear, any implant should be removed. Once the infection has resolved, the implant can be reinserted when oedema and induration have settled—usually after several months.

Necrosis Ischaemic necrosis with loss of the skin, breast tissue or part of the nipple areolar complex is a severe complication of breast surgery. Infection exacerbates the effect of ischaemia causing more severe skin loss.

Figure 17.8
Expanding haematoma of the left breast. All the dressings must be removed to inspect skin and nipple viability. Surgical drainage is essential to avoid delayed healing.

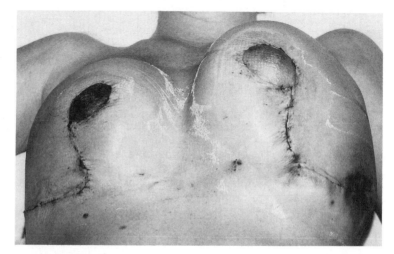

Diagnosis. Necrosis should be suspected at an early stage if there is severe pain or swelling and tenseness of the breast. All dressings should be removed to allow inspection of the skin for quality of circulation and loss of capillary flow.

Surgical management depends on the stage at which necrosis is discovered.

1 At operation, good planning and careful technique should prevent flap or nipple ischaemia. However, if the circulation appears compromised or the closure is tight, the wound must not be sutured completed. It can be left open or a graft can be applied to the defect. The skin graft can be excised later to improve the scarring. An implant should not be inserted if it causes undue tension. Once healing has taken place, the implant can be inserted, if necessary after tissue expansion.
2 In the early postoperative phase, incipient necrosis in a prejudiced flap may be prevented by removal of tight sutures, release of haematoma or removal of the implant.
3 Once established necrosis has occurred, residual infection should be drained and slough removed either by conservative management using repeated dressings or by surgical debridement. Later suture or graft repair should be limited to simple measures aimed only at closing the wound. After healing is obtained, all oedema and induration should be allowed to settle for a considerable time before definitive reconstruction is attempted.

Sensory loss Some degree of sensory loss of the nipple is almost inevitable when a major segment of breast tissue is removed. The patient must be warned of the risk prior to surgery. The sensation may recover spontaneously in the first few months after surgery, but recovery is by no means the rule. Nothing can be done to speed or improve recovery.

Pain There is inevitably a considerable degree of postoperative pain in the skin wound and in relation to movement of the pectoralis major muscles until healing is complete. Mastectomy with immediate reconstruction is not a good operation for treatment of breast pain, and recurrence is likely.

Patient dissatisfaction After most types of breast surgery, a small number of patients confess dissatisfaction even if the result is technically perfect. Most will settle into and accept the change in shape after a while. Discussion and showing the patient the pre-operative photographs may help. If the patient's true wishes have been misinterpreted, re-operation to correct the deficit may be possible, but should be delayed for a few months until oedema has settled.

Augmentation mammoplasty

Augmentation methods

Dermal fat grafts were used up to the 1950s but have now been abandoned. Shrinkage of the graft with fat necrosis causes loss of volume. Late complications include calcification, giving rise to hardness, irregularity and asymmetry (Fig. 3.13).

Fat flap repair is not usually used for augmentation, but in reconstructive surgery post-mastectomy a vast range of procedures has been developed, some of which use buried de-epithelialized flaps for volume replacement without the need for implants. Omental fat methods have potential major abdominal complications and are rarely used.

Subcutaneous injection of various substances, such as paraffin, has been abandoned because the inevitable result is infection, fat necrosis and sinus formation. Inert substances such as free liquid silicone are not used, because they tend to shift and migrate to the abdominal wall.

Implants. The early synthetic sponge implants have been abandoned. Fibrous-tissue infiltration gives rise to extreme hardness of the breasts.

The modern silicone gel implants and inflatable fluid-filled silicone implants have proved to be a major advance in augmentation or reconstructive mammaplasty. Polyurethane sponge-coated silastic implants are also available. Their advocates claim less capsule formation but, if infection occurs, it is more difficult to remove the implant.

Capsule formation

It is normal and inevitable for the body to produce a biological reaction at an interface with an implant or any other foreign body. Capsule formation around a breast implant almost certainly occurs, to some extent, in all patients, as part of the normal process of healing and walling-off of the implant pocket. It is not a problem in the majority of patients, but in a variable proportion of breasts the capsule can contract to give a hard, globular deformity that in the worst cases can be seen as well as felt (Fig. 17.9).

Capsule contracture can be unilateral or more rarely bilateral, but is frequently unequal, giving rise to asymmetry. It may occur early but usually develops some months postoperatively.

Predisposing factors

1 Haematoma or seroma formation at the time of surgery or in the postoperative phase may predispose to early capsule formation. On rare occasions, late trauma with bruising can give rise to onset of capsule contracture.

Figure 17.9
Severe bilateral
capsule contracture
with impending
extrusion of the right
implant following
subcutaneous
mastectomy with
immediate
reconstruction.

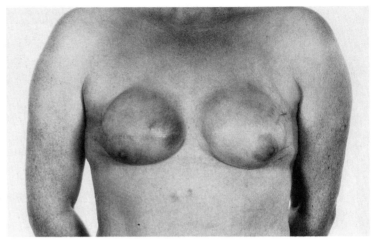

Figure 17.9
Severe bilateral
capsule contracture
with impending
extrusion of the right
implant following
subcutaneous
mastectomy with
immediate
reconstruction.

2 Infection is a potent stimulant for excessive scarring, but it seems unlikely that prophylactic antibiotics will prevent capsule contracture, as it often occurs late, many months after wound healing.

3 A foreign body such as glove powder or surgical suture materials may initiate a reaction leading to capsule contracture. Traumatic surgical technique, causing tissue damage, may stimulate excessive scar formation (Fig. 17.10).

4 Rupture of an implant is frequently associated with capsule formation. However, it is not certain whether the rupture causes the capsule, since capsular contraction can fold the implant shell, giving rise to fatigue fracture (Fig. 17.11). Gel bleed, the diffusion of silastic through the outer covering, may be an important factor.

Figure 17.10
Severe capsule
contracture after
augmentation for
Poland's syndrome.
When the capsule was
explored, a retained
swab left in at the
operation 10 years
previously was found.
The foreign body
reaction could well
have initiated the
capsule contracture.

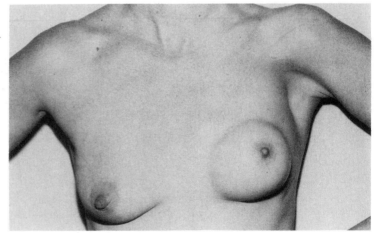

Figure 17.11
(a) Lateral X-ray of severe capsule contracture, which developed quite suddenly 14 years after breast augmentation. The implant has ruptured and a separate gel fragment can be seen at the lower pole. (b) Result six months after capsulectomy and replacement of the implants, showing an improved breast shape.

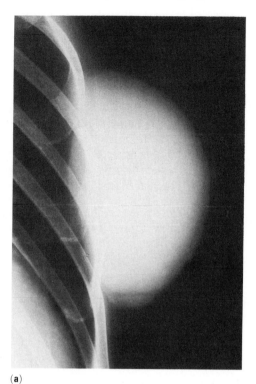

(**a**)

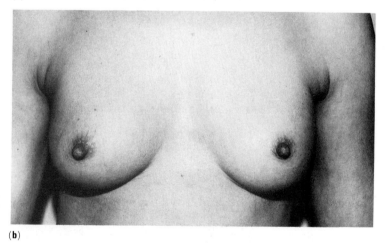

(**b**)

Prevention 1 The precise cause of capsule contraction is not known, but all factors likely to cause an inflammatory reaction must be avoided. Powder-free gloves are preferable. Glove powder must be washed off the gloves of surgeon and assistants prior to surgery.

2 Steroid installation into the pocket or in the inflation fluid is

not used in Great Britain as there is a definite incidence of steroid complications such as local tissue atrophy. Antibiotics should not be injected into a prosthesis, because of the risk of allergy.

3 Polyurethane-coated or 'low-bleed' gel prostheses may be less likely to develop capsular contracture, but inflatable prostheses can cause severe capsule contraction (Fig. 17.12).

4 Submuscular placement of an implant seems to give rise to less firm capsule formation than submammary placement. This may be because of the pressure effect of the muscle keeping the pocket dilated or it may be an illusion, with the greater thickness of muscle disguising the deformity to some extent (Fig. 17.13).

5 Postoperative pressure dressings or exercises to keep the pocket dilated appear to be useful. There is a tendency for implants to displace superiorly, so that compression exercises should concentrate on pressing the implant downwards and medially.

Management Treatment should only be considered if the patient has symptoms or is dissatisfied with the results. Slight capsular contraction gives more prominence of the breasts and some patients prefer this. It is important not to advise surgery if the patient is satisfied, even if the surgeon is disappointed, because the results of treatment are extremely variable and cannot be guaranteed. If the capsule contracture is mild, with minimal symptoms, conservative management is indicated. Pressure exercises or the patient's lying prone may help to stretch the capsule.

Closed capsulotomy has been very popular in the past and can be performed without an anaesthetic as an out-patient procedure. There are many complications, including irregular capsule rupture causing distortion, haemorrhage, rupture of the prosthesis,

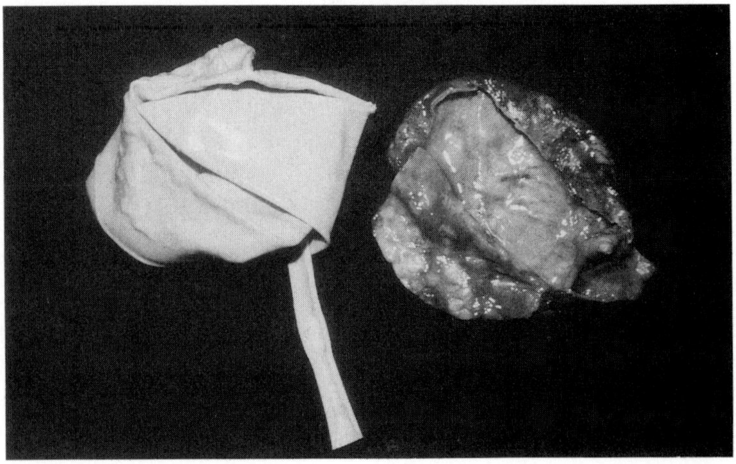

Figure 17.12
Following severe capsule contracture, this inflatable implant ruptured. The excised capsule shows calcification.

Figure 17.13
The submuscular
position for a breast
implant puts the
prosthesis in a more
protected, padded
position, particularly
over the upper half of
the breast.

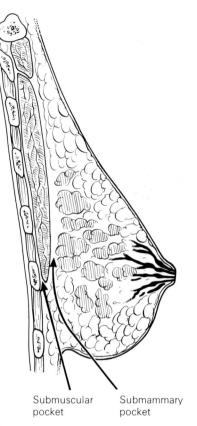

Submuscular   Submammary
pocket   pocket

and gel migration to nipple or axilla. This procedure should not
be performed under general anaesthetic in case excessive force
is used.

Open capsulotomy is more successful in the short term to correct
contraction. It has the added advantage of allowing inspection
of the prosthesis for leakage, and the prosthesis can then be
replaced if necessary.

If the prosthesis is submammary, changing placement to a
submuscular pocket is frequently successful.

In resistant cases or when the prosthesis has been in place for
many years, microcalcification in the capsule is a common
problem. Capsulectomy with replacement of the implants will be
needed (Figs. 17.11, 17.12).

Removing a 'slick' (smooth-gel-filled) prosthesis and substi-
tuting a polyurethane-coated implant decreases the subsequent
incidence of contracture. Capsulectomy is not required.

When capsule contracture is severe, with symptoms such as
pain, the only cure is to remove the implants.

Rupture of the prosthesis

Inflatable prostheses commonly rupture or leak at the valve or side-tubing. Modern designs have better valves that may decrease this problem. Gel prostheses with fixation patches should not be used, because they cause a weak spot as well as being palpable if the implant shifts before it has settled into place.

Extrusion

Early-extrusion occurs if there is wound breakdown or flap necrosis. In the absence of infection, the prosthesis can be removed, the cavity irrigated and the prostheses returned. Prophylactic antibiotic is essential, but the chances of success are not high. It is better to remove the prosthesis, wait for wound healing and re-insert it later.

Late extrusion can occur many years postoperatively. Capsule contraction with atrophy of subcutaneous tissues or the scar is the cause even in the absence of trauma (Fig. 17.14). The implant can be reinserted deep to muscle or deep to the posterior part of the capsule.

Displacement of the implant

The implant can shift its position in the immediate postoperative phase, especially in breast reconstruction if large flaps have been used with wide dissection of pockets or tunnels. These spaces should be closed with tacking sutures if possible. Careful dressing and avoidance of excessive exercise will help to prevent the problem.

Downward displacement of the implant is more common when the implant is in the submammary position, and can lead to extrusion.

Figure 17.14
Late extrusion of this breast implant following capsular contraction occurred through the peri-areolar scar.

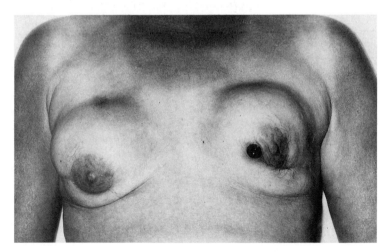

When the implant is placed subpectorally, there is a tendency for it to move superiorly, particularly if capsule contracture develops. Division of the lower fibres of pectoralis major from their origin on the ribs, will help to prevent this complication. Once it has developed, open capsulotomy with division of these fibres is indicated.

Ptosis

Careful preoperative selection is required to prevent this undesirable result. If there is ptosis pre-operatively, with the nipple below the inframammary fold, a mastopexy is essential in addition to augmentation mammaplasty. In some patients, the mastopexy alone may suffice, avoiding implants.

Inevitably, with aging, the patient's breast tissue will become more lax. Submammary prostheses give rise to a characteristic 'ball in a sock' deformity (Fig. 17.15), whereas, in submuscular

Figure 17.15 Progressive ptosis following augmentation mammaplasty with the implants in a submammary pocket. (a) Preoperative appearance showing considerable ptosis. Ideally a mastopexy should have been performed. (b) One year following augmentation the result is acceptable. (c) Ten years later, with further ptosis, the typical ball-in-a-sock deformity has developed.

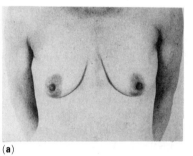

(a)

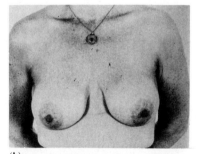

(b)

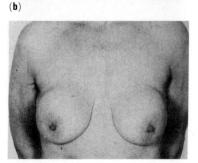

(c)

implants, the breast appears to fall off the implant (Fig. 17.16). These appearances vary with the position of the body and breast support will disguise the deformity. Treatment requires mastopexy with or without removal and repositioning of the prosthesis.

Reduction mammaplasty and mastopexy

Reduction mammaplasty and mastopexy are closely related and considered together because they can be regarded as parts of the same spectrum of breast surgery. Mastopexy is the repositioning of the ptotic breast and alters breast shape by tightening the skin and breast tissue. Reduction mammaplasty implies diminution of the volume of the breast, but this cannot be achieved without tightening of the skin envelope if ptosis is to be prevented. Recurrent ptosis after mastopexy is common if the breast is left too large. Combinations of varying degrees of reduction and mastopexy are required in the majority of patients.

Prevention of complications

Pre-operative assessment, planning and discussion with the patient must be performed well in advance of the surgery. It is vital to know what the patient hopes or expects as a result of treatment. The appropriate technique can then be tailored to suit these requirements.

Planning is best done by marking on the skin with the patient upright, as symmetry is judged most easily in this position. The site for the nipple areolar complex must be marked with the patient in the anatomical position with the arms symmetrically

Figure 17.16
After submuscular placement of the implant, ptosis of the patient's own breast gives rise to the appearance of the breast sliding off the implant.

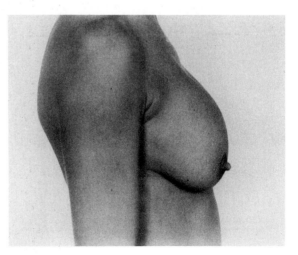

at the side. If one arm is elevated, the skin on that side will also be raised and the subsequent nipple position will be too low (Figs. 17.17, 17.18).

Necrosis   Methods of breast reduction bearing the nipple areolar complex on dermal flaps have reduced the incidence of nipple, skin and breast parenchyma necrosis. However, if the breast hypertrophy

Figure 17.17
Diagram of the relationship of nipple position to the chest wall. The suprasternal notch and both nipples lie at the corners of an equilateral triangle.

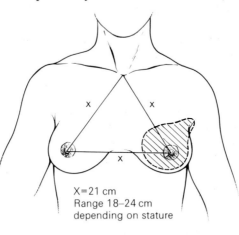

Figure 17.18
The ideal site for this nipple reconstruction should be marked in a symmetrical position measured from the suprasternal notch, disregarding the asymmetry of the underlying sternum. Otherwise the nipple would be placed too far laterally.

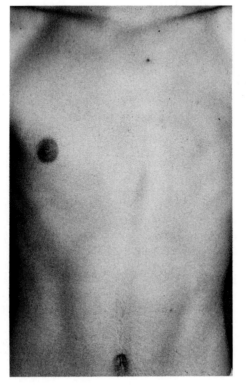

is massive in the older or obese patient, or when there are multiple scars of the breast, amputation reduction with free graft of the nipple is preferable.

During operation, any resected skin should be kept moist and sterile so that it can be replaced as a graft if necessary. If the planned closure is too tight, so that nipple or skin flap circulation is compromised, a change to excision of the nipple with free grafting should be considered or the resected skin can be inserted as a free graft.

Postoperatively, minor skin necrosis can be treated conservatively with dressings. Major skin or nipple loss is best treated by surgical debridement, once the demarcation of necrotic tissue has declared itself. Temporary skin grafts applied to aid healing can be resected later. Nipple reconstruction is performed later as necessary and loss of breast substance can be disguised by insertion of an implant.

Asymmetry Estimation of volume is very important pre-operatively, particularly when there is asymmetry, so that the comparative amounts to be removed can be judged (Fig. 17.19). Minor discrepancies in breast volume are common after breast reduction and do not usually require correction. If the patient insists on treatment, it must be delayed until full resolution of postoperative oedema has taken place, as the size and shape of the breasts will fluctuate after surgery for several months.

Major differences in breast volume should be prevented by careful pre-operative assessment and removal of the correct amount of tissue. If secondary surgery is needed, it is usually better to reduce the large breast further rather than put an implant in the smaller breast, unless the discrepancy is gross.

Nipple position *Asymmetry* can be caused by faulty pre-operative planning and operative or postoperative problems.

1 If the breasts are symmetrical pre-operatively, make sure that the plan and marking are equal on the two sides.
2 When one breast is larger pre-operatively, the skin will be more tightly stretched. This must be taken into consideration when marking the proposed nipple position. It must be sited lower to compensate for the elevation once the excess breast tissue is removed (Fig. 17.19a).
3 Nipple position varies slightly with the height of the patient, but it is rare that the measurement from suprasternal notch to nipple centre is less than 21 cm. Check the marking carefully if this happens, as the postoperative nipple position could be too high. A good check of the new nipple position is to transpose the inframammary fold level onto the anterior breast skin. This is usually the ideal nipple position for a reduction mammoplasty (Fig. 17.20).

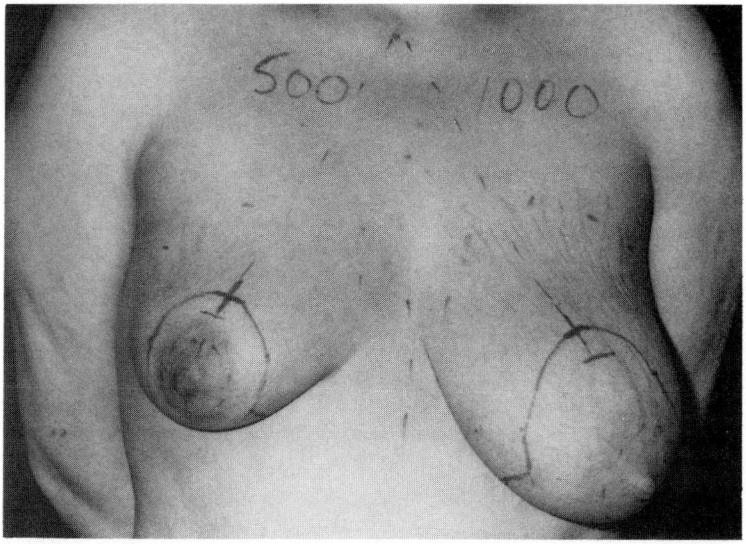

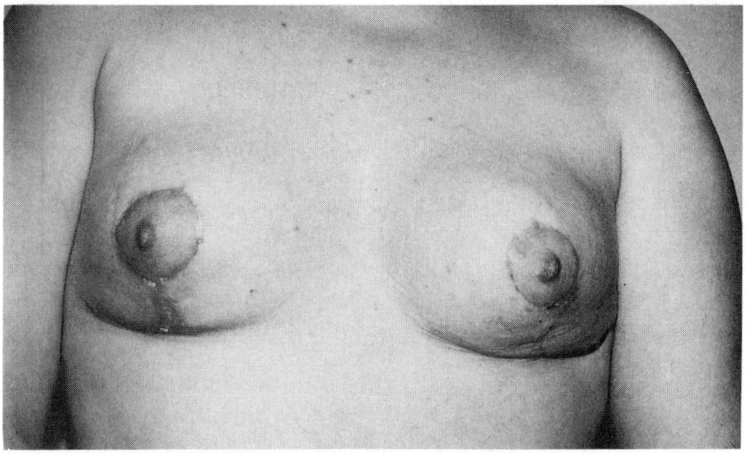

Figure 17.19
Patient with breast asymmetry. The breast volumes are measured pre-operatively and marked on the skin (a). Five hundred grams of breast tissue was excised from the left side to restore symmetry (b). Note that the nipple position is marked slightly lower on the left side as the skin is relatively stretched by the excess weight of the larger breast and after reduction the nipple will rise.

(**b**)

Treatment of the nipple placed too high is very difficult. If the error is only minor, further reduction of breast substance or excision of an inframammary ellipse of skin will lower the nipple slightly. Gross malposition requires excision and suture of the nipple site and regrafting in a lower position, but it leaves very unsightly scars. A nipple that is too low is more easily elevated because the resulting scar is placed in the lower half of the breast (Fig. 17.21).

Late ptosis   Recurrent droop of the breasts is inevitable, under the influence of gravity, if the breasts are left substantial in size. The only method to prevent late loss of shape is to reduce the breasts to an

Figure 17.20
Diagram to show a useful practical technique for estimating the new nipple position.

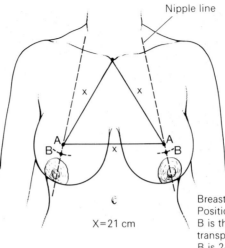

Nipple line

X = 21 cm

Breast reduction:
Position A will make the nipple too high.
B is the level of the inframammary fold transposed to the front of the breast.
B is 2–3 cm below A.

A-cup size or smaller! Weight loss by the patient postoperatively causes ptosis to recur.

Treatment is by a mastopexy, re-tightening the breast envelope and re-positioning the nipple higher if necessary.

Dermatochalasis can affect the breasts severely, in some cases producing gross ptosis. These patients should be warned that recurrent ptosis is common and that a second stage of retightening may be required (Fig. 17.22).

Scars   All the techniques of breast reduction cause scars. There are guidelines that can help to minimize scarring.

Figure 17.21
Nipples placed too far laterally and inferiorly following reduction mammaplasty. Correction is easily obtained by moving them superiorly and medially on a subcutaneous pedicle. The inverted T-shaped reduction mammaplasty with the scars joining at the mid-line has inevitably caused symmastia with loss of the cleavage.

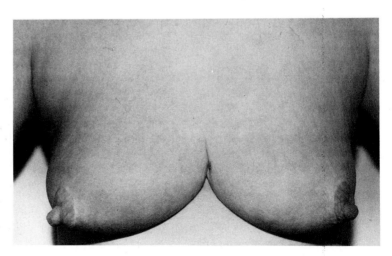

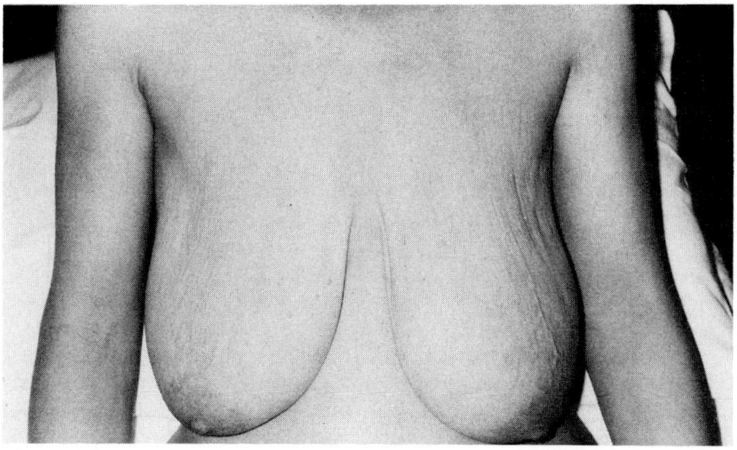

Figure 17.22
(a) Severe ptosis in a girl 18 years of age with dermatochalasis. (b) Three months following mastopexy there has been stretching of the inferior skin, and further tightening of the skin below the nipple is required.

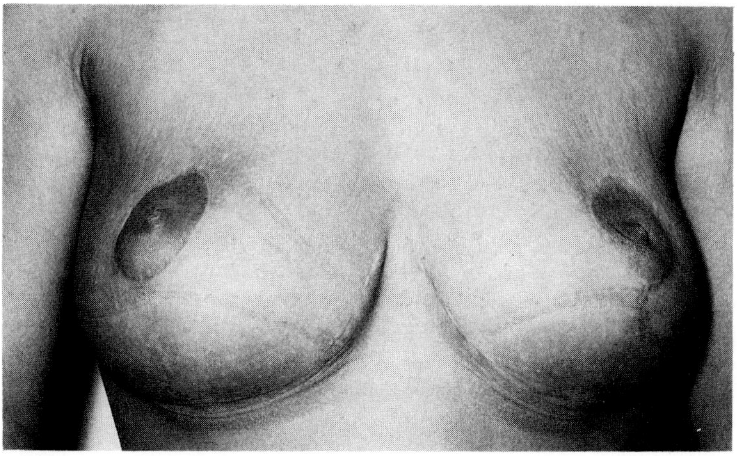

(**a**)

(**b**)

1 A previous history of hypertophic or keloid scarring should make patient and surgeon consider carefully whether reduction mammaplasty is justifiable.

2 In susceptible individuals, the practice of scratching the marking on the skin with the back of a scalpel to prevent them being washed away during the operation should be avoided, as deep scratches can cause hypertrophic scars.

3 Scars must be kept as short as possible. In the traditional inverted-T incision, great care must be taken to ensure that the incisions do not approach the midline or meet each other. Severe problems of webbing and symmastia will result (Fig. 17.21).

4 Lateral reduction methods avoiding any medial element to the inframammary fold scar give more pleasing results in all except massive reduction operations.

Subcutaneous mastectomy

Subcutaneous mastectomy with immediate reconstruction has a high incidence of complication and unsatisfactory results. The main initial causes of problems are the general complications of breast surgery, principally ischaemic necrosis of the skin and nipple areolar complex. Later problems mainly relate to implant complications such as capsule contracture.

Choice of operation
The chief determining factor is the size of the breast pre-operatively.

1 In a small breast, a peri-areolar incision extending in a curve out into the lateral half of the breast gives excellent access and preserves vascularity of the skin flaps. A wedge excision of the skin will tighten the skin envelope if there is ptosis. A transverse inframammary incision with undermining of the whole breast skin and nipple puts the flap on the lower half of the breast at risk.
2 When more than 500 g of breast tissue has to be removed, or if there is severe scarring from previous surgery, simple mastectomy with free grafting of the nipple should be considered. When there is scarring from previous breast surgery, the same approach should again be considered.

   If there is any doubt about skin viability, the implants should be inserted at a second operation, although there are problems of skin puckering and wrinkling if the implants are delayed. Implants placed beneath pectoral and serratus muscle flaps, so that they are not in contact with the subcutaneous wound, have a lower incidence of infection, extrusion and capsule formation.

Breast reconstruction

The complications of breast reconstruction are many and varied because of the wide variety of methods used. Principal complications arise in five main ways.

1 General complications of breast surgery.
2 Complications of implants.
3 Complications of the flap methods used to reconstruct skin cover.
4 Nipple areolar reconstruction complications.
5 Aesthetic problems of symmetry.

Prevention of complications
Prevention of complications depends on careful evaluation of what is missing and replacement of the deficit in quantity and

quality. The aim is to restore the three missing elements—skin cover, volume, and nipple areolar complex—in a pleasing symmetrical arrangement. Wide experience of reconstructive techniques is essential for coping with the frequent unexpected problems that occur during surgery. Good surgical technique, with particular attention to gentle tissue-handling, haemostasis and careful flap planning and execution are required.

Choice of operation (*see* Table 17.1)
The precise technique should be tailored to suit the particular patient's problem. The 'single-technique' approach, in which all breasts are reconstructed in a basic repetitive manner, is not likely to be adaptable enough to construct the diverse variety of different breast sizes and shapes in the population.

It is extremely difficult to match breast size and shape exactly. A planned, two stage, reconstruction allows adjustment of the contralateral breast at the same time as nipple areolar complex reconstruction is performed. Adjustment of the opposite breast by reduction or augmentation is required in about 40% of cases.

Skin cover

Predisposing factors
The amount of skin cover provided must be carefully tailored to the size of breast needing to be reconstructed. Too much skin produces ptosis, with the skin and subcutaneous tissue gradually drooping under the influence of gravity (Figs. 17.22, 17.27). Skin deficiency prevents the development of a normal size and contour of the reconstructed breast (Fig. 17.23). The placement of too large a prosthesis under a tight skin cover can delay wound healing, cause skin necrosis, and lead to extrusion of the implant. Previous radiotherapy is a potent cause of this problem.

Prevention of complications
The most important factor in planning breast reconstruction is to decide at the outset the size of reconstruction required. The decision can only be made with the full knowledge and consent of the patient after evaluation of her wishes and examination of the mastectomy site and the other breast. Factors that must be taken into account are the patient's age, general body shape, and availability of donor sites.

In general, it is easier to reconstruct a medium-sized breast of A or B cup. Therefore, if the normal breast is very large, reduction should be offered; if it is very small, augmentation may be preferable, rather than trying to perform the difficult task of matching the reconstruction to the large or small normal breast. The patient may herself decide that an augmentation to give equal volume is all that she desires to avoid the need for an external prosthesis (Fig. 17.24). This request must be respected, particularly as an alteration to this decision can be made at a later stage.

Table 17.1 Flow chart: Breast reconstruction

Stage 1

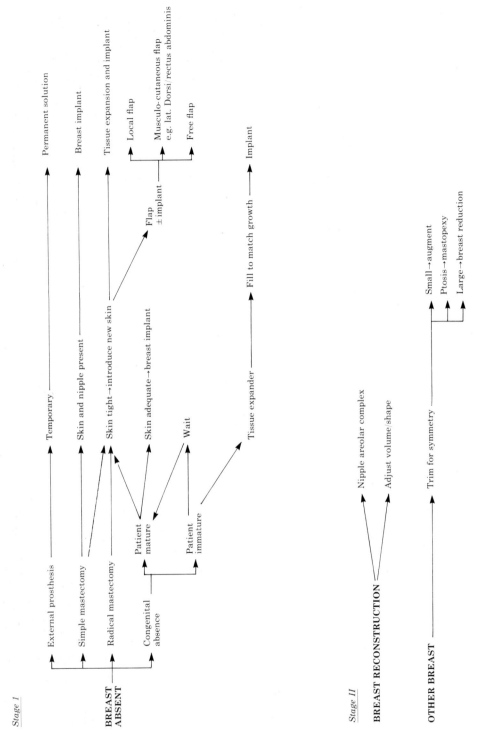

Stage II

BREAST RECONSTRUCTION ────────→ Nipple areolar complex

────────→ Adjust volume/shape

OTHER BREAST ────────→ Trim for symmetry ────────→ Small→augment

Ptosis→mastopexy

Large→breast reduction

Figure 17.23
Inadequate reconstruction of the left breast, which lacks skin and soft tissue, has been exaggerated following mammoplasty on the right side by the patient putting on weight. Correction will require repeat reduction on the right side or increased augmentation and skin provision on the left.

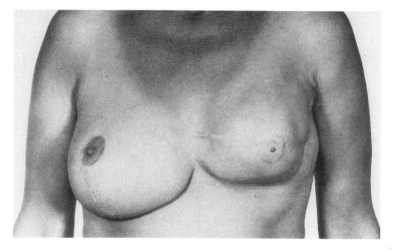

If a moderate-sized breast is wanted, extra skin cover is not usually required. Additional skin can be provided, where necessary, by tissue expansion or skin flap.

Tissue expansion has become a very popular method for providing increased skin cover in breast reconstruction. Complications are few under favourable circumstances: if the remaining breast skin is of good quality with a few scars and if there has been no radiotherapy. At each expansion injection, the implant must not be inflated so far that pain is caused or the skin is blanched. Skin necrosis and extrusion of the implant may occur if the expansion has been too rapid. In the rare event of infection around the prosthesis, it must be removed. Once the wound has

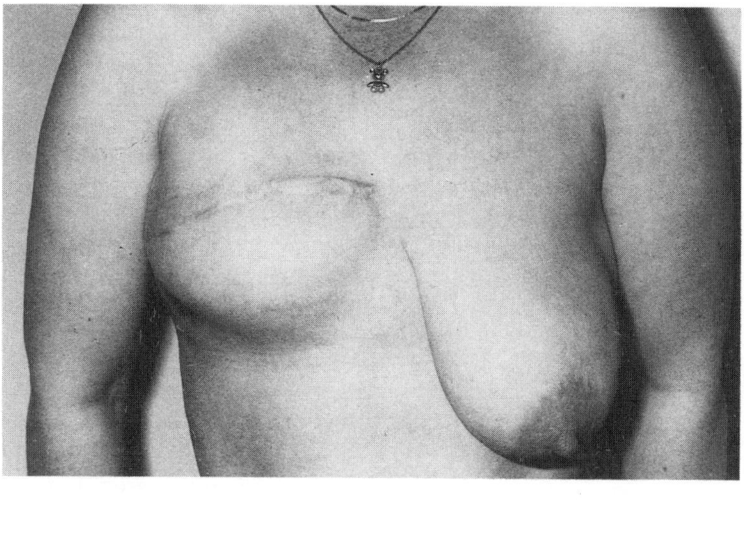

Figure 17.24
Simple augmentation to give volumetric symmetry is requested by many patients. The result looks satisfactory when the patient is wearing a brassiere. A decision to perform a mastopexy can be easily made at a later stage.

healed and infection has settled, the prosthesis can be reinserted.

Tissue expansion is contra-indicated after radiotherapy. The
complication rate is much higher, the skin does not expand
readily and flap repair to introduce non-irradiated skin is
preferable.

A potentially serious complication of tissue expansion over
the chest wall is the pressure effect on the ribs, which can cause
deformation and a depression. Fractured ribs may occur. Once
the expander is removed, a larger than expected implant will be
required.

In order to give a more natural slightly ptotic shape to the
reconstructed breast, it is best to overinflate the expander and
hold it at this size for a few weeks before replacing it with an
implant. Correct siting of the expander at the initial insertion is
obviously vital, since once the expansion has taken place it is
very difficult to readjust the position for the implant at a later
stage.

Flap repair inevitably causes additional scarring around the
edge of the flap and therefore it is best to place any introduced
skin into the lower half of the reconstructed breast. Local flaps
will have a better colour and consistency match but the main
difficulty is that the maximum area of flap required is at the
centre of the breast and local flaps that have to be obtained from
the edge of the defect may be inadequate in size (Fig. 17.25).

The direction of the mastectomy scar determines to a considerable extent the type of local flap selected. If the scar is
transverse, a sliding advancement flap from the axillary tail
(which is usually available in the fuller-busted or more obese
patient (Fig. 17.26)), or a direct upward advancement flap of the
upper abdominal wall, are suitable. When the mastectomy scar
is more vertical, a transposition flap from the axillary tail or a
lateral pectoral flap of the same or contralateral side will be
required.

Musculocutaneous flaps have the advantage that their longer
pedicle allows larger areas of skin to be introduced from a more
distant site such as the back by the latissimus dorsi flap or from
the lower abdomen by the rectus abdominis flap. The donor scar
of the latter flap can be sited quite low and combined with an
abdominal lipectomy. The donor site of the latissimus dorsi flap
can be placed transversely or obliquely and the choice should be
discussed with the patient prior to surgery to choose a suitable
scar that can be covered by her preferred style of clothing. Free
microvascular flaps can also be used.

Treatment of
complications
Once the breast has been reconstructed at the first stage, any
minor adjustments of the skin cover can be made later at the
second stage. Excess skin can be trimmed or the implant can be
changed for a larger one, depending on the effect required

Figure 17.25
(a) A poorly designed local flap in this patient broke down and the implant was extruded. (b) A latissimus dorsi musculocutaneous flap was introduced into the lower half of the breast and the implants were re-inserted deep to muscle on each side.

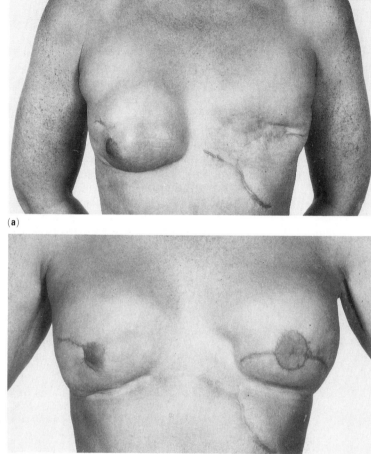

(a)

(b)

Figure 17.26
When the mastectomy scar is placed transversely, a sliding advancement flap from the lateral chest wall provides good, soft skin cover.

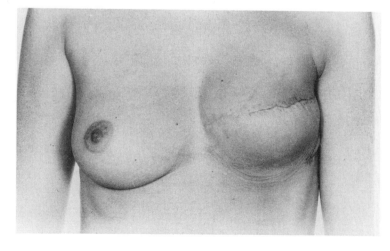

(Fig. 17.27). The most common error is to make the breast too small and the most effective solution is to reduce the size of the normal breast. However if the skin cover is adequate, a larger implant can be inserted.

Breast volume

Estimation of the size of implant is more difficult in reconstruction work than in cosmetic augmentation. The volume of the imported flap must be taken into account. However, as the flap may be under more tension it will be thinner and an underestimate of the volume is the more common error. Any implant used should be of a generous size. It can easily be changed for a smaller one at a second stage. If the reconstruction is too small, it is more difficult to enlarge it later.

Figure 17.27 (a,b) Poor result following subcutaneous mastectomy with immediate reconstruction. The excess skin should have been excised by performing a mastopexy at the original operation.

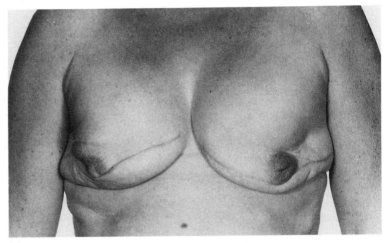

(a)

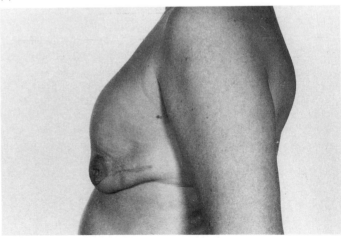

(b)

The commonest method used to augment the reconstructed breast is a silastic implant; the complications of silastic implants have been discussed earlier in this chapter. Fat or dermal fat grafts should not be used, because of the very high complication rate. If a flap from a fatty donor site is used, the volume may be sufficient to augment the breast to the desired volume without the use of an additional implant, thereby avoiding the complications of an implant. This method is not suitable in the thin patient. The omental fat flap is also not usually suitable in the thin patient.

Nipple areolar complex

Prevention of complications

Careful planning of the site for the reconstruction is vital. The most reliable method is to decide on the correct placement after the first stage of the reconstruction. A temporary nipple prosthesis can be worn by the patient. In some patients this becomes their preferred method and reconstruction is not requested subsequently. The appropriate site can be readjusted as the breast reconstruction matures into its permanent shape, so that the final accurate placement can be made at the second stage.

If the breast has been removed for malignant disease, it is important not to store the nipple as a graft in a different site, since malignant disease has been transferred to this temporary site in some patients (Fig. 17.5).

The colour match required determines the donor site used for the areolar reconstruction. A brown skin graft can be obtained from the upper thigh. The tip of the opposite nipple provides a good graft for the nipple.

Treatment of complications

Once the nipple is sited incorrectly, it is extremely difficult to reposition it and unless the discrepancy is gross it is better to leave it. Excision and suture with transfer to another site is possible, but leaves scarring in the old nipple site that will be difficult to camouflage.

If the areolar reconstruction fades in colour, it can be made browner by ultraviolet light, or tattooing can be used. Loss of nipple prominence can be helped by placing a small cartilage graft under it or by use of de-epithelialized flaps turned under the central area.

Recurrent carcinoma

There is no evidence that reconstruction of the breast removed for the treatment of cancer causes recurrence of breast cancer. However, it is obviously vital to exclude local recurrence before undertaking reconstruction. If at operation any suspicious area is encountered, frozen-section biopsy must be performed to exclude recurrence before proceeding. The presence of malignant disease elsewhere, however, is not necessarily a contraindication to breast reconstruction. Patients with recurrent carcinoma must not be denied the opportunity of reconstruction if they desire it strongly.

If local recurrence occurs it can be treated by further excision or radiotherapy as necessary. The placement of an implant deep to muscle in the reconstructed breast makes management of subsequent local recurrence much easier, as wider excision can be performed without having to remove the implant.

Gynaecomastia

Planning A full evaluation must be made including physical examination to look for lumps in the breast, liver disease or testicular tumours. Liver function studies and hormone assays should be performed.

The amount and type of tissue—gland, skin and fat—that has to be removed must be determined. Most males have large pectoral muscles and this must be pointed out to the patient or he might be disappointed by the result.

Incision Unless there is gross increase in size, a simple mastectomy performed through a lower peri-areolar incision gives the best results.

Contour deformity The most common complaint is failure to remove enough tissue. Minor re-excision can be carried out under local anaesthetic. If there is a peripheral rim of fatty tissue causing a saucer shaped deformity, it can be thinned by suction lipectomy, leaving minimal scarring. Suction lipectomy is not effective in removing breast tissue, as it is too fibrous to aspirate.

Persisting controversies
- Prevention and treatment of capsular contracture around an implant.
- Does the foam-covered prosthesis perform well in the long term?
- Do 'low-bleed' prostheses cause less contracture?
- Choice of breast reconstruction method.

Further reading
Ward, C.M. (1986) Reconstruction of the Breast after Mastectomy. In: *Current Operative Surgery: Plastic and Reconstructive Surgery*, Ed. I.F.K. Muir. London: Baillière Tindall.

Regnault, P.F. & Daniel R.K. (Eds) (1984) *Aesthetic Plastic Surgery: Principles and Technique*. Boston: Little Brown.

18 Pressure Sores

Referrals of patients with pressure sores to the plastic surgeon is a common occurrence. Often they have been present for many weeks or months, unresponsive to various conservative methods of management and as a last resort referred for surgical opinion.

The extent of the problem is not widely appreciated. Many studies have been done to find out the incidence of pressure sores and figures ranging from 3% to 8.8% of the general hospital in-patient population have been reported. Many more patients have signs of early skin problems that may or may not progress to a full-blown pressure sore. The annual cost to the British National Health Service is staggering—£160 million. Many of these can be prevented by simple measures and a considerable part of the discussion in this chapter will concentrate on prevention. Before discussing the management, however, a brief outline and understanding of the mechanism of formation of pressure sores is essential.

Adverse factors contributing to pressure sore formation

By definition, pressure sores occur when the soft tissues are compressed, usually between a bony prominence such as the ischium, trochanter or sacrum and a supporting structure, e.g. a bed or wheelchair. Shearing and friction forces can accentuate this.

Two processes, which may occur concurrently or separately, are thought to occur in the formation of bed sores. Firstly, exclusion of blood from the skin of immobilized patients owing to sustained pressure in excess of the mean capillary systolic pressure. The wound is initially superficial and then extends deeply. Secondly, damage to the endothelial cells of the blood vessels supplying the soft tissues. The wound here tends to be a full-thickness one from the start. Many other factors contribute to the formation of the sore and its healing, including general nutrition, drug therapy (e.g. corticosteroids), care of the pressure areas, etc. The tissues of the skin are able to survive ischaemia for a limited period of time when blood has been excluded by pressure alone, but there are limits. Prolonged unconsciousness, enforced immobility as a result of injury, paraplegia, arthritis, etc., will obviously aggravate the situation. In chair-ridden patients, the skin over the coccyx and ischial tuberosities is partially at risk, the latter in wheelchair patients particularly.

In the second type of pressure sore, the process is initiated by endothelial damage with subsequent thrombosis in the micro-circulation. Destruction occurs first in the fat and deeper tissues; the skin sloughs secondarily—there may be a pinhole defect with a large cavity. Precipitating factors include bacter-aemia, endotoxins, metabolic acidosis (e.g. renal disease), diabetes, dehydration and other systemic toxic conditions. It has been suggested that endotoxins may be released when the cavity of the sores—if they are growing large numbers of Gram-negative bacteria such *E. coli*, *Pseudomonas*, etc.—is irrigated with hypochlorite solutions such as Eusol.

The early clinical signs of a pressure sore are erythema, oedema and punctate haemorrhages. The overlying skin subsequently sloughs and there may be a zone surrounding the area of cellulitis. Several days following this, a well-defined central area of necrosis results. Secondary infection may occur and considerable undermining of the surrounding skin may result. Systemic infection may supersede and an offensive discharge ensue.

Complications of pressure sores

Infection
Infection in a pressure sore is common, not unnaturally. Localized infection will result in an offensive odour from the sore. However, septicaemia may result and this can cause death in the patient. In these systemic cases, endocarditis is common.

Predisposing causes
1 *Necrotic tissue* in the sore is a ready-made culture medium for many organisms and the warm, moist environment due to prolonged pressure in the area aids this process.
2 *Soiling.* Many of these incapacitated patients are incontinent of urine and of faeces, which causes further contamination of the sore.

Treatment
Treatment consists of appropriate antibiotics and dressings to the sore as well as general measures such as relieving pressure to the area. Any pus present should be drained as for any abscess, and necrotic tissue should be excised.

Antibiotics have little place when the infection is confined to the sore because penetration through the dead eschar is usually very limited. Povidone Iodine is useful and should be packed into the wound and changed three or four times per day until the sore is clean. The use of hypochlorite solutions such as Eusol may cause endotoxin release from several organisms, as already mentioned. The effect of this varies from mild pyrexic episodes to acute oliguric renal failure.

Haemorrhage

An infected, deep sore may erode through a blood vessel resulting in haemorrhage. This is not very common but must be dealt with urgently.

Predisposing causes

1 *Infection.*   Spontaneous haemorrhage from a pressure sore is almost always associated with infection.
2 *Trauma.*   Any irritation to the area can result in haemorrhage.

Treatment

Urgent treatment may be necessary. The wound should be packed. Any infection should be treated with appropriate antibiotics. The vessel causing the bleeding can be identified readily. It may be possible to cauterize, ligate or transfix it. Following these emergency measures, particularly if the haemorrhage is recurrent, more definite management of the sore must be considered. When possible, the sore should be excised and the defect repaired with a skin flap.

Erosion

In erosion the sore extends with wide undermining of the surrounding tissues (Fig. 18.1). Around the perineum, erosion

Figure 18.1
Extensive undermining
of pressure sore.

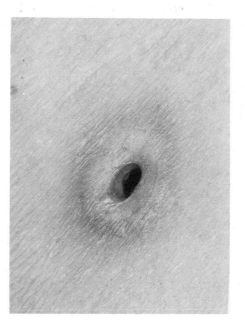

may occur into the genital tract or rectum. Joints can be involved and secondary infection may supervene.

Predisposing causes
Continued pressure over the area of the sore, infection or general malaise of the patient either from malnutrition, anaemia, etc., can all contribute to extension of the sore (Fig. 18.2).

Treatment
The management is to recognize this high-risk group of patients and to instigate corrective measures, most importantly to relieve pressure on the affected area and correct any anaemia, together with adequate feeding, either with a high-protein, high-calorie diet when the patient can tolerate this, or with parenteral nutrition or even intravenous hyperalimentation.

It is important to recognize that just as a sore can initially occur within only a few hours, so it can extend similarly in a matter of hours with further more widespread necrosis developing.

Delayed rehabilitation
Delayed rehabilitation is a very important consideration, particularly in the younger paraplegic patient in whom motivation must be encouraged and on whose morale prolonged treatment, often with frequent dressings and possibly surgery, can have a very negative effect.

Predisposing causes
Infection, haemorrhage and erosion will all contribute to this problem. Low morale from these complications or simply related to slow progress in healing, can influence the patient's own motivation in caring for his skin and general hygiene.

Figure 18.2
Extension of pressure sore contributed to by pressure of dressing.

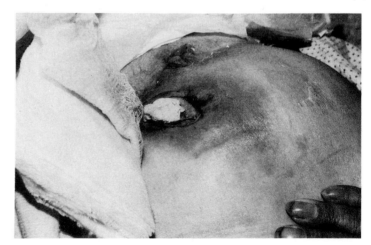

Treatment

Aggressive treatment of these complications, together with encouragement to the patient, will help in the management.

Amyloidosis

Amyloid is recognized as a complication of sepsis from pressure sores, particularly in paraplegic patients. In a study in which the cause of death in paraplegic patients with pressure sores was studied, a significant number of patients were found to have amyloid disease, and the exclusive source of amyloid sepsis was found to be the pressure sore. The immediate causes of death in these patients were hypoproteinaemia, septicaemia, haematemesis, cardiac infarction and end-stage renal failure. Amyloidosis can, of course, still be a cause for the patient's demise even after the sore has healed.

Predisposing factors of pressure sores

Surgical management of pressure sores is difficult and is associated with recognized complications, not least of which is recurrence of the sore or development of new ones. Prevention is therefore all important, not only in the patient who has not previously had a pressure sore but also in those who have had pressure sores in the past.

As in all preventive medicine, a knowledge of the 'at-risk' group is vital and this group of patients is well recognized. In an article by Bliss (*Care—Science and Practice*, Vol. 1, No. 1, July 1981) a scoring system was devised (see Fig. 18.3). From this helpful guide, the following factors seem to be important.

Figure 18.3
Scoring system for patients at risk of developing pressure sores.

THE PRESSURE SORE SCORE

A method of estimating which patients are likely to develop pressure sores *before they appear,* so that preventive measures can be instituted.

- Decide which grade in each category.
- Add up the corresponding numbers to give the total score.

General condition	Mental state	Activity	Mobility in bed	Incontinence
0. Good	0. Alert	0. Ambulant	0. Full	0. Not
1. Fair	1. Confused	1. Walks with help	1. Slightly limited	1. Occasionally
2. Poor	2. Apathetic	2. Chairfast	2. Very limited	2. Usually/urine
3. Bad	3. Stuporose	3. In bed all day	3. Immobile	3. Doubly

Patients with a score of 8 or over are liable to develop pressure sores, especially if their condition is deteriorating.

1 *General condition.* Although this is a rather difficult category to define, the initial impression of the patient's overall condition is important. The clinically cachectic patient is an obvious example.

2 *Mental state.* Trying to educate patients with regard to nutrition and diet, position in which they lie or sit, and mobility will depend on their mental state. Thus the patient at greatest risk is one who is very confused or even stuporous. These patients are unable to help themselves and therefore are 'at risk'.

3 *Activity.* Generally speaking, patients who are ambulant are at much less risk of developing sores and will also have the best chance of healing.

4 *Mobility.* This reflects the patient's ability to move about the bed or chair so as to relieve pressure on different areas of the skin.

5 *Incontinence.* When the skin is constantly moist, maceration and breakdown are more likely, together with secondary infection made more likely when the patient is incontinent of both urine and faeces.

On the basis of this scoring system, any patient with a score of 8 or over is liable to develop pressure sores, especially if his or her condition is deteriorating.

Other predisposing factors include the following.

Age. The older the patients, the more frail they tend to be, being less mobile and frequently undernourished, all of which can predispose to pressure-sore formation.

Paraplegia, multiple sclerosis, etc. Reduced activity and poor mobility make these patients often at higher risk of developing sores.

Diabetes. In diabetics, angiopathy together with the greater risk of minor wounds and abrasions becoming infected, coupled with neuropathy (associated with diabetes), again make this group of patients more susceptible to developing pressure sores.

Drugs. Long-term corticosteroid use causes the skin to become thin, more readily breaking down when subjected to pressure and shearing forces.

Prevention

The importance of this has already been mentioned but its importance cannot be overemphasized, particularly in the group with a high 'at-risk' score. When the patient is in the supine position, the skin over the sacrum is at greatest risk. Figure 18.4

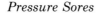

Figure 18.4
Pressure areas at risk
of breaking down in
incapacitated patient.

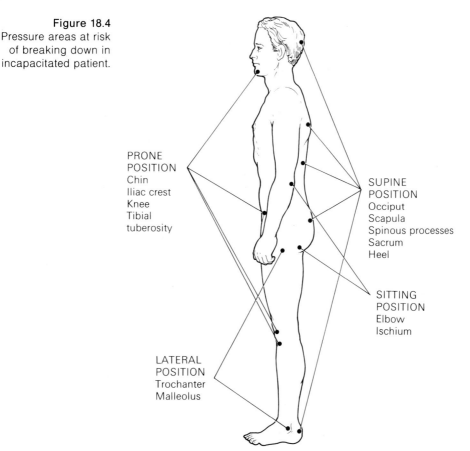

PRONE
POSITION
Chin
Iliac crest
Knee
Tibial
tuberosity

SUPINE
POSITION
Occiput
Scapula
Spinous processes
Sacrum
Heel

SITTING
POSITION
Elbow
Ischium

LATERAL
POSITION
Trochanter
Malleolus

shows other areas that are at risk in different positions. In the sitting position, the skin over the ischial tuberosities is at greatest risk, together with the elbow and sacrum. In the lateral position, the skin over the greater trochanter and lateral malleolus is at greatest risk and in the prone position, the skin over the iliac crest, knee, pretibial tuberosity and chin are at risk.

The basic principle of all preventive measures is to reduce the pressure over the bony prominences by reducing the time the patient is lying in the one position and/or by increasing the 'spread area of the load'. Generally speaking, nursing care (turning, etc.) helps with the former, whereas different types of cushions and beds help with the latter, but both forms of management are important in the prevention of pressure sores.

Nursing care

Turning The patient confined to bed who is at risk should be turned two-hourly, round the clock. This obviously requires a large number of staff, particularly when the patient is heavy. The state of the skin should be carefully noted at each turn, to see whether there is any deterioration. Although this measure of turning appears in principle simple enough, it is demanding on nursing time and personnel and in a busy unit can easily be delayed or overlooked. The technique of turning the patient is important in avoiding back-strain on the nurses' part. The patient should be positioned so that the weight of the body is distributed over the largest possible area. Localized pressure is minimized by proper body alignment and the careful placement of sheepskin covers, cushions and pillows.

It is important to emphasize to the patient in a wheelchair the importance of repositioning himself or elevating himself for approximately 1 minute in every 15 minutes.

Patients in bed should be provided with 'monkey poles' and encouraged where possible to lift themselves up on these to relieve pressure on the skin and also as an aid to repositioning themselves.

When the patient is turned, it is important to ensure that the bedclothes are not wrinkled and are kept clean and dry at all times. Anything that might cause localized pressure must be avoided, e.g. buttons, clips, and so on.

Skin care   It is essential to keep the skin clean and dry at all times. This is obviously a particular problem in patients who are incontinent of urine, faeces or both. The skin in the 'at-risk' areas should be washed with a bland soap and carefully dried at least twice per day and when soiled. The use of a fine talcum powder applied to the dry skin is helpful and a barrier cream such as zinc and castor oil is helpful in patients who tend to be incontinent.

The use of sheepskin rugs is also helpful.

Catheterizing of the incontinent patient should only be done if it proves impossible to keep the area reasonably dry, because it often proves extremely difficult, particularly in geriatric patients to restore good bladder control and enable rehabilitation to take place later.

Beds and cushions

A great deal of research has been done in recent years to devise a bed suitable for patients at risk of developing pressure sores that will reduce the localized pressure on susceptible areas and also the need for frequent turning of the patient. It is important to recognize, however, that they only reduce the pressure, they do not eliminate it, and each bed has its own potential complication. Regular inspection of the skin must still be carried out, combined with the nursing procedures already mentioned, as required.

Ripple mattresses   Ripple mattresses may be large- or small-celled and work on the principle of two interdigitating systems of cells that inflate and deflate alternately every 10 minutes underneath the patient, lifting him off the surface of the mattress and supporting his weight on one set of cells and then on the other, thus alternating the points of pressure on the body. These have proved in clinical practice to be effective in preventing pressure sores in susceptible patients, but care must be taken in the proper maintenance and servicing, with correct adjustment of the pressure in the cells, for them to be fully effective (see Fig. 18.5).

Complications
Obstruction to the normal inflation/deflation cycle.

Prevention
Care must be taken to prevent any folds in the sheets or clothes that may cause obstruction to the normal cycle.

Water beds Water beds are also effective in distributing the patient's weight evenly. However, they are heavy and difficult to move and store. Lifting a patient on and off a water bed may also be very difficult. They are effective only when the patient is lying down all the time.

Complications
1 *Cooling* of the patient (if the water cools down too much).
2 Many patients complain of *nausea* similar to 'seasickness'.

Figure 18.5
Use of ripple mattress.

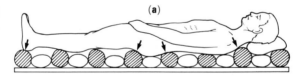

(a)

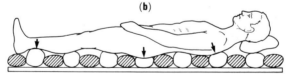

(b)

Showing normal change in pressure points during a 7-minute cycle of a large-celled ripple bed. Alternating pressure in cells distributes pressure on skin.

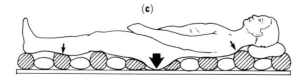

(c)

Faulty large-celled ripple mattress showing area of constant pressure.

3 *Pressure* over the bony prominences may be too great in a shallow water bed. The patient needs to be 'fully immersed' for the bed to be effective. The covering must be very loose to prevent a 'hammock effect'.

4 *Burn*—the water temperature must obviously not be too high, otherwise a burn to the skin may occur.

Prevention
The temperature of the water must be controlled accurately, as should the volume.

Net suspension bed   In this type of bed, the patient lies in a hammock that is suspended from rollers fixed on a frame above the bed. The rollers have handles so that one nurse can turn a patient easily for dressing, etc. The net conforms to the shape of the body and distributes the weight evenly. These are relatively inexpensive.

Complications
1 *Position.* Not all patients find this bed comfortable, especially the elderly. There is a tendency to fall into the middle of the net.
2 *Contracture.* This type of bed can discourage patients from moving themselves. Flexion contractures may, therefore, be at greatest risk of development.
3 *Excess pressure.* This may result from the tension in the net being too great if it is stretched when turning the handles.

Prevention
Assessment of patient compatibility with this type of bed is important. Excess tension in the net when winding the handles should be avoided.

Rotary beds   Rotary beds work on the principle of constant movement of the bed from side to side and are also effective in reducing localized pressure on the skin over pressure points.

Complications
Failure through breakdown of the motor will render this bed useless in redistributing pressure.

Prevention
Regular maintenance of the motor is important.

Mediscus low-airloss bed   The low-airloss bed consists of a continuously inflated air mattress that not only supports the patient evenly and in comfort but ventilates the skin as well. The bed is in sections and one of its great advantages is that the position of patients can be altered so that they can sit up as well as lie down. It is very acceptable to patients and is relatively easy to store when the air cushions are deflated. Although they are expensive, when the overall saving on nursing time and cost of the management of pressure sores is taken into consideration, a more accurate perspective is obtained.

Complications
Inadequate relief of pressure may be given to some patients, e.g. bilateral amputees.

Prevention
The relief of pressure points offered by this bed may need to be supplemented with regular turning by the nursing staff.

Fluidized bead bed In the fluidized bead bed, warm filtered air is passed into a tank of beads (tiny glass microspheres), which then act like a fluid. The patient 'floats' in this, partially immersed in a warm, dry fluid with a stream of warm air blowing imperceptibly over the skin. This type of bed is again expensive and a further complication is that the patient has to lie flat for it to be fully effective.

Complications
Pressure on the buttock area may result if the patient is propped up on this sort of bed.

Prevention
This type of bed is very good where the patient is lying flat for prolonged periods of time.

All these beds are effective in reducing localized pressure over the bony prominences and reducing the need for turning by the nursing staff. They are expensive and require maintenance, particularly the more complex types, for effective use but they are certainly an advance in the management of this condition.

Cushions Cushions are also important for use with wheelchairs in preventing sores, particularly over the ischial tuberosities. It is very important to emphasize that, when attempting to reduce both the pressure on these parts and the shearing forces to which they are subject (both of which will contribute to the formation of pressure sores), the wheelchair and cushion must be taken into consideration together.

Brattgard (1977) found that by correct adjustment of the arm rests on the wheelchair the pressure over the ischial tuberosities could be reduced by 25–30%; lowering the backrest from 90° to 115° reduced the pressure by 25%; and allowing the lower legs and feet to hang freely instead of being supported by footrests reduced the pressure by 20%. This last, however, is obviously dangerous and impractical.

The second point to make about wheelchairs and cushions is that no cushion has been shown to reduce the pressure to a level of less than 40 mm of mercury (i.e. to allow normal skin perfusion) and therefore the patient still needs to employ pressure-relieving manoeuvres on a regular basis to prevent tissue necrosis.

Many different types of cushions are available—water filled, particle filled, air cushions (e.g. Roho), alternating pressure, foam cushions and gel-filled cushions. Standard foam cushions are probably the most widely used and, provided the patient finds them comfortable and there is no sign of danger to the skin, this is a perfectly satisfactory cushion to use. The foam should, however, be checked approximately every six months to ensure that it has not degraded and, if it has, a new cushion must be provided.

If this is not satisfactory, then the particular needs of the patient must be carefully considered. Some cushions are better suited to particular requirements of the patient than others, as the following list illustrates.

- *Pressure.* For patients who cannot or will not lift themselves, it is better to use a cushion that 'flows' and uses some other method to equalize pressure, e.g. gel, water-filled, or a Roho.
- *Shear.* A Roho cushion is designed to have minimum shear. A sheepskin on top of a conventional cover will also minimize shear.
- *Temperature.* Gel-filled cushions keep the temperature fairly constant, whereas water cushions tend to lower the skin temperature.
- *Moisture.* If this is a problem, it may be because the interface temperature is too great. Otherwise, sheepskin has very good moisture-absorbing qualities, though it may get too hot to sit on.
- *Stability.* Foam is probably the most stable, tending to mould to the body contours. Some gel and water cushions feel very unstable.
- Patients who are underweight will generally need more padding the more pronounced are the bony prominences.
- *Portability.* If the patient is to be moved about frequently, in a car for example, the weight of the cushion will be important—foam cushions being the lightest.
- *Simplicity.* This is important if patients have to place the cushion themselves at home. Their mental state, age, etc, must be taken into account if it is to be used correctly.
- *Flammability.* Most cushions are now fireproof, but this should be checked together with the nature of the fabric cover. This is obviously particularly a danger in a wheelchair-bound patient who smokes.
- *Cover* must be extensive to prevent a hammock effect with increasing pressure.

Once the type of cushion has been chosen, the correct size must be obtained by careful measurement, and this should be done at the same time as the measurements for the wheelchair are carried out.

Nutrition

The patient at risk of developing pressure sores should be maintained on a high-protein, high-calorie diet. This may need to be administered via a nasogastric tube or even intravenously in seriously ill patients. Zinc and vitamin supplements should also be given as these too affect skin healing

Management of the established pressure sore

Pressure sores need not occur and where adequate prophylactic measures are in operation they should not occur. In considering the management of an established sore, three aspects should be considered:

1 correction of the cause;
2 conservative measures;
3 surgery.

Correction of the cause It is important to get a history of the events leading up to the development of the sore—for example, debilitating illness in a frail patient; a change of wheelchair and/or cushion which has been incorrectly matched with the size of the patient; breakdown of the normal nursing supervision in a bed-ridden patient, etc. Once this is established, the intercurrent illness is actively treated or the necessary preventive measures are instigated, so that when the pressure sore is healed the risk of further breakdown can be reduced. This is extremely important. The risk factor in each individual patient should be recognized as outlined previously and the necessary curative and preventive measures should be started.

Conservative measures Many small pressure sores will heal with dressings only but most others will require considerable time pre-operatively with appropriate dressings. These have the function of cleaning the wound and chemically debriding any slough in the base of the sore. Many different materials have been used for this function. For grossly infected sores, dressings three or four times per day with Providone Iodine are very effective and these may be combined with systemic antibiotics if there is surrounding cellulitis or evidence of more systemic infection. De-sloughing the wound with Eusol is again helpful though the potential danger of using this has already been mentioned. Any loose slough at the time of dressing change should be simply excised in the ward. As the wound becomes cleaner, the dressings can be changed to saline soaks. Many new dressings have recently been publicized as having a beneficial effect on these type of wounds.

A particular feature is that they are non-adherent, so epithelization is not interfered with at dressing changes. However, they tend to be very expensive, and overall have not been widely accepted for routine use in this condition to date. However, several papers have shown the value of a foam elastomer dressing in which a silastic bung is prepared to fit the wound exactly. The patient can remove and replace this himself at home, after cleaning the area or bathing once or twice per day and he then attends the clinic weekly when a new bung is made as the wound closes itself. This has many advantages, particularly in the patient who is mobile and able to do this himself, thereby saving the district nurse frequent home visits to carry out conventional dressings.

Surgery Larger sores will usually require surgical treatment. This should only be carried out after the cause has been carefully investigated and the wound properly prepared.

Prevention of complications—general factors

Good nutrition
The patient should be given a high-protein, high-calorie diet with vitamin supplements as required. Preferably this should be given orally but if necessary by nasogastric tube or even parenterally. Failure to recognize this will result in poor healing and early breakdown.

Clean wound
It is often difficult to achieve a completely sterile wound, but swabs should be clear of β-haemolytic streptococci or heavy contamination by *Pseudomonas*, etc., and dressings should be aimed at cleaning up gross infection prior to surgery.

Complete excision
It is important that the whole cavity of the pressure sore be excised (Fig. 18.6). This is often difficult in very deep sores and staining the lining at the start of the operation with methylene blue will help to define the limits of the cavity and ensure the completeness of the excision during the dissection.

Excision of bony prominences
This need not be radical but any sharp bony prominence or exostosis should be excised or filed down. This will reduce the risk of further breakdown if pressure is applied to the overlying tissue on a subsequent occasion.

Viable skin coverage
The resulting cavity must carefully be checked for haemostasis and closed using viable tissue, either by apposition of the surrounding tissue (or skin graft) if the defect is small or using various skin and/or muscle flaps if it is larger.

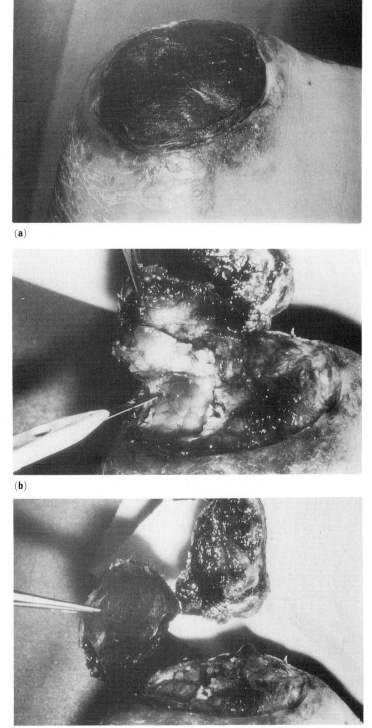

Figure 18.6
(a) Black eschar;
(b) surgical
debridement; (c) large
cavity.

(a)

(b)

(c)

Suction drainage
This is important. Suction drains should be used to prevent collection of fluid at the site of excision. As these sores are frequently round the perineum and likely to be contaminated, any collection of fluid or seroma developing in the wound is likely to get infected. Suction drainage should be maintained for a minimum of 7–10 days postoperatively.

Control of spasms
Spasms may cause rubbing of the skin against clothes, bed sides, etc., with a tendency to form sores. The lateral thigh is particularly at risk. Every effort should be made to reduce or eliminate spasms prior to surgery being carried out. Apart from the increased risk of sores in patients who have spasms, where a muscle or myocutaneous flap is used for the reconstruction the muscle may pull away from its bed and thereby interfere with healing. Several drugs that can help control spasms are available, the two being used most commonly are probably diazepam and dantrolene. The dose should be increased gradually over several weeks until the spasms are controlled. Severe spasms not responding to drug therapy may need surgical treatment, e.g. anterior rhizotomy.

Flap reconstruction
Occasionally small shallow sores can be skin grafted or closed directly. However, most, after the excision of the sore, will require a skin flap.

Prevention of complications
As in all skin defects a very large number and variety of flaps is available for reconstruction. In choosing, several important points should be borne in mind in the special situation of pressure sores to minimize the risk of complication.

1 The flap should be of sufficient size to fill the defect, should sit in place without tension and be well vascularized.
2 It should provide good padding over the bony surface.
3 It should be planned as far as possible so that the scars resulting will not exclude local tissue being used for any subsequent flap procedure if a further sore should develop at the same site (Fig. 18.7). This is a very important consideration, e.g. if a gluteus maximus muscle or musculocutaneous flap is used for a sacral pressure sore without due consideration for the skin incision, this incision may well prevent a large skin-only rotation flap being used on a subsequent occasion (Figs. 18.8, 18.9). It should also be planned so as to avoid the donor site scar lying over another potential pressure area, e.g. planning a posterior thigh flap for an ischial defect results in the donor scar in the posterior thigh well away from bony prominences.
4 Caution should be exercised when considering the use of a

Figure 18.7
Use of large flaps that
can be readvanced.

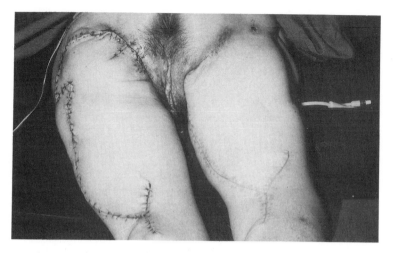

muscle flap in a patient in whom spasms are not well controlled. A large muscle or musculocutaneous flap may tend to
pull away from the bed in which it has been placed. Again,
caution should be exercised in deciding to use a large muscle
or musculocutaneous flap in a non-paraplegic patient in case
function is interfered with.

5 Where skin (without muscle) flaps are planned, the deep fascia
should be included in the flap whenever possible. (See Chapter
4 on fasciocutaneous flaps.)

6 *Drainage.* It is imperative to insert a drain before suturing
these wounds. The wound is potentially contaminated and
often there has been considerable undermining of adjacent
tissues in raising the flap. This resulting dead space will
predispose to infection, particularly if any haematoma or

Figure 18.8
Planning incision—
how to do and not to
do it.

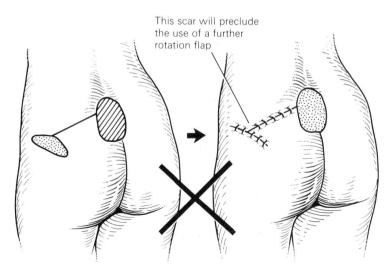

This scar will preclude
the use of a further
rotation flap

Figure 18.9
(a) Planning incision;
(b) gluteus maximus
flap with graft to
sacral sore. Patient
has had a previous left
trochanteric sore
repaired with a tensor
fascia lata flap.

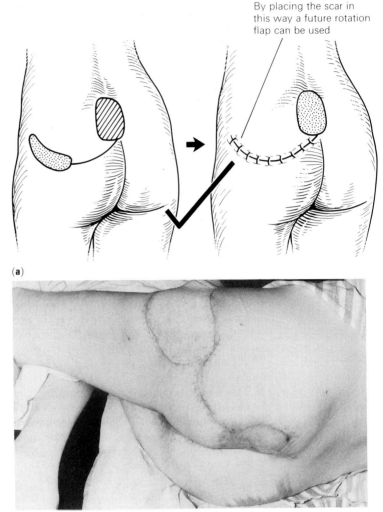

By placing the scar in
this way a future rotation
flap can be used

(a)

(b)

seroma is allowed to develop. The author uses closed suction drainage, which has worked well. It should be left in place for at least 7 days.

Choice of procedure In *sacral* sores, where the defect is shallow with no exposed bone and in a patient with sensation present, skin grafts may be suitable. Buttock rotation flaps can be used or the transverse back flap or small local transposition flaps for smaller defects. Of the muscle and musculocutaneous flaps, those based on the gluteus maximus (upper or lower parts) have proved of most value. Various designs of flaps based on this muscle have been described.

For *ischial* sores, skin grafts rarely have any part to play. The most widely used flap is probably a large posterior thigh advancement/rotation flap, based medially. This is a safe flap and has the great advantage of being raised on subsequent occasions and readvanced to fill-in the defect over the ischium should this recur. Biceps femoris may be detached distally, deep to the flap, and folded up on itself to give extra padding over the ischium. Gluteus maximus flaps have also been used here, as have inferior gluteal thigh flaps (based on the deep branch of the inferior gluteal artery).

For *trochanteric* sores, grafts again have little place. Tensor fasciae latae flap has proven of great value in this situation. A flap based on the vastus lateralis muscle can also be used, as can the gluteal thigh flap.

These three groups comprise the majority of sores encountered in practice, but Mathes and Nahai's book *Clinical Applications for Muscle Musculocutaneous Flaps* (see Further Reading) gives an excellent account of the various flaps that can be used, together with their limitations.

Complications of surgery and their management

1 *Infection.* This is always a risk given the nature of a pressure sore, the risk of soiling from the patients themselves, etc. Various measures to try and reduce the risk have already been mentioned in this chapter.

  If infection develops postoperatively, it should be actively treated with a suitable antibiotic.

2 *Haematoma.* Particularly when a large flap has been raised, the risk of haematoma is present. Careful haemostasis and suction drainage will help to reduce the risk of haematoma.

  If it does occur, it should be drained without delay and the patient treated with antibiotics.

3 *Necrosis.* This is more likely to occur in frail patients, but in diabetics small vessel disease may result in poor perfusion at the end of a large flap. Poor design of flap may also be the cause, as might failure to take account of previous scars. Pressure over the flap area in the postoperative period may also cause necrosis and should be avoided.

  Treatment. This should generally be conservative unless there is a massive necrosis of the flap, in which case it will have to be excised and an alternative used. Small areas of marginal necrosis, with careful nursing care, will often heal spontaneously. One advantage of the musculocutaneous flaps is that if necrosis does occur, it may be confined to the cutaneous part of the flap, and if the muscle survives it may subsequently be grafted.

4 *Recurrence.* This is always a risk and hence the importance of preventive measures at all times. The patient must be educated in skin care; at the first sign of pressure damage to the skin, extra precautions should be taken to avoid pressure

Figure 18.10
Pressure changes in
skin flap developing
within 24 hours of
discharge from
hospital.

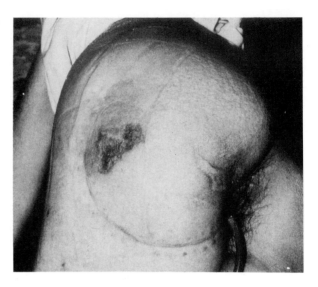

Figure 18.10 Pressure changes in skin flap developing within 24 hours of discharge from hospital.

to the area. As most of these patients will be discharged home, the patients' families and relatives should also know the importance of skin care. District nurses, social workers, etc., must be encouraged in the active treatment to prevent recurrence of the pressure sore (Fig. 18.10).

Persisting
controversies
- Use of prophylactic antibiotics in the surgery of pressure sores.
- Choice of flap for reconstruction.
- Optimum bed for prevention.

Further reading
Bliss, (1981). *Care—Science and Practice*, 1, (1)
Mathes, S.J. & Nahai, F. (1982). *Clinical Applications for Muscle and Musculocutaneous Flaps*. St Louis, Toronto, London: Mosby.
Brattgard, (1977). See *Care 1*:1 (1981), further reading.

Index